T0359064

Alcohol-Associated Liver Disease

Editor

ASHWANI K. SINGAL

CLINICS IN LIVER DISEASE

www.liver.theclinics.com

Consulting Editor
NORMAN GITLIN

November 2024 • Volume 28 • Number 4

ELSEVIER

1600 John F. Kennedy Boulevard • Suite 1800 • Philadelphia, Pennsylvania, 19103-2899

http://www.theclinics.com

CLINICS IN LIVER DISEASE Volume 28, Number 4
November 2024 ISSN 1089-3261, ISBN-13: 978-0-443-24670-8

Editor: Kerry Holland
Developmental Editor: Akshay Samson

Clinics in Liver Disease (ISSN 1089-3261) is published quarterly by Elsevier Inc., 360 Park Avenue South, New York, NY 10010-1710. Months of issue are February, May, August, and November. Business and Editorial Offices: 1600 John F. Kennedy Blvd., Ste. 1800, Philadelphia, PA 19103-2899. Customer Service Office: 3251 Riverport Lane, Maryland Heights, MO 63043. Periodicals postage paid at New York, NY and additional mailing offices. Subscription prices are $339.00 per year (U.S. individuals), $100.00 per year (U.S. student/resident), $447.00 per year (international individuals), $200.00 per year (international student/resident), $405.00 per year (Canadian individuals), $100.00 per year (Canadian student/resident). For institutional access pricing please contact Customer Service via the contact information below. Foreign air speed delivery is included in all *Clinics* subscription prices. All prices are subject to change without notice. Orders, claims, and journal inquiries: Please visit our Support Hub page https://service.elsevier.com for assistance.

Reprints. For copies of 100 or more of articles in this publication, please contact the Commercial Reprints Department, Elsevier Inc., 360 Park Avenue South, New York, NY 10010-1710. Tel.: 212-633-3874; Fax: 212-633-3820; E-mail: reprints@elsevier.com.

Clinics in Liver Disease is covered in *MEDLINE/PubMed (Index Medicus)*, Science Citation Index Expanded, Journal Citation Reports/Science Edition, and Current Contents/Clinical Medicine.

Contributors

CONSULTING EDITOR

NORMAN GITLIN, MD, FRCP (London), FRCPE (Edinburgh), FAASLD, FACP, FACG
Head of Hepatology, Southern California Liver Centers, San Clemente, California, USA

EDITOR

ASHWANI K. SINGAL, MD, MS, FACG, FAASLD, AGAF
Professor, Department of Medicine, Division of Gastroenterology Hepatology and
Nutrition, University of Louisville School of Medicine; Transplant Hepatology and Staff
Physician, University of Louisville Health Jewish Hospital and Trager Transplant Center;
Director, Clinical Trials in Hepatology, University of Louisville; Research Scientist, Rob
Rexley VA Medical Center, Louisville, Kentucky, USA

AUTHORS

RUCHITA AGRAWAL, MD
Assistant Professor, Department of Psychiatry and Behavioral Sciences, Seven Counties
Services, Inc, Louisville, Kentucky, USA

IBRAHIM MUNAF AHMED, MD
Clinical Instructor, Department of Internal Medicine, University of South Dakota Sanford
School of Medicine, Sioux Falls, South Dakota, USA

DYLAN ROSE BALTER, BA
Research Assistant, Medical and Public Health Student, Yale School of Medicine, New
Haven, Connecticut, USA

NEERAJ BHALA, DPhil, MSc, FRCP, FRCPE
Clinical Associate Professor, Nottingham Digestive Diseases Centre, Translational
Medical Sciences, NIHR Nottingham Biomedical Research Centre, Nottingham University
Hospitals NHS Trust and the University of Nottingham School of Medicine, Queens
Medical Centre, University of Nottingham, Nottingham, United Kingdom; Division of
Gastroenterology and Hepatology, Mayo Clinic, Rochester, Minnesota, USA

HYE YOUNG CHOI, MPH
Research Assistant, Medical Student, Yale School of Medicine, New Haven, Connecticut,
USA

ERIN G. CLIFTON, PhD
Clinical Assistant Professor, Department of Psychiatry, University of Michigan, Ann Arbor,
Michigan, USA

ANNE C. FERNANDEZ, PhD
Associate Professor, Department of Psychiatry, University of Michigan, Ann Arbor,
Michigan, USA

PEGAH GOLABI, MD
Fellow, Beatty Liver and Obesity Research Program, Inova Health System, Falls Church, Virginia, USA

ELLEN W. GREEN, MD, PhD
Fellow, Division of Gastroenterology and Hepatology, University of North Carolina, Chapel Hill, North Carolina, USA

NGHIEM B. HA, MD, MAS
Assistant Professor, Liver Transplant, Department of Medicine, University of California, San Francisco, San Francisco, California, USA

LAMIA Y. HAQUE, MD, MPH
Assistant Professor, Department of Internal Medicine - Section of Digestive Diseases, Core Faculty, Yale Program in Addiction Medicine, Yale School of Medicine, New Haven, Connecticut, USA

JOSIAH E. HARDESTY, PhD
Assistant Professor, Department of Pharmacology and Toxicology, University of Louisville School of Medicine, Division of Gastroenterology, Hepatology, and Nutrition, Department of Medicine, University of Louisville, Louisville, Kentucky, USA

RYUKI HASHIDA, MD, PhD
Visiting Scholar, Beatty Liver and Obesity Research Program, Inova Health System, Falls Church, Virginia, USA; Division of Rehabilitation, Kurume University Hospital, Department of Orthopedics, Kurume University School of Medicine, Kurume, Japan

JIANNAN HUANG, MD
Clinical Instructor, Department of Internal Medicine, University of South Dakota Sanford School of Medicine, Sioux Falls, South Dakota, USA

PATRICK S. KAMATH, MD
Professor, Department of Medicine, Mayo Clinic, Rochester, USA

TAKUMI KAWAGUCHI, MD, PhD
Professor, Division of Gastroenterology, Department of Medicine, Kurume University School of Medicine, Division of Rehabilition, Kurume University Hospital, Kurume, Japan

ANAND V. KULKARNI, MD, DM
Senior Consultant, Department of Hepatology, AIG Hospitals, Hyderabad, India

LORENZO LEGGIO, MD, PhD
Clinical Director, Deputy Scientific Director, Chief, Clinical Psychoneuroendocrinology and Neuropsychopharmacology Section, Translational Addiction Medicine Branch, National Institute on Drug Abuse Intramural Research Program and National Institute on Alcohol Abuse and Alcoholism Division of Intramural Clinical and Biological Research, National Institutes of Health, Baltimore, Maryland, USA; Department of Behavioral and Social Sciences, Center for Alcohol and Addiction Studies, School of Public Health, Brown University, Providence, Rhode Island, USA; Division of Addiction Medicine, Department of Medicine, School of Medicine, Johns Hopkins University, Baltimore, Maryland, USA; Department of Neuroscience, Georgetown University Medical Center, Washington, DC, USA

ANDRÁS H. LÉKÓ, MD, PhD
Fellow, Clinical Psychoneuroendocrinology and Neuropsychopharmacology Section, Translational Addiction Medicine Branch, National Institute on Drug Abuse Intramural Research Program and National Institute on Alcohol Abuse and Alcoholism Division of

Intramural Clinical and Biological Research, National Institutes of Health, Baltimore, Maryland, USA; Department of Psychiatry and Psychotherapy, Semmelweis University, Budapest, Hungary

ALEXANDRE LOUVET, MD, PhD
Professor, Service des Maladies de L'appareil Digestif, Hôpital Huriez, Lille, France

ABHISHEK MANDAL, PhD
Post Doctoral Associate, Department of Medicine, University of Massachusetts Chan Medical School, Worcester, Massachusetts, USA

PRANOTI MANDREKAR, PhD, FAASLD
Professor, Department of Medicine, University of Massachusetts Chan Medical School, Worcester, Massachusetts, USA

CRAIG J. McCLAIN, MD
Professor, Department of Pharmacology and Toxicology, University of Louisville School of Medicine, Division of Gastroenterology, Hepatology, and Nutrition, Department of Medicine, University of Louisville, Robley Rex Veterans Medical Center, University of Louisville Alcohol Center, University of Louisville Hepatobiology and Toxicology Center, Louisville, Kentucky, USA

JESSICA L. MELLINGER, MD, MSc
Assistant Professor, Departments of Psychiatry and Internal Medicine, University of Michigan, Ann Arbor, Michigan, USA

CHRISTOPHE MORENO, MD, PhD
Professor, Department of Gastroenterology, Hepatopancreatology and Digestive Oncology, Hôpital Universitaire de Bruxelles, C.U.B. Hôpital Erasme, Laboratory of Experimental Gastroenterology, Universite Libre de Bruxelles, Brussels, Belgium

TIMOTHY R. MORGAN, MD
Chief, Hepatology, Medical Service, Gastroenterology, VA Long Beach Healthcare System, Long Beach, California, USA; Professor, Department of Medicine, University of California, California, Irvine, Irvine, California, USA

JANUS ONG, MD, MPH
Professor (Associate), College of Medicine, University of the Philippines, Manila, Philippines

LUKAS OTERO SANCHEZ, MD, PhD
Postdoctoral Research Fellow, Department of Gastroenterology, Hepatopancreatology and Digestive Oncology, Hôpital Universitaire de Bruxelles, C.U.B. Hôpital Erasme, Laboratory of Experimental Gastroenterology, Université Libre de Bruxelles, Brussels, Belgium

PONNI PERUMALSWAMI, MD
Associate Professor of Medicine, Gastroenterology Section, Veterans Affairs, Ann Arbor Healthcare System, Department of Internal Medicine, University of Michigan, Ann Arbor, Michigan, USA

SHIV KUMAR SARIN, MD, DM, DSc
Senior Professor, Department of Hepatology, Chancellor and Director, Institute of Liver and Biliary Sciences, New Delhi, India

BERND SCHNABL, MD
Professor, Department of Medicine, University of California San Diego, La Jolla, Department of Medicine, VA San Diego Healthcare System, San Diego, California, USA

VIJAY H. SHAH, MD
Carol M. Gatton Professor, Division of Gastroenterology and Hepatology, GI Research Unit, Mayo Clinic, Rochester, Minnesota, USA

SAGGERE MURALIKRISHNA SHASTHRY, MD, DM
Additional Professor, Department of Hepatology, Institute of Liver and Biliary Sciences, New Delhi, India

ASHWANI K. SINGAL, MD, MS, FACG, FAASLD, AGAF
Professor, Department of Medicine, Division of Gastroenterology Hepatology and Nutrition, University of Louisville School of Medicine; Transplant Hepatology and Staff Physician, University of Louisville Health Jewish Hospital and Trager Transplant Center; Director, Clinical Trials in Hepatology, University of Louisville; Research Scientist, Rob Rexley VA Medical Center, Louisville, Kentucky, USA

KINZA TAREEN, MD
Clinical Assistant Professor, Department of Psychiatry, University of Michigan, Ann Arbor, Michigan, USA

VATSALYA VATSALYA, MD
Assistant Professor, Department of Medicine, Division of Gastroenterology, Hepatology, and Nutrition, University of Louisville, Louisville, Kentucky, USA

TIAN WANG, MD
Assistant Professor of Neurology, Georgetown University, Attending Physician of Neurology, Comprehensive Epilepsy Center, MedStar Georgetown University Hospital, Georgetown Unviersity Medical Center, Washington, DC; Division Chief of Neurology, MedStar Southern Maryland Hospital Center, Clinton, Maryland

GERALD SCOTT WINDER, MD, MSc
Associate Clinical Professor, Departments of Psychiatry, Surgery, and Neurology, University of Michigan, Ann Arbor, Michigan, USA

KATIE WITKIEWITZ, PhD
Distinguished Professor of Psychology and Director, Center on Alcohol, Substance Use, and Addictions, University of New Mexico, Albuquerque, New Mexico, USA

ROBERT J. WONG, MD, MS
Clinical Associate Professor, Stanford University School of Medicine, Division of Gastroenterology and Hepatology, Veterans Affairs Palo Alto Helath Care System, Palo Alto, California

CHENCHENG XIE, MD, FACP
Assistant Professor, Department of Internal Medicine, University of South Dakota Sanford School of Medicine, Attending Physician, Division of Hepatology, Avera McKennan Hospital and University Health Center, Sioux Falls, South Dakota, USA

YONGQIANG YANG, PhD
Fellow, Department of Medicine, University of California San Diego, La Jolla, California, USA

FRANCIS YAO, MD, FAASLD
Professor of Medicine and Surgery, Director, Hepatology, Liver Transplant, Division of Gastroenterology and Hepatology, Department of Medicine, University of California, San Francisco, San Francisco, California, USA

ZOBAIR M. YOUNOSSI, MD, MPH
Professor and Chairman, Beatty Liver and Obesity Research Program, Inova Health System, Falls Church, Virginia, USA

WEI ZHANG, MD, PhD
Hepatologist, Gastroenterology Unit, Massachusetts General Hospital, Boston, Massachusetts, USA

Contents

> Alcohol use disorder (AUD) is a chronic medical condition that affects over 29.5 million people and accounts for $249 billion in social and health care costs annually. Prevalence is higher among young adults, males, sexual and gender minorities, American Indians and Alaska Natives, and the uninsured. Despite its high prevalence and societal impact, AUD is often overlooked in health care settings. This has resulted in insufficient implementation of AUD screening as well as low levels of treatment uptake. Addressing these challenges requires recognition of the current epidemiology of AUD and role of social determinants of health.

> Alcohol-associated liver disease (ALD) was already on the rise globally when the advent of coronavirus disease 2019 further accelerated this trend. ALD has emerged as the leading cause for liver transplantation in the United States. The pandemic has not only intensified the prevalence of ALD but has also highlighted significant disparities in its impact, particularly, among young adults and women. This review aims to dissect the complex landscape of ALD, focusing on gender, race, and emerging risk factors in the context of the current global health crisis.

> Alcohol-related liver disease and metabolic-dysfunction-associated steatotic liver disease are the most common causes of chronic liver disease. Globally, alcohol intake, and metabolic syndrome driven by excessive caloric intake and sedentary lifestyle have steadily increased over the past decades. Given the high prevalence rates of both excessive alcohol consumption and components of metabolic syndrome, both can frequently coexist in the same individuals and impact their lives. In this article, we review the impact of alcohol and metabolic syndrome on liver-related outcomes.

Alcohol-associated liver disease (AALD) is a global health problem with increasing incidence with associated high morbidity and mortality. Patients with AALD have varied clinical presentation encompassing a spectrum ranging from alcoholic steatosis, alcoholic steatohepatitis to alcohol-associated fibrosis/cirrhosis, which can be either compensated or decompensated. We need uniformity in defining each of the stages of AALD, which will help in both research and patient care. Algorithmic approach using noninvasive tests like enhanced liver fibrosis score, elastography, and fibrosis-4 scores can help in early diagnosis in addition to the presence of any red flags (low albumin, low platelet count, and raised transaminases).

Alcohol-associated liver disease (ALD) poses a significant risk for hepatocellular carcinoma (HCC), comprising various liver conditions from steatosis to cirrhosis. Despite accounting for a third of global HCC cases and deaths, ALD-related HCC lacks characterization compared to viral hepatitis-related HCC. Proposed mechanisms for ALD-related HCC include acetaldehyde toxicity, increased reactive oxygen species, and inflammation. This review examines ALD-associated HCC epidemiology, co-factors like viral hepatitis and metabolic syndrome, surveillance, and treatment challenges. Despite advances in screening and management, ALD-related HCC often presents at advanced stages, limiting treatment options and survival.

The pathogenesis of alcohol-associated liver disease (ALD) is complex and multifactorial. Several intracellular, intrahepatic, and extrahepatic factors influence development of early fatty liver injury leading to inflammation and fibrosis. Alcohol metabolism, cellular stress, and gut-derived factors contribute to hepatocyte and immune cell injury leading to cytokine and chemokine production. The pathogenesis of alcohol-associated hepatitis (AH), an advanced form of acute-on-chronic liver failure due to excessive chronic intake in patients with underlying liver disease, is not well understood. While pathogenic mechanisms in early ALD are studied, the pathogenesis of AH requires further investigation to help design effective drugs for patients.

Alcohol-associated liver disease (ALD) poses a significant global public health challenge, with high patient mortality rates and economic burden. The gut microbiome plays an important role in the onset and progression of alcohol-associated liver disease. Excessive alcohol consumption disrupts the intestinal barrier, facilitating the entry of harmful microbes and their products into the liver, exacerbating liver damage. Dysbiosis, marked by imbalance in gut bacteria, correlates with ALD severity. Promising microbiota-centered therapies include probiotics, phages, and fecal microbiota transplantation. Clinical trials demonstrate the potential of these interventions to improve liver function and patient outcomes, offering a new frontier in ALD treatment.

Alcohol use, while commonly associated with liver damage, also has significant neurologic implications, which often mimic hepatic encephalopathy and complicate diagnosis and management. Alcohol mediates its acute central nervous system effects by altering neurotransmitter balance, notably between gamma-aminobutyric acid and glutamate. Its chronic neurotoxicity, compounded by thiamine deficiency, results in chronic neurologic complications. Clinically, alcohol-related neurologic disorders present a spectrum from acute intoxication and withdrawal to chronic conditions like Korsakoff syndrome, dementia, cerebellar degeneration, and peripheral neuropathy. This review underscores differentiating these conditions from hepatic encephalopathy and highlights the importance of history-taking and physical examination in clinical practice.

Harmful alcohol use and alcohol use disorder (AUD) are common worldwide, and rates of alcohol-associated liver disease (ALD) are also increasing. AUD is a disease that is treatable and can be diagnosed and managed, and recovery from AUD through abstinence or reductions in drinking is possible. Management of AUD among individuals with ALD is increasingly being addressed via integrated medical and psychosocial treatment teams that can support reductions in drinking and prevent progression of liver disease. Early diagnosis of AUD and ALD can improve lives and reduce mortality.

Alcohol-associated liver disease (ALD) remains a significant public health concern, accounting for at least half of cirrhosis cases in Europe. Historically, liver biopsy has been considered the gold standard method for both diagnosing and staging ALD. However, in the past 3 decades, there has been a growing interest in developing noninvasive biomarkers for identifying high-risk patients prone to develop liver-related complications, including elastography methods or blood-based biomarkers. This review aims to summarize currently available noninvasive testing methods that are clinically available for assessing patients with ALD, including notably steatosis and fibrosis.

of training and discomfort in managing patients with AUD. There are system-level barriers, including challenges related to insurance-based health care systems, and the general reluctance to invest in AUD by organizations focused on for-profit milestones. Therefore, it is imperative to develop multidisciplinary hepatology/addiction integrated care approaches.

Alcohol-associated liver disease (ALD) is the most common cause of liver disease and an indication for liver transplantation. Identification of ALD at an earlier stage and treatment of concomitant alcohol use disorder (AUD) could potentially prevent or delay the progression to advanced stages of ALD like alcohol-associated cirrhosis and alcohol-associated hepatitis. However, screening for alcohol use is often not performed and treatment of AUD is rarely administered in ALD patients, due to several barriers at the level of patients, clinicians, and administrative levels.

Alcohol-associated liver disease is a well-validated indication for liver transplantation and recent data have refined the patterns of alcohol consumption and their impact on the pre-LT and post-LT periods. The selection process is a multidisciplinary approach that integrates liver and addiction parameters. The present review analyzes the drivers of outcome and alcohol relapse and focuses on the changing paradigm in terms of access to the waiting list.

Artificial intelligence (AI) has the potential to aid in the diagnosis and management of alcohol-associated liver disease (ALD). Machine learning algorithms can analyze medical data, such as patient records and imaging results, to identify patterns and predict disease progression. Newer advances such as large language models (LLMs) can enhance early detection and personalized treatment strategies for individuals with chronic diseases such as ALD. However, it is essential to integrate LLMs and other AI tools responsibly, considering ethical concerns in health care applications and ensuring an evidence base for real-world applications of the existing knowledge.

Liver is the most common organ affected by alcohol misuse. The spectrum of alcohol-associated liver disease (ALD) ranges from simple steatosis to cirrhosis and its complications. The unique clinical phenotype of alcohol-associated hepatitis has a risk for high short-term mortality. Several gaps exist with respect to epidemiology, noninvasive testing, prognostication, and treatment of ALD. Most studies focus on short-term survival as the ideal endpoint and ignore other aspects of alcohol-use disorder and ALD. In this review, the authors discuss the existing knowledge gaps, enumerate ongoing clinical trials, and highlight the research priorities and future landscape of clinical trials.

CLINICS IN LIVER DISEASE

SERIES OF RELATED INTEREST

Gastroenterology Clinics of North America
https://www.gastro.theclinics.com

THE CLINICS ARE AVAILABLE ONLINE!
Access your subscription at:
www.theclinics.com

Preface

Alcohol-Associated Liver Disease: Treatment and Prevention

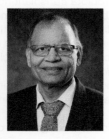

Ashwani K. Singal, MD, MS
Editor

Recent developments in "Alcohol-Associated Liver Disease (ALD)" over the last few years led to planning this focused issue of the *Clinics in Liver Disease*, with a total of 18 articles covering various aspects of ALD. On behalf of Dr Norman Gitlin and his team at *Clinics in Liver Disease*, I would like to thank the experts for their respective contributions.

The first article, by *Dr Lamia Haque* and team (Drs Hye Young Choi and Dylan Balter), elaborates on the current and increasing global and US health care burden of alcohol use disorder (AUD), the most important risk factor for the development of ALD. This is followed by a comprehensive review by *Dr Robert Wong* on the current epidemiology and economic burden of ALD, especially the changing landscape and demographics, with increasing burden in younger individuals and in women. In the background of the increasing prevalence of obesity and metabolic syndrome, and the changing nomenclature of nonalcoholic fatty liver disease to metabolism-associated steatotic liver disease, *Dr Zobair Younossi* discusses the interaction of alcohol use and metabolic syndrome on the risk and severity of ALD, with a special emphasis on MetALD. *Dr Shiv Sarin* along with Dr S.M. Shasthry describes the whole spectrum of ALD in a separate article from early ALD (steatosis ± steatohepatitis) to advanced ALD with cirrhosis and/or clinical symptomatic alcohol-associated hepatitis (AH). This article also covers the more severe form of ALD of acute-on-chronic liver failure with multiorgan failure. Hepatocellular carcinoma in ALD is a separate article written by *Dr Francis Yao* to highlight its unique features related to pathogenesis, comorbid liver conditions as etiology, pathologic features, and management.

As alcohol-induced damage may involve several organs in the body, *Dr Chencheng Xie* and team (Drs Jiannan Huang, Ibrahim Ahmed, and Tian Wang) comprehensively discuss extrahepatic neurologic issues caused by alcohol, which are relevant in

Clin Liver Dis 28 (2024) xvii–xix
https://doi.org/10.1016/j.cld.2024.08.006
1089-3261/24/© 2024 Published by Elsevier Inc.

distinguishing from hepatic encephalopathy in a patient with advanced ALD. *Dr Pranoti Mandrekar* along with Dr Abhishek Mandal from her laboratory team discusses the pathways and mechanisms of ALD, including the role of alcohol metabolism, gut-liver axis, innate and adaptive immunity in causing hepatic and systemic inflammation, oxidative stress, and hepatic fibrosis. As the altered gut microbiome plays a critical role in the pathogenesis of ALD, a separate article contributed by *Dr Bernd Schnabl* describes gut microbiome (bacterial, viral, and fungal) changes in ALD and highlights how this can be modulated, especially with the use of fecal microbiota transplant not only to help the liver disease but also to work as a dual target in benefiting the second pathology of AUD in patients with ALD. The next two articles discuss the diagnostic aspects, the first one by *Dr Katie Wikiewitz* on the diagnosis of AUD and of ALD in a patient presenting with suspected liver disease. This is followed by an important article by *Dr Christophe Moreno* with coauthor Dr Lukas Otero Sanchez, who provide a detailed algorithmic approach on screening for ALD in at-risk individuals and identify those with advanced fibrosis using noninvasive tests (serologic and radiologic) in clinical practice.

This focused issue highlights the critical component of AUD in the management of any spectrum of ALD. *Dr Gerald Scott Winder* and team (Drs Kinza Tareen, Erin Clifton, Jessica Mellinger, and Ponni Perumalswami) very eloquently describe the management of AUD, including behavioral and pharmacologic therapies, with a section on the rarity of implementing this in ALD patients in the real-world practice. The next article, by *Dr Lorenzo Leggio* with coauthor Dr Andras Leko, elucidates clinical, patient, and system level barriers to treatment of AUD in ALD patients, highlighting a need for an integrated multidisciplinary treatment approach to overcome several of these barriers. *Dr Ashwani K. Singal* and team (Drs Ruchita Agarwal and Vatsalya Vatsalya) expand upon in a separate article this integrated approach to manage AUD in ALD patients, especially its role and structure in the liver transplant (LT) setting.

Pharmacologic therapies and LT are two main modes of treating any liver disease, including ALD. *Dr Craig McClain* and coauthor Dr Josiah Hardesty review the current role of corticosteroids and nutritional supplementation, with an algorithmic approach to manage patients with AH. The authors highlight the limitations of current therapies, recognizing an urgent need for effective therapies. A separate article by Dr. Timothy Morgan discusses promising targets like fecal microbiota transplantation, G-CSF, interleukin-22, and DUR-928, all of which are currently in phase 2 or phase 3 clinical trials. *Dr Alexandre Louvet* discusses the status of LT in ALD on the role of early LT (with <6 months of sobriety) for select patients, candidate selection for LT, and monitoring recipients for recurrence of alcohol use. Additionally, two important articles are included, with the first one by *Dr Vijay Shah* with coauthor Dr Neeraj Bhala on the emerging data on artificial intelligence and machine learning in the management of ALD and in prognosticating the outcomes to improve upon existing prognosis scores in AH patients. The second one, by *Dr Ashwani K. Singal* with team (Drs Anand Kulkarni and Patrick Kamath), is on the integrated approach in clinical research and trials for ALD patients, especially adaptive and SMART design clinical trials to manage the ALD and AUD components with the primary endpoint of improving liver-related outcomes.

As the Guest Editor, I would like to thank *Clinics in Liver Disease* for deciding to bring about this special issue on ALD. I hope that this issue will benefit the readers and encourage researchers to take the clinical unmet needs into their respective research agenda to fill these knowledge gaps and help the long-term goal of the World Health Organization to reduce the disease burden of ALD.

ACKNOWLEDGMENTS

The author acknowledges the use of the facilities at the University Louisville School of Medicine and the Clinical Translational Alcohol Research Centre in Louisville, Kentucky, USA.

Ashwani K. Singal, MD, MS
University of Louisville School of Medicine
505 South Hancock Street
Louisville, KY 40202, USA

E-mail address:
ashwanisingal.com@gmail.com

Epidemiology and Health Care Burden of Alcohol Use Disorder

Hye Young Choi, MPH[a,1], Dylan Rose Balter, BA[a,1],
Lamia Y. Haque, MD, MPH[b,*]

KEYWORDS

- Alcohol use disorder • Prevalence • Epidemiology • Disease burden
- Health care utilization • Health care costs • Health disparities

KEY POINTS

- Alcohol use disorder (AUD) is one of the most prevalent substance use disorders (SUDs) in the United States, with over 10% of people aged 12 or older reporting a past-year diagnosis.
- Prevalence of AUD is greater among young adults, males, sexual and gender minorities, American Indians and Alaska Natives, and the uninsured.
- AUD frequently co-occurs with other SUDs, medical comorbidities, and psychiatric conditions and is associated with increased risk of suicide.
- AUD is associated with a high societal cost in the United States, including $249 billion in decreased workplace productivity and increased law enforcement and health care expenditures annually.
- Levels of screening and treatment of AUD remain low.

INTRODUCTION

Alcohol use disorder (AUD) stands as one of the most frequently diagnosed substance use disorders (SUDs) in the United States, impacting around 10% of individuals aged 12 or above, or approximately 29.5 million people. It is causally linked to over 60 diseases and accounts for half of all morbidity and mortality related to alcohol use.[1] Beyond its significant health implications, AUD also bears a substantial economic burden of $249 billion annually, and associated gaps in prevalence, screening, and treatment rates perpetuate social inequality.

[a] Yale School of Medicine, 333 Cedar Street, New Haven, CT 06510, USA; [b] Department of Internal Medicine - Section of Digestive Diseases, Yale Program in Addiction Medicine, Yale School of Medicine, 40 Temple Street, Suite 1A, New Haven, CT 06510, USA
[1] Both authors contributed equally to this work.
* Corresponding author. 40 Temple Street, Suite 1A, New Haven, CT 06510.
E-mail address: lamia.haque@yale.edu

Clin Liver Dis 28 (2024) 577–588
https://doi.org/10.1016/j.cld.2024.06.006
liver.theclinics.com
1089-3261/24/© 2024 Elsevier Inc. All rights reserved, including those for text and data mining, AI training, and similar technologies.

AUD is defined by the Diagnostic and Statistical Manual of Mental Disorders, Fifth Edition (DSM-5) as a pattern of alcohol use leading to behavioral, psychosocial, and physical impairment or distress.[2] Since 2013, AUD has subsumed 2 previously separate diagnoses including "alcohol abuse" and "alcohol dependence," and can be specified as mild, moderate, or severe AUD based on the number of specific DSM-5 criteria present.[2]

Of note, AUD is a chronic medical condition based on past-year symptoms whereas "excessive alcohol use," "heavy alcohol use," "binge drinking," and other forms of at-risk alcohol use are defined based on the quantity of alcohol consumption, and all fall under the category of "unhealthy alcohol use" along with AUD.[3] Specifically, excessive alcohol use includes: binge drinking, defined as having greater than or equal to 4 drinks on one occasion for women and greater than or equal to 5 drinks for men or as a level of alcohol intake that leads to a blood alcohol concentration of greater than or equal to 0.08%; heavy alcohol use, defined as having greater than or equal to 4 drinks per day or greater than or equal to 8 drinks per week for women and greater than or equal to 5 drinks per day or greater than or equal to 15 drinks per week for men; underage drinking, defined as any alcohol use by individuals less than 21 year old; and pregnant drinking, defined as any alcohol use by pregnant individuals.[3] A standard drink is defined as 14 g of alcohol in the United States, which amounts to 12 ounces of beer, 5 ounces of wine, or 1.5 ounces of distilled spirits.[3] At-risk alcohol use, including binge drinking and heavy alcohol use, may increase risk for AUD.[3] However, the majority of those reporting excessive drinking do not meet criteria for AUD.[4] While all forms of unhealthy alcohol use are of public health importance, the remainder of this article will primarily focus on the epidemiology of AUD and its health care burden.

EPIDEMIOLOGY

Among all the substances included in the 2022 National Survey of Drug Use and Health (NSDUH) SUD measures, alcohol ranks first in use and misuse in the United States, with over 29.5 million people or 10.5% of people aged 12 or older reporting a past year AUD.[5] Within this group, 17 million have mild AUD, 6 million have moderate AUD, and 6.1 million have severe AUD.[6] Overall, the prevalence of AUD surpasses the prevalence of all drug use disorders combined, including marijuana, cocaine, heroin, hallucinogens, inhalants, methamphetamine, or prescription drug use disorders, comprising 60.6% of all SUDs.[5]

Across the lifespan, there are roughly 4 times the number of adults aged 26 or older with AUD relative to young adults aged 18 to 25 and adolescents aged 12 to 17. However, young adults are proportionally at the greatest risk of AUD, with over 5.7 million or 16.4% of the age group reporting a past year diagnosis. In comparison, roughly 23.1 million or 10.4% of adults aged 26 or older and less than 753,000 or 2.9% of adolescents aged 12 to 17 have AUD.

While adolescents comprise a small fraction of those with AUD and underage alcohol use has been declining by 50% to 70% since 2002, high-risk adolescents may be important targets for prevention, as 15% of all lifetime AUD cases are known to develop before age 18.[7,8] Indeed, earlier age at first drink of alcohol is associated with increased risk of developing AUD and youth are particularly vulnerable to other forms of unhealthy alcohol use, particularly binge drinking.[9,10] According to the NSDUH from 2022, among 5.8 million people aged 12 to 20 who reported past-month drinking, more than half, or 3.2 million people, reported binge drinking.[7] In addition to elevated risk for developing AUD in adulthood, binge drinking is associated with additional adverse outcomes such as suicide, substance use, and risky sexual behaviors.[10]

By gender, AUD has consistently predominated among males compared with females. Yearly NSDUH estimates show males continue to report higher rates of AUD than females, with 17.4 million or 12.6% of male respondents reporting AUD versus 12.2 million or 8.5% of female respondents in 2022. The prevalence of AUD increased for both males and females at a similar rate between 2019 and 2021, consistent with reports of increased alcohol consumption and disruptions in AUD treatment during the coronavirus disease 2019 (COVID-19) pandemic.[11,12] In the most recent NSDUH estimates from 2022, females returned to pre-pandemic levels of prevalence while males demonstrated a constant rate of increase (**Fig. 1**). While men comprise the majority of individuals with AUD, a review of 51 studies published between March 2020 and July 2022 found cisgender women suffered higher rates of alcohol use and alcohol-related harms than cisgender men.[13]

Among gender diverse people, comprehensive epidemiology of AUD is lacking, as annual NSDUH surveys do not include gender categories beyond male and female. However, existing literature suggests that on average, gender diverse individuals may suffer from higher rates of AUD. In the largest national cross-sectional study of SUD diagnoses among transgender (n = 15,637) and cisgender (n = 46,911) individuals, transgender participants had significantly higher rates of AUD than their cisgender counterparts across all age groups and geographic regions.[15] Similarly, a retrospective cohort study of gender diverse (n = 293) and cis (n = 1698) patients at a single site from 2013 to 2021 revealed a significantly higher proportion of AUD diagnoses among gender diverse patients.[16]

For lesbian, gay, and bisexual (LGB) populations, NSDUH data span from 2015 to 2022. Since 2015, LGB adults have reported higher rates of AUD than their heterosexual counterparts across all age strata in each year. However, similar to heterosexual individuals, LGB young adults aged 18 to 25 were at greatest risk for AUD, with over 1.5 million or 20% reporting a past year AUD in 2022.[17] This period of heightened

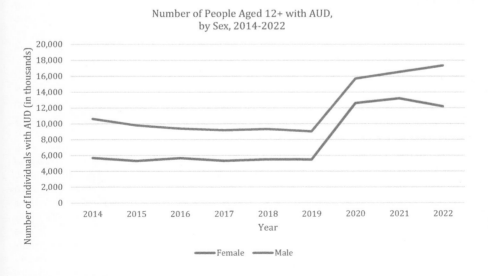

Fig. 1. Number of people aged 12+ with alcohol use disorder (AUD) from 2014 to 2022, by sex.[14]

risk has been estimated to decrease after age 28 in LGB adults versus age 23 in heterosexual adults.[18]

One of the prevailing theories for heightened risk of AUD among sexual and gender minorities (SGM) includes the minority stress theory, which states that stress and stigma associated with sexual orientation and gender identity leads to adverse health outcomes. Numerous insults including internalized stigma, discrimination, abuse, violence, and victimization have been linked to increased odds of excessive alcohol use, AUD, and alcohol-related consequences among LGBTQ people.[19]

Across race and ethnicity categories specified in the NSDUH, American Indians and Alaska Natives (AIANs) had the highest proportion of AUD with 280,000 people or 15.9% of the population reporting a past year diagnosis in 2021. In 2022, the proportion of AIANs with AUD decreased to 10.5%, a rate comparable to other racial and ethnic groups, with the exception of Asians who had an AUD prevalence of 5.6% (**Fig. 2**). NSDUH data show that Asians are significantly less likely than all other racial and ethnic groups to have an AUD. However, prevalence of AUD varies widely upon disaggregation by nativity, in which Korean Americans (13.1%) demonstrate highest prevalence of AUD.[20] Regardless of race or ethnicity, minoritized groups exhibit a dose-dependent association between frequency of discriminatory experiences and severity of AUD.[21]

Heritability of AUD varies between 12% and 50% depending on methodology, with recent twin-studies yielding the highest proportions of variance explained by genes.[22] Large-effect alleles associated with increased risk of AUD include variants of genes responsible for alcohol metabolism such as *ADH* and *ALDH*. However, AUD traits are mostly explained by thousands of small-effect alleles, which are under-researched compared to the polygenicity of less severe alcohol use behaviors.[23] While ongoing genome and epigenome wide association studies, identification of single-nucleotide polymorphisms, and aggregation of polygenic risk scores continue to elucidate biological risk factors and potential pharmacologic interventions for AUD, the environment and gene-environment interactions constitute key modifiable contributors of AUD risk.

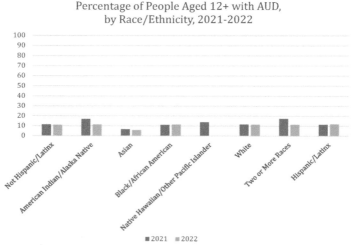

Fig. 2. Percentage of people aged 12+ with AUD from 2021 to 2022, by race/ethnicity.[14]

Socioeconomic status (SES) is measured in NSDUH primarily through educational attainment, poverty level, and employment status. In 2022, those with some college or an associate's degree reported the highest proportion of AUD at 12.4%, followed by college graduates at 11.6%, high school graduates at 10.1%, and those with less than a high school education at 9.5%. Among 3 poverty strata, the greatest proportion of AUD was observed among those over 200% below the federal poverty level (FPL) at 10.8%. Those less than 100% below the FPL had AUD rates of 10.5%, and those within 100% to 199% of the FPL had AUD rates of 9.4%. AUD prevalence also varies by employment status, with unemployed individuals having the highest proportion at 15.5%, full-time employees at 14.1%, part-time employees at 12.3%, and people not in the labor force at 6.8%. NSDUH data do not point to an obvious relationship between SES and prevalence of AUD. Indeed, studies show people with higher SES consume similar or greater amounts of alcohol compared to people with lower SES, but the latter group suffers a disproportionate burden of negative alcohol-related consequences.[24] This phenomenon, also known as the Alcohol Harm Paradox, has been observed internationally across multiple measures of SES since 1980, but its causal factors beyond individual risk behaviors remain understudied.[25]

Finally, in terms of health insurance status, individuals without coverage exhibited the highest proportion of AUD at 13.1%, surpassing the rates among privately insured individuals at 10.6%, Medicaid enrollees at 9.9%, and others (such as Medicare and military personnel) at 7.3%. Recent Kaiser Family Foundation statistics show the uninsured population is predominantly young adults, individuals with lower SES, AIANs, and non-US citizens.[26] Notably, this demographic aligns closely with the aforementioned populations that are disproportionately impacted by AUD, and these social determinants may contribute to worse AUD-related consequences.

Psychiatric conditions as well as other SUDs and medical illnesses frequently co-occur with AUD. NSDUH data show among those with AUD, 42.2% had a mental illness in the past year and 37% had a comorbid SUD.[14] In the Epidemiologic Catchment Area Study (ECA, 1980–1985), one of the most extensive national investigations of the prevalence of mental illnesses, those with AUD exhibited a wide distribution of comorbid mental illnesses. Among them, antisocial personality disorder was the most prevalent at 14.3%, followed by any affective disorder at 13.4%, and schizophrenia at 3.8%.[27] Globally, the longitudinal association between AUD and psychiatric comorbidity based on pooled estimates from meta-analyses ranged from 2.00 to 2.09 for major depressive disorder, 1.35 to 1.74 for attention-deficit hyperactivity disorder, 1.5 to 1.61 for anxiety disorder, 0.7 to 5.43 for post-traumatic stress disorder, and 1.5 to 1.6 for psychotic experiences.[28]

The National Epidemiologic Survey on Alcohol and Related Conditions (NESARC III, 2012–2013) revealed that adults with AUD had 3.3 times the odds of another SUD, 1.9 times the odds of borderline personality disorder, 1.6 times the odds of antisocial personality disorder, 1.3 times the odds of any anxiety disorder, and 1.2 times the odds of major depressive disorder.[27] Based on NESARC II and III data, increased severity of AUD also correlated with more intense manifestations of psychopathology.[29] Furthermore, alcohol use is known to independently increase risk for suicide, which is further pronounced with added psychiatric conditions. For instance, among individuals with comorbid AUD and borderline personality disorder, lifetime prevalence of suicide attempts is known to range from 21% to 42%.[30] Finally, AUD is associated with a litany of medical conditions, some of which include cancers, cardiovascular disease, cognitive impairment, liver disease, pancreatic disease, infectious diseases, and traumatic injuries.[3]

Given the powerful association between SUDs and mental illnesses and increased risk for poorer outcomes with co-occurring disorders, researchers and clinicians have developed integrated treatment models to facilitate concurrent substance use and mental health interventions. Integrated care models in which AUD is treated along with co-occurring medical conditions have also shown promise. Integrated treatment is the best practice of care for people with co-occurring disorders and has been effective in diverse populations across different treatment settings.[31]

THE ECONOMIC, SOCIETAL, AND HEALTH CARE BURDEN OF ALCOHOL USE DISORDER

Excessive alcohol use also has a substantial impact on economic, societal, and health care costs. In 2010, the economic cost of unhealthy alcohol use in the United States totaled $249 billion.[32] These costs were predominantly driven by decreased workplace productivity, increased health care and law enforcement expenditures, and expenses due to motor vehicle crashes (MVC).[32] One study in Minnesota found that the economic cost of unhealthy alcohol use was almost $8 billion, or the equivalent of $1383 per state resident.[33] The greatest contributor to these economic costs was decreased productivity, which accounted for $5.59 billion. Reasons for decreased productivity included compromised performance at work, lost productivity secondary to premature mortality, and greater rates of absenteeism. Additionally, this study found that binge drinking was the costliest drinking pattern, as it was associated with 40% of health care expenditures, 72.4% of decreased productivity costs, and 97.2% of other societal expenses.[33] A similar study in North Carolina found that excessive alcohol consumption reached $9.72 billion. Of this $9.72 billion, the state government paid $4.43 billion, individuals who drink alcohol in North Carolina paid $3.76 billion, and those who do not drink alcohol in North Carolina paid $1.53 billion.[34] Thus, unhealthy alcohol use results in significant expenditures among not only federal and state governments, but also individuals.

In addition to staggering economic costs, excessive alcohol use has also contributed to significant societal costs. In 2021, alcohol was involved in 13,384 MVC deaths, which equates to 31% of all MVC fatalities.[35] Furthermore, there is a significant interplay between alcohol and mental health emergencies. The Centers for Disease Control and Prevention estimates that 21% of people who die by suicide have elevated blood alcohol concentrations and that approximately 25% of people who die by suicide have AUD.[35]

Excessive alcohol use has also substantially impacted the health care system and exacerbated health care expenditures. Among a population of 162 million individuals with employer-sponsored health insurance, the total annual health care cost associated with AUD was $10.2 billion.[36] Additionally, research has found that having a diagnosis secondary to excessive alcohol use is associated with higher yearly personal health care expenses by $14,918 and $4823 for individuals with commercial and Medicaid insurance, respectively.[37] The majority of these costs were due to heart disease, stroke, malignancies, and liver, gallbladder, and pancreas pathologies, all of which were secondary to excessive alcohol use.[37]

While heavy alcohol use has exacerbated health care expenditures at large, it has particularly impacted the emergency department (ED) setting. From 2006 to 2014, the ED saw a 47% increase in alcohol-associated visits.[38] This increase equates to 210,000 additional ED visits, as well as a 272% rise in health care costs, from $4.1 billion to $15.3 billion. Notably, the rate of chronic alcohol-associated ED visits increased more than that of acute alcohol-associated visits (57.9% vs 40%).

Additionally, there was a greater annual percent change in rates of alcohol-associated ED visits for females versus males (5.3% vs 4.0%).[38] The ED has also experienced an increase in co-morbid alcohol and opioid-related events—in 2020, it is estimated that alcohol was involved in 7.1% of ED visits and 17.4% of fatalities attributable to opioid overdoses.[35]

Moreover, it is important to acknowledge the role of the COVID-19 pandemic in augmenting the economic, societal, and health care burden of AUD. A cross-sectional study of individuals during the COVID-19 pandemic found that 60% of individuals reported increased alcohol consumption compared to before the pandemic. Those who endorsed stress related to the pandemic reported an increase in both amount and frequency of drinking.[11] As rates of alcohol consumption climbed during the COVID-19 pandemic, alcohol sales likewise increased. In 2020, alcohol sales rose by 2.9%, reflecting the greatest annual sales increase in 50 years.[39,40] Such increases in both alcohol consumption and sales have further contributed to the societal burden of AUD. Data from the National Highway Traffic Safety Administration found a 14% increase in alcohol-involved traffic deaths in 2020, following years of decreasing fatality rates.[39,41] The pandemic also perpetuated AUD's health care burden, as ED visits for alcohol withdrawal increased by 34% in 2020 compared to 2019.[39,42] Alcohol-related deaths at large also rose during the pandemic. From 1997 to 2017, the rate of deaths involving alcohol increased by an average of 2.2% per year. However, the COVID-19 pandemic rapidly accelerated these deaths rates, with an estimated increase of 25% from 2019 to 2020. While death rates increased across all age groups, individuals aged 25 to 44 experienced the largest increase.[43] Alcohol consumption during this time was associated with male sex and recent unemployment due to the pandemic.[44] Predictive models estimate that increases in alcohol use during the COVID-19 pandemic will result in a lower life expectancy, an additional 295,000 hospitalizations, and an associated cost of $5.4 billion during the next 5 years.[44] Thus, the pandemic reflects one important driver of increasing rates of alcohol use and disease burden. Although the relationship between the pandemic and alcohol use has not been fully elucidated, research suggests that heightened emotional and financial stress, increased availability of alcohol, unprecedented social isolation, and the large mental health toll of the pandemic have contributed to alcohol's increasing health care burden.[11,45]

Beyond the COVID-19 pandemic, alcohol's increasing health care burden is also a reflection of significant barriers to both AUD screening and treatment within our health care system. Despite the high rates of AUD-related morbidity and mortality, unhealthy alcohol use is frequently overlooked in health care settings, thereby leading to significant gaps in health care quality for individuals with AUD.[46] Currently, the United States Preventive Services Taskforce (USPSTF) recommends that all adults aged 18 or older receive screening for unhealthy alcohol use in the primary care setting.[47,48] Although individuals with AUD have high rates of health care engagement, studies have found that there has been poor implementation of validated screening for unhealthy alcohol use in the primary care setting.[46,49] This lack of formal screening may prevent appropriate subsequent interventions and treatment.[50]

For patients who screen positive for unhealthy alcohol use, USPSTF advises brief behavioral counseling interventions, which have been shown to decrease number of weekly drinks, the proportion of individuals surpassing recommended alcohol limits, and the proportion of individuals reporting an episode of heavy alcohol use.[47,48,51] Notwithstanding the effectiveness of these interventions, data from the 2015 to 2019 NSDUH show that only 14.6% of people with AUD reported receiving a brief intervention in the past year.[49] Qualitative studies of patients and providers have found that some barriers to screening and brief interventions in primary care include societal stigma, as well as lack of time, resources, and provider knowledge and training.[50,52,53]

Similarly, there are astonishingly low AUD treatment rates.[54] Gold-standard treatment for AUD consists of a combination of evidence-based behavioral and pharmacotherapy modalities.[46] NSDUH data from 2022 estimate that 7.6% of adults with AUD received treatment in the past year, and only 2.2% specifically received medication treatment for AUD in the past year.[54] Several barriers may contribute to these low treatment rates, including limited health care training and emphasis on AUD treatment, as well as stigma attached to addiction and its treatment.[55–59]

Thus, AUD is associated with an increasing economic, societal, and health care burden. Though not exhaustive, some important drivers of this increasing burden include the COVID-19 pandemic as well as inadequate implementation of AUD screening and treatment within our health care system. It is critical to further explore such drivers and health care gaps to reduce future health care burden of AUD.

SUMMARY

AUD is rising in prevalence and is one of the most common SUDs. Although AUD occurs more frequently in males, the prevalence among females and some minoritized populations, who are more likely to experience harmful effects and consequences of AUD, has risen. Despite the high morbidity, mortality, acute health care utilization, and societal cost associated with AUD, multiple barriers to AUD treatment exist along the cascade of AUD care, leading to insufficient screening and low levels of evidence-based treatment uptake. Innovative interventions that involve patient-centered multidisciplinary care models as well as public health and policy measures to prevent and treat AUD are needed.

CLINICS CARE POINTS

- AUD is more prevalent among young adults, males, some minoritized racial/ethnic groups, sexual and gender minorities, and the uninsured.
- Clinicians should assess for comorbid SUD as well as medical and psychiatric conditions that can co-occur with AUD.
- Clinicians should screen for unhealthy alcohol use in the primary care setting using a validated screening tool.
- Alcohol use is associated with significant societal, economic, and health care costs.

DISCLOSURE

The authors have no relevant commercial or financial conflicts of interest. This work is supported in part by NIAAA Career Development Award K23AA031334 (L.Y. Haque).

REFERENCES

1. Connor JP, Haber PS, Hall WD. Alcohol use disorders. Lancet 2016;387(10022): 988–98. https://doi.org/10.1016/S0140-6736(15)00122-1.
2. Alcohol use disorder: a comparison between DSM–IV and DSM–5 | national institute on alcohol abuse and alcoholism (NIAAA). Available at: https://www.niaaa. nih.gov/publications/brochures-and-fact-sheets/alcohol-use-disorder-comparison-between-dsm. [Accessed 7 August 2023].

3. Donroe JH, Edelman EJ. Alcohol use. Ann Intern Med 2022;175(10):ITC145–60. https://doi.org/10.7326/AITC202210180.

4. Esser MB. Prevalence of alcohol dependence among US adult drinkers, 2009–2011. Prev Chronic Dis 2014;11. https://doi.org/10.5888/pcd11.140329.

5. Substance Abuse and Mental Health Services Administration. (2023). Key substance use and mental health indicators in the United States: Results from the 2022 National Survey on Drug Use and Health (HHS Publication No. PEP23-07-01-006, NSDUH Series H-58). Center for Behavioral Health Statistics and Quality, Substance Abuse and Mental Health Services Administration. Available at: https://www.samhsa.gov/data/report/2022-nsduh-annual-national-report   (Accessed 25 February 2024).

6. Section 5 PE tables – results from the 2022 national survey on drug use and health: detailed tables, SAMHSA, CBHSQ. Available at: https://www.samhsa.gov/data/sites/default/files/reports/rpt42728/NSDUHDetailedTabs2022/NSDUHDetailedTabs2022/NSDUHDetTabsSect5pe2022.htm. [Accessed 7 January 2024].

7. Underage drinking in the United States (ages 12 to 20) | national institute on alcohol abuse and alcoholism (NIAAA). Available at: https://www.niaaa.nih.gov/alcohols-effects-health/alcohol-topics/alcohol-facts-and-statistics/underage-drinking-united-states-ages-12-20. [Accessed 25 February 2024].

8. Glantz MD, Bharat C, Degenhardt L, et al. The epidemiology of alcohol use disorders cross-nationally: findings from the World Mental Health Surveys. Addict Behav 2020;102:106128. https://doi.org/10.1016/j.addbeh.2019.106128.

9. Quigley J, Committee on substance use and prevention, Ryan SA, et al. Alcohol use by youth. Pediatrics 2019;144(1):e20191356. https://doi.org/10.1542/peds.2019-1356.

10. Siqueira L, Smith VC, et al. Committee on substance abuse. Binge drinking. Pediatrics 2015;136(3):e718–26. https://doi.org/10.1542/peds.2015-2337.

11. Grossman ER, Benjamin-Neelon SE, Sonnenschein S. Alcohol consumption during the COVID-19 pandemic: a cross-sectional survey of us adults. Int J Environ Res Publ Health 2020;17(24):9189. https://doi.org/10.3390/ijerph17249189.

12. Schmidt RA, Genois R, Jin J, et al. The early impact of COVID-19 on the incidence, prevalence, and severity of alcohol use and other drugs: a systematic review. Drug Alcohol Depend 2021;228:109065. https://doi.org/10.1016/j.drugalcdep.2021.109065.

13. Veldhuis C. Are cisgender women and transgender and nonbinary people drinking more during the COVID-19 pandemic? It depends. ARCR 2023;43(1):05. https://doi.org/10.35946/arcr.v43.1.05.

14. NSDUH national releases. Available at: https://www.samhsa.gov/data/nsduh/national-releases. [Accessed 13 September 2023].

15. Hughto JMW, Quinn EK, Dunbar MS, et al. Prevalence and Co-occurrence of alcohol, nicotine, and other substance use disorder diagnoses among US transgender and cisgender adults. JAMA Netw Open 2021;4(2):e2036512. https://doi.org/10.1001/jamanetworkopen.2020.36512.

16. McDowell MJ, King DS, Gitin S, et al. Alcohol use disorder treatment in sexually and gender diverse patients: a retrospective cohort study. J Clin Psychiatry 2023;84(5):48739. https://doi.org/10.4088/JCP.23m14812.

17. Delphin-Rittmon ME. 2022 National Survey on Drug Use and Health: Among the Lesbian, Gay, or Bisexual (LGB) Population Aged 12 or Older.

18. Peralta RL, Victory E, Thompson CL. Alcohol use disorder in sexual minority adults: age- and sex- specific prevalence estimates from a national survey,

2015-2017. Drug Alcohol Depend 2019;205:107673. https://doi.org/10.1016/j. drugalcdep.2019.107673.

19. Crane PR, Swaringen KS, Foster AM, et al. Alcohol use disorders among sexual and gender minority populations. In: Rothblum ED, editor. The oxford handbook of sexual and gender minority mental health. New York, NY: Oxford University Press; 2020. https://doi.org/10.1093/oxfordhb/9780190067991.013.9.

20. Hai AH, Lee CS, John R, et al. Debunking the myth of low behavioral risk among Asian Americans: the case of alcohol use. Drug Alcohol Depend 2021;228: 109059. https://doi.org/10.1016/j.drugalcdep.2021.109059.

21. Glass JE, Williams EC, Oh H. Racial/ethnic discrimination and alcohol use disorder severity among United States adults. Drug Alcohol Depend 2020;216: 108203. https://doi.org/10.1016/j.drugalcdep.2020.108203.

22. Friedel E, Kaminski J, Ripke S. Heritability of alcohol use disorder: evidence from twin studies and genome-wide association studies. In: el-Guebaly N, Carrà G, Galanter M, et al. editors. Textbook of addiction treatment: international perspectives. Milano, Italy: Springer International Publishing; 2021. p. 21–33. https://doi. org/10.1007/978-3-030-36391-8_3.

23. Genetics of substance use disorders in the era of big data | Nature Reviews Genetics. Available at: https://www.nature.com/articles/s41576-021-00377-1. [Accessed 13 January 2024].

24. Collins SE. Associations between socioeconomic factors and alcohol outcomes. Alcohol Res 2016;38(1):83–94.

25. Boyd J, Sexton O, Angus C, et al. Causal mechanisms proposed for the alcohol harm paradox—a systematic review. Addiction 2022;117(1):33–56. https://doi. org/10.1111/add.15567.

26. Tolbert J, Drake P, Published AD. Key facts about the uninsured population. KFF. 2023. Available at: https://www.kff.org/uninsured/issue-brief/key-facts-about-the-uninsured-population/. [Accessed 15 January 2024].

27. Zaorska J, Wojnar M. Comorbidity of alcohol use disorders with substance use disorders and psychiatric disorders. In: Mueller S, Heilig M, editors. Alcohol and alcohol-related diseases. Cham, Swizerland: Springer International Publishing; 2023. p. 289–307. https://doi.org/10.1007/978-3-031-32483-3_17.

28. Castillo-Carniglia A, Keyes KM, Hasin DS, et al. Psychiatric comorbidities in alcohol use disorder. Lancet Psychiatr 2019;6(12):1068–80. https://doi.org/10. 1016/S2215-0366(19)30222-6.

29. Helle AC, Trull TJ, Watts AL, et al. Psychiatric comorbidity as a function of severity: DSM-5 alcohol use disorder and HiTOP classification of mental disorders. Alcohol Clin Exp Res 2020;44(3):632–44. https://doi.org/10.1111/acer. 14284.

30. Esang M, Ahmed S. A closer look at substance use and suicide. American Journal of Psychiatry Residents' Journal 2018;13(6):6–8. https://doi.org/10.1176/appi. ajp-rj.2018.130603.

31. TIP 42. Substance use treatment for persons with Co-occurring disorders | SAMHSA publications and digital products. Available at: https://store.samhsa. gov/product/tip-42-substance-use-treatment-persons-co-occurring-disorders/p ep20-02-01-004. [Accessed 30 January 2024].

32. Excessive drinking is draining the U.S. Economy. 2022. Available at: https://www. cdc.gov/alcohol/features/excessive-drinking.html. [Accessed 7 August 2023].

33. Gloppen KM, Roesler JS, Farley DM. Assessing the costs of excessive alcohol consumption in Minnesota. Am J Prev Med 2022;63(4):505–12. https://doi.org/ 10.1016/j.amepre.2022.04.031.

34. Gora Combs K, Fliss MD, Knuth KB, et al. The societal cost of excessive drinking in North Carolina, 2017. N C Med J 2022;83(3):214–20. https://doi.org/10.18043/ncm.83.3.214.

35. National Institute on Alcohol Abuse and Alcoholism. Alcohol-related emergencies and deaths in the United States. 2023. Available at: https://www.niaaa.nih.gov/alcohols-effects-health/alcohol-topics/alcohol-facts-and-statistics/alcohol-related-emergencies-and-deaths-united-states.

36. Li M, Peterson C, Xu L, et al. Medical costs of substance use disorders in the US employer-sponsored insurance population. JAMA Netw Open 2023;6(1):e2252378. https://doi.org/10.1001/jamanetworkopen.2022.52378.

37. Ozluk P, Cobb R, Sylwestrzak G, et al. Alcohol-attributable medical costs in commercially insured and Medicaid populations. AJPM Focus 2022;1(2):100036. https://doi.org/10.1016/j.focus.2022.100036.

38. White AM, Slater ME, Ng G, et al. Trends in alcohol-related emergency department visits in the United States: results from the nationwide emergency department sample, 2006 to 2014. Alcohol Clin Exp Res 2018;42(2):352–9. https://doi.org/10.1111/acer.13559.

39. Deaths involving alcohol increased during the COVID-19 pandemic | National Institute on Alcohol Abuse and Alcoholism (NIAAA). Available at: https://www.niaaa.nih.gov/news-events/research-update/deaths-involving-alcohol-increased-during-covid-19-pandemic. [Accessed 27 February 2024].

40. Surveillance report #120 | national institute on alcohol abuse and alcoholism (NIAAA). Available at: https://www.niaaa.nih.gov/publications/surveillance-reports/surveillance120. [Accessed 27 February 2024].

41. Stewart T. Overview of motor vehicle crashes in 2020 (Report No. DOT HS 813 266). National Highway Traffic Safety Administration. 2022.

42. Sharma RA, Subedi K, Gbadebo BM, et al. Alcohol withdrawal rates in hospitalized patients during the COVID-19 pandemic. JAMA Netw Open 2021;4(3):e210422. https://doi.org/10.1001/jamanetworkopen.2021.0422.

43. White AM, Castle IJP, Powell PA, et al. Alcohol-related deaths during the COVID-19 pandemic. JAMA 2022;327(17):1704–6. https://doi.org/10.1001/jama.2022.4308.

44. Killgore WDS, Cloonan SA, Taylor EC, et al. Alcohol dependence during COVID-19 lockdowns. Psychiatry Res 2021;296:113676. https://doi.org/10.1016/j.psychres.2020.113676.

45. Yue Y, Wang S, Smith E, et al. Alcohol consumption and mental health during the COVID-19 pandemic. Alcohol Alcohol 2023;58(3):247–57. https://doi.org/10.1093/alcalc/agad011.

46. Cohen SM, Alexander RS, Holt SR. The spectrum of alcohol use: epidemiology, diagnosis, and treatment. Med Clin North Am 2022;106(1):43–60. https://doi.org/10.1016/j.mcna.2021.08.003.

47. US Preventive Services Task Force, Curry SJ, Krist AH, et al. Screening and behavioral counseling interventions to reduce unhealthy alcohol use in adolescents and adults: US preventive Services task force recommendation statement. JAMA 2018;320(18):1899. https://doi.org/10.1001/jama.2018.16789.

48. Screening and behavioral counseling interventions to reduce unhealthy alcohol use in adolescents and adults: recommendation statement. afp 2019;99(12). online-online.

49. Mintz CM, Hartz SM, Fisher SL, et al. A cascade of care for alcohol use disorder: using 2015–2019 National Survey on Drug Use and Health data to identify gaps in

past 12-month care. Alcohol Clin Exp Res 2021;45(6):1276–86. https://doi.org/10.1111/acer.14609.

50. Chatterton B, Agnoli A, Schwarz EB, et al. Alcohol screening during US primary care visits, 2014–2016. J Gen Intern Med 2022;37(15):3848–52. https://doi.org/10.1007/s11606-021-07369-1.

51. Bertholet N, Daeppen JB, Wietlisbach V, et al. Reduction of alcohol consumption by brief alcohol intervention in primary care: systematic review and meta-analysis. Arch Intern Med 2005;165(9):986–95. https://doi.org/10.1001/archinte.165.9.986.

52. McNeely J, Kumar PC, Rieckmann T, et al. Barriers and facilitators affecting the implementation of substance use screening in primary care clinics: a qualitative study of patients, providers, and staff. Addict Sci Clin Pract 2018;13:8. https://doi.org/10.1186/s13722-018-0110-8.

53. Johnson M, Jackson R, Guillaume L, et al. Barriers and facilitators to implementing screening and brief intervention for alcohol misuse: a systematic review of qualitative evidence. Journal of Public Health 2011;33(3):412–21. https://doi.org/10.1093/pubmed/fdq095.

54. National Institute on Alcohol Abuse and Alcoholism. Alcohol treatment in the United States: age groups and demographic characteristics 2023. Published online.

55. Abraham AJ, Andrews CM, Harris SJ, et al. Availability of medications for the treatment of alcohol and opioid use disorder in the USA. Neurotherapeutics 2020;17(1):55–69. https://doi.org/10.1007/s13311-019-00814-4.

56. Rieckmann T, Muench J, McBurnie MA, et al. Medication-assisted treatment for substance use disorders within a national community health center research network. Subst Abuse 2016;37(4):625–34. https://doi.org/10.1080/08897077.2016.1189477.

57. Williams EC, Gupta S, Rubinsky AD, et al. Variation in receipt of pharmacotherapy for alcohol use disorders across racial/ethnic groups: a national study in the U.S. Veterans Health Administration. Drug Alcohol Depend 2017;178:527–33. https://doi.org/10.1016/j.drugalcdep.2017.06.011.

58. Williams EC, Achtmeyer CE, Young JP, et al. Barriers to and facilitators of alcohol use disorder pharmacotherapy in primary care: a qualitative study in five va clinics. J Gen Intern Med 2018;33(3):258–67. https://doi.org/10.1007/s11606-017-4202-z.

59. Leggio L, Falk DE, Ryan ML, et al. Medication development for alcohol use disorder: a focus on clinical studies. In: Nader MA, Hurd YL, editors. Substance use disorders: from etiology to treatment. Handbook of experimental pharmacology. Cham, Switzerland: Springer International Publishing; 2020. p. 443–62. https://doi.org/10.1007/164_2019_295.

Epidemiology of Alcohol-Associated Liver Disease Including Increasing Burden in Young Adults and Females Especially Since Covid-19 Pandemic

Wei Zhang, MD, PhD[a], Robert J. Wong, MD, MS[b],*

KEYWORDS

- Alcohol-associated liver disease • Alcohol-associated hepatitis • Cirrhosis
- Steatosis • Liver transplantation

KEY POINTS

- The rising clinical and economic burden of alcohol-associated liver disease (ALD) has been exacerbated by the surge in high-risk alcohol use during and following the onset of the coronavirus disease 2019 pandemic.
- The rise in ALD and ALD-related morbidity and mortality has particularly affected young adults, women, and ethnic minority populations.
- This observed rise in ALD is paralleled by the increasing prevalence of metabolic dysfunction-associated steatotic liver disease (MASLD), which is especially concerning given that high-risk alcohol use in MASLD is associated with worse outcomes.

EPIDEMIOLOGY OF ALCOHOL-ASSOCIATED LIVER DISEASE

Alcohol-associated liver disease (ALD) encompasses a range of liver pathologies resulting from excessive alcohol consumption. This spectrum begins with alcohol-associated steatosis (AS) (fatty liver), may progress to alcohol-associated steatohepatitis (ASH), and can lead to alcohol-associated hepatitis (AH) or cirrhosis (AC), and

[a] Gastroenterology Unit, Massachusetts General Hospital, 55 Fruit Street, Boston, MA 02114, USA; [b] Division of Gastroenterology and Hepatology, Veterans Affairs Palo Alto Healthcare System, Stanford University School of Medicine, 3801 Miranda Avenue, GI-111, Palo Alto, CA 94304, USA
* Corresponding author. Division of Gastroenterology and Hepatology, Veterans Affairs Palo Alto Healthcare System, Stanford University School of Medicine, 3801 Miranda Avenue, GI-111, Palo Alto, CA 94304.
E-mail address: Rwong123@stanford.edu

Clin Liver Dis 28 (2024) 589–600
https://doi.org/10.1016/j.cld.2024.06.001
liver.theclinics.com
1089-3261/24/© 2024 Elsevier Inc. All rights reserved, including those for text and data mining, AI training, and similar technologies.

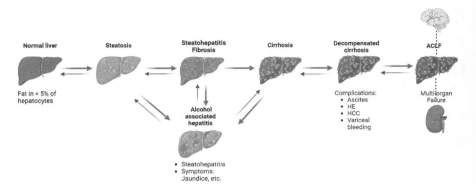

Fig. 1. Progression of alcohol-associated liver disease.

ultimately result in decompensation of the cirrhosis and acute on chronic liver failure (ACLF) (**Fig. 1**).[1] The Global Burden of Disease project estimated 1256900 deaths globally in 2016 due to cirrhosis and chronic liver diseases, with 334900 (27%) attributable to alcohol.[2] In the United States (US), the estimated prevalence of ALD was about 8%, based on data from 3 national databases spanning from 2001 to 2016.[3] Along with these trends, ALD has emerged as the leading cause for liver transplantation in the US.[4] Even before the onset of the coronavirus disease 2019 (COVID-19) pandemic, ALD was already on the rise globally.[5,6] The COVID-19 pandemic has further impacted these figures, with age-adjusted mortality rates for ALD rising by 23.4% from 6.4 to 7.0 per 100000 people.[7] A predictive modeling study, utilizing data from multiple national databases, suggests that if current alcohol consumption trends continue, the age-standardized death rates for ALD could increase from 8.2 deaths per 100000 patient per year in 2019 to 15.2 by 2040. Similarly, the age-standardized incidence of decompensated AC in the US is projected to rise by 77%, from 9.9 cases per 100000 patient per year in 2019 to 17.5 by 2040.[8] In addition to the increasing prevalence of ALD resulting from the pandemic, significant disparities have also been observed on the impact of alcohol use disorder (AUD) and ALD, particularly among young adults and women.[9] These epidemiologic changes are shaped by the pandemic's influence on alcohol consumption patterns, as well as the rise of metabolic risk factors and comorbidities, such as metabolic syndrome and obesity.[9,10] The recent adoption of the term 'metabolic dysfunction-associated ALD' represents a notable advancement in the conceptualization and categorization of the disease.[11,12]

ALCOHOL-ASSOCIATED STEATOSIS

AS can be identified on sonography, computed tomography (CT), or MRI of the liver.[13] While liver biopsy is the "gold standard" for histologic confirmation of steatosis, advancements in non-invasive radiographic techniques can often avert the need for biopsy for detection of hepatic steatosis. The American College of Gastroenterology guidance defines AS based on imaging studies or elevated liver enzymes (aspartate aminotransferase>alanine aminotransferase), serum bilirubin less than 3 mg per dL, and the absence of other causes of liver disease.[14] It is estimated that AS develops in 90% of the patients who drink at least 4 to 5 standard drinks a day.[10] Based on the 2001 to 2016's National Health and Nutrition Examination Survey (NHANES) data, the prevalence of AS was about 4.3% to 4.7% among the US adults.[15] The accurate prevalence of AS is difficult to ascertain and is probably underreported and under diagnosed. This under-estimation may occur because patients with this condition can go undetected by imaging modalities, and liver enzyme tests may not always show abnormalities. While AS was once thought to be a benign condition reversible through abstinence from alcohol, recent research indicates that with continued drinking, it can progress to advanced fibrosis and cirrhosis, leading to heightened morbidity and mortality.[16] It is estimated that about 10% to 35% of patients will develop ASH, and 8% to 20% of these will go on to develop AC with continued heaving drinking.[13] In addition, a meta-analysis of biopsy proven AS patients estimated an annual mortality rate of approximately 6%, with deaths from non-liver-related causes exceeding those from liver-related complications.[17] Another study from Sweden, utilizing biopsy-confirmed cases, demonstrated that individuals with AS had an increased risk of cardiovascular disease (subdistribution hazard ratio [sHR], 1.46; 95% confidence interval [CI], 1.17–1.82) compared to a matched general population group.[18] We have recently found that patients with AS have a higher 30-day mortality risk (HR 2.84, $P<.001$), increased overall mortality (HR 1.40, $P<.001$), and a greater likelihood of readmission (HR 1.21, $P<.01$) compared to those without AS.[19] In another unpublished study by our group that identified AS through imaging studies, we observed that patients with AS had a notably higher risk of progressing to advanced ALD with HR of 2.0 ($P<.001$), underscoring the substantial risk AS poses for advancing to advanced ALD. Despite these findings, AS remains understudied.

ALCOHOL-ASSOCIATED HEPATITIS

AH is a clinical syndrome characterized by jaundice and liver failure in the setting of recent heavy alcohol use. The histopathologic counterpart, ASH, is a specific finding on liver biopsy but is not solely sufficient for a clinical diagnosis of AH without the presence of corresponding clinical symptoms.[13] The National Institute of Alcohol Abuse and Alcoholism-funded Alcohol Associated Hepatitis Consortia has proposed criteria to clinically define AH, which have been widely adopted for both clinical practice and research. Patients with AH are classified by severity, with severe AH typically defined by a Maddrey Discriminant Function score of 32 or higher or a Model for End-Stage Liver Disease score of 20 or above.[20] While moderate AH was once considered relatively benign, recent studies have revealed that its associated risks and mortality rates have been underestimated. Mortality rates for moderate AH are reported to be 3% to 7% in the short-to-medium term (1–3 months) and 13% to 20% at 1 year.[21] It has been observed that patients with AH tend to experience the most rapid progression of fibrosis, contributing to the increased mortality risk.[22] The overall prevalence of AH is 17% among hospitalized patients with ALD-related ACLF.[23] In addition, the rate of readmission was notably high. The data from the Nationwide Readmissions Database indicated that, out of 61750 patients admitted with a diagnosis of AH, 23.9% were readmitted within a 30-day period.[24] Furthermore, a recent international multicenter cohort study demonstrated that the 90-day mortality rate for patients with AH ranges from 20% to 50%.[25]

ALCOHOL-ASSOCIATED CIRRHOSIS

Alcohol-associated cirrhosis (AC) represents the most advanced stage of ALD and may co-occur with AH. Literature indicates that among patients hospitalized for AH, the prevalence of concomitant AC ranges from approximately 70% to 90%.[26–28] Globally, in 2017, there were 23.6 million cases of alcohol-associated compensated cirrhosis, with a stable prevalence rate of approximately 288 per 100000, consistent since 1990. This is despite an increase in absolute numbers from 13.5 million in

1990. Conversely, the number of decompensated AC cases rose from 1.10 million to 2.46 million during the same period, with the age-standardized prevalence rate increasing from 25.3 (23.9–26.7) to 30.0 (28.2–31.8) per 100000.[29] In the US, the data from the NHANES study indicated that the prevalence of advanced fibrosis or early cirrhosis increased significantly from 2.2% in 2001 to 2002 to 6.6% in 2015 to 2016. Hospitalizations for AC also saw a substantial increase of 32.8% from 2007 to 2014.[3] Furthermore, in 2019, alcohol was implicated in 25% of cirrhosis-related deaths globally. The highest regional mortality rates were in Europe (42%) and the Americas (35%), with the Eastern Mediterranean region reporting the lowest (8%). Additionally, the global age-standardized death rate for AC was estimated at 4.5 per 100000 population.[30]

IMPACT OF CORONAVIRUS DISEASE 2019 ERA ON ALCOHOL USE DISORDER AND ALCOHOL-ASSOCIATED LIVER DISEASE TRENDS AMONG WOMEN AND YOUNG ADULTS

During the COVID-19 pandemic, there was a significant escalation in the incidence of AUD and ALD. An online survey conducted from February to April 2020, shortly after the onset of the pandemic, revealed a 26% increase in overall alcohol consumption. This included rises in binge drinking, daily alcohol intake, and the proportion of individuals exceeding safe drinking guidelines. Notably, the increase in exceeding drinking limits was more pronounced in women than men ($P=.026$) and in Black, non-Hispanic individuals compared to White, non-Hispanic individuals ($P=.028$).[31] Retail sales of alcohol and tobacco during the early phase of the COVID-19 pandemic increased by 34% and 13%, respectively, compared to the same period in the previous year.[32] Women experienced a greater overall percentage increase in alcohol consumption, while men exhibited increased risky drinking behaviors and higher overall alcohol consumption.[33]

In terms of ALD, the pandemic exacerbated an already increasing prevalence. A study from 3 major hospitals in California indicated a 51% rise in hospital admissions for AH from 2019 to 2020, with the most significant increases observed in women and adults under 40 years of age.[34] Additionally, multiple studies have shown that patients with ALD are at an increased risk of severe illness and death from COVID-19.[35] ALD-related mortality also rose during the pandemic, with a 21% increase in males and 27% in females from 2019 to 2020, particularly affecting females and young adults.[6] Data from the Centers for Disease Control and Prevention's Wide-Ranging Online Data for Epidemiologic Research revealed that among 626090 chronic liver disease-related deaths between 2010 and 2021, age-standardized mortality rates (ASMRs) for ALD significantly increased between 2010 to 2019 and 2020 to 2021, with an annual percentage change (APC) from 3.5% to 17.6% ($P<.01$). The rise in ASMRs for ALD was most pronounced in non-Hispanic Whites, Blacks, and Alaska Indians or Native Americans (APC: 11.7%, 10.8%, 18.0%, all $P<.05$). The increase was particularly severe in the 25 to 44 age group (APC: 34.6%, compared to 13.7% and 12.6% for the 45–64 and >65 age groups, respectively, all $P<.01$), which were all higher than pre-COVID-19 rates.[36]

RISK FACTORS FOR ALCOHOL-ASSOCIATED LIVER DISEASE
Alcohol

A dose-response relationship has been established between alcohol consumption and the risk of developing ALD (**Table 1**).[22] Epidemiologic evidence suggests that alcohol use markedly increases the risk of liver disease mortality by a factor of 260,

Table 1
A summary of risk factors for alcohol-associated liver disease

Risks / Disease	ALD
Alcohol	1. Most important risk factor, dose-dependent 2. There may not be "liver-safe drinking" 3. AUD or at risk drinking can both cause ALD
Genetics	1. ALDH2, ADH1B, ADH1B and ADH1C are related to AUD 2. PNPLA3, TM6SF2, and MBOAT7 are the most studies genetic risk factors
Gender	1. Women are more likely to develop ALD with the same amount of alcohol consumption 2. There is increased drinking, including at risk drinking and associated AUD in women 3. There is increased incidence of ALD in women
Metabolic Risk Factors	1. Synergistic with alcohol drinking in causing ALD 2. There is increased prevalence of metabolic syndrome and obesity 3. Threshold for safe drinking may not be present as even low alcohol drinking is associated with increased risk for ALD 4. The new nomenclature of Met-ALD will enhance our understanding of the synergistic effects of ALD and MASLD
Race/Ethnicity	1. Hispanic and African American have higher risk for ALD compared to White 2. There is increased prevalence of ALD in Hispanic and African American population
Age	1. Age is an independent risk factor for ALD mortality 2. There is increased prevalence and mortality of young patients aged 25–34 with ALD
COVID-19	COVID-19 increased the risk of AUD, ALD and mortality

compared to a 3.2-fold increase for cardiovascular mortality and a 5.1-fold increase for cancer mortality.[37] Chronic heavy alcohol consumption, defined as intake exceeding 40 g of pure alcohol per day over several years, is associated with the highest risk of ALD. Globally, alcohol accounts for approximately 21% of cases of prevalent compensated cirrhosis.[29] In particular, heavy drinking contributes to over half of the attributable fraction for cirrhosis, with the highest rates observed in North America (62%) and Europe (60%).[38]

A systematic review encompassing 7 cohort studies and 2 case-control studies, with a total of 2629272 participants and 5505 cirrhosis cases, found that the risk of cirrhosis becomes significant at consumption levels as low as 1 drink per day when compared to long-term abstainers. The risk escalates with increased alcohol intake. For instance, consuming greater than or equal to 5 drinks per day is associated with a markedly elevated risk for both women (RR = 12.44, 95% CI: 6.65–23.27 for 5–6 drinks; RR = 24.58, 95% CI: 14.77–40.90 for $\geq$7 drinks) and men (RR = 3.80,

95% CI: 0.85–17.02; RR = 6.93, 95% CI: 1.07–44.99, respectively).[39] The pattern of alcohol consumption also influences cirrhosis risk. For example, a Danish study indicated that daily alcohol consumption in men is associated with a higher risk of AC compared to drinking 2 to 4 days per week. Additionally, the type of alcoholic beverage may play a role; wine consumption has been associated with a lower risk of AC compared to beer and spirits.[40] Further research suggests that the prevalence of cirrhosis among individuals who have consumed more than 10 drinks per day for over 15 years is 3.1% for men and 4.7% for women by the age of 40 years.[41] Currently, no liver-safe limit of alcohol consumption has been firmly established. Despite these associations, it is noteworthy that only 10% to 20% of individuals with chronic heavy alcohol use develop AC or AH, underscoring the importance of other contributing factors to the pathogenesis of these conditions[1]

Age

The relationship between age and the progression of ALD remains somewhat ambiguous. Research has shown that age is an independent risk factor for mortality in cases of advanced liver disease confirmed through biopsy. This implies a more severe disease course or poorer prognosis with increasing age.[42] However, contrasting to this trend, there has been a notable increase in alcohol consumption and associated ALD among younger individuals. An observational study done in 2017 estimated the highest average annual percentage change (AAPC) in mortality from cirrhosis of any cause in patients aged 25 to 34 from year 2009 to 2016 was 10.5% with CI of 8.9%–12.2% around AAPC.[43] Further supporting this, data from NHANES database indicated a rise in the incidence of ALD in the US, especially among young people. This shift is particularly concerning as it affects individuals in their most productive years, spanning ages 15 to 44. The increasing burden of ALD in this younger population not only presents a public health challenge but also has broader social and economic implications, affecting individuals in their prime working years.[44]

These findings collectively suggest a dual trend in ALD progression: while older age is associated with higher mortality, there is an emerging and significant burden of the disease among younger adults, warranting attention, and targeted interventions.

Gender

It is well-known that women have a significantly higher relative risk of developing ALD than men for any given level of alcohol intake.[45] A meta-analysis showed that consumption of 1 drink per day in comparison to long-term abstainers showed an increased risk for liver cirrhosis in women, but not in men.[39] This appears to be related to higher blood alcohol concentrations in women than men who ingest the same amount of alcohol due to that women have lower body weight than men.[46] Moreover, women have decreased gastric and slower gastric emptying of alcohol resulting in poorer first-pass metabolism and increased bioavailability of alcohol compared with men. Similarly, women who drank the same average daily amount as men had significantly higher mortality rates with the relative risk for 5 drinks per day for women was 14.7 [95% CI: 11.0, 19.6],while for men the relative risk was 7.0 [95% CI: 5.8, 8.5].[9] The data from 3 national databases spanning from 2001 to 2016 showed increased admissions from women than men (33.5% vs 14.7).[3] A study that included 43093 participants in the National Epidemiologic Survey on Alcohol and Related Conditions showed that between 2001 to 2002 and 2012 to 2013, 12-month alcohol use, high-risk drinking, and DSM-IV AUD increased more significantly in women than men.[47]

Genetics

Genetics can predispose to AUD and the development of ALD. Patients with severe ALD, particularly AC, often have a family history of AUD and ALD. Twin studies have further underscored the importance of genetic factors in the risk for ALD.[48] Recent advancements in genome-wide association studies (GWAS) have identified specific genetic markers, such as single nucleotide polymorphisms (SNPs), in genes encoding alcohol-metabolizing enzymes, cytokines, and antioxidant enzymes that are associated with AUD and ALD.[49] Several meta-analyses and studies focusing on populations with well-defined phenotypes have revealed genome-wide significant associations between variants in genes related to AUD. Notably, variants in ALDH2 and ADH1B are associated with AUD in East Asian ancestry populations, while ADH1B and ADH1C are linked in European, African, and East Asian ancestry populations.[50] In the context of AC, GWAS have identified PNPLA3, TM6SF2, and MBOAT7 as risk loci.[51] More recently, using 2 independent Genome ALC datasets (Genome ALC-1 and Genome ALC-2) along with the data from the United Kingdom Biobank (UKB), researchers developed a polygenic risk score combining 3 SNPs (PNPLA3:rs738409, SUGP1-TM6SF2:rs10401969, HSD17B13:rs6834314). In patients with diabetes, those with high-risk scores exhibited Odds Ratios (ORs) of 14.7 (95% CI: 7.69–28.1) in the GenomALC-1 dataset and 17.1 (95% CI: 11.3–25.7) in the UKB, compared to those without diabetes and with low-risk scores.[52] These findings are instrumental in uncovering new pathways and genetic associations involved in the pathogenesis of ALD.

Metabolic Factors

The available evidence suggests that both alcohol consumption and metabolic factors play independent and combined roles in the development of chronic liver disease. For instance, a Finnish study found that individuals in the general population who engaged in moderate or risky drinking and metabolic syndrome had a higher 10-year cumulative risk for incident advanced liver disease compared to those without metabolic syndrome. The risk increased from 0.3% to 1.4% for moderate drinking and from 0.8% to 2.4% for at-risk drinking.[53] Similarly, a recent French study on individuals hospitalized with diabetes revealed that 57% of liver-related complications were attributable to AUD, while less than 10% were attributed to obesity or metabolic syndrome.[54] Another study conducted with the UKB demonstrated that individuals who were both obese and engaged in at-risk drinking had the highest excess cumulative incidence of ALD at 1.83% compared to those with a normal body mass index and safe drinking habits.[55] Additionally, a Swedish study found that patients with non-alcoholic fatty liver disease who consumed moderate amounts of alcohol (less than 140 g per week) had an increased risk of significant fibrosis progression compared to those who abstained or consumed less alcohol.[56] Although earlier studies suggested that mild to moderate drinking could reduce the risk of metabolic syndrome-related phenotypes, recent research has shown that even low alcohol intake in steatotic liver disease is associated with an increased risk for advanced liver disease.[57]

Race or Ethnicity

Findings from various studies highlight significant racial and ethnic differences in AUD and ALD. Hispanic populations are at a higher risk of harmful drinking and tend to experience more advanced ALD.[44] Notably, Hispanic patients often develop ALD at younger ages, typically 4 to 10 years earlier, compared to Black or White patients.[58] Additionally, Black and Hispanic patients with ALD generally have higher levels of liver enzymes than White patients who consume equivalent amounts of alcohol.[59]

A recent comprehensive study, utilizing the administrative data from multiple US health care systems and spanning from 1999 to June 2021, examined 8445720 patients, found that Black patients were significantly more likely than White patients to be diagnosed with AH, with an OR of 2.63 and a 95% CI of 2.46 to 2.81.[60]

Studies also have underscored an overall increase in alcohol consumption across all racial and ethnic groups. Between 2001 and 2013, there was a 27% increase in past 12-month alcohol use among Native Americans, a 17% increase among Hispanics, and a 24% increase among Black individuals, compared to an 8% increase among Whites. More strikingly, the rates of AUD, which represents the most severe form of alcohol misuse, increased dramatically among Black (93% increase) and Hispanic Americans (52% increase), in contrast to a 47% increase among White Americans. These findings indicate significant difference in the prevalence and severity of alcohol-related health issues across different racial and ethnic groups.[47]

Trends of Alcohol-Associated Liver Disease as an Indication for Orthotopic Liver Transplantation

The only curative therapy for decompensated ALD is liver transplantation. The traditional 6-month abstinence rule for ALD patients evaluated for transplantation has been under scrutiny due to weak supporting evidence. A pivotal 2011 randomized clinical trial in France demonstrated that early liver transplantation significantly enhances survival in patients with AH showing a survival rate of 77 ± 8% compared to 23 ± 8% in those who did not undergo transplantation.[61] Despite these successes, the issue of alcohol relapse post-transplantation remains significant. Recent studies, including a French clinical trial, have indicated a higher frequency of high alcohol intake following early liver transplantation.[62]

Further research, including a clinical trial in the US, has also suggested that a 6-month period of abstinence may not be necessary for successful outcomes.[63] Epidemiologic studies reveal a substantial increase in the proportion of liver transplants for ALD, doubling from 15.3% in 2002 to 30.6% in 2016.[64] This trend, which predates the COVID-19 pandemic, has been further accelerated by the pandemic, leading to increased referrals, waitlist registrations, and transplantations for ALD.[65,66] The most significant rise in ALD has been observed in young adults, with a 33% increase.[65] The number of liver transplants for AH has also risen dramatically, from 28 in 2014 to 138 in 2019, a 5-fold increase.[67] The COVID-19 pandemic has further intensified this trend, with a 325% increase in AH patients added to the waiting list and a 269% increase in liver transplants compared to expected rates.[68]

SUMMARY

Prior to the COVID-19 pandemic, there was already a notable rise in the prevalence of ALD, particularly among younger individuals and females. Ethnic groups such as Hispanics, Blacks, and Native Americans were disproportionately affected by AUD and ALD. The pandemic further fueled these trends. Additionally, the escalating rates of obesity and metabolic syndrome, in conjunction with alcohol consumption, are anticipated to lead to even higher incidences of ALD. The introduction of a new category, Met-ALD, is expected to enhance our understanding of the synergistic effects of ALD and MASLD. There has been a significant increase in early liver transplantation for ALD, although concerns about alcohol relapse post-transplantation remain prevalent. Early detection and treatment are crucial in managing this condition, which holds significant public health benefits.

CLINICS CARE POINTS

- The prevalence of ALD is on the rise due to increased level of high risk alcohol use, emphasizing the importance of routine assessment of alcohol use with prompt referral to resources for those with unhealthy alcohol use.
- ALD can co-exist in patients underlying MASLD and metabolic disease co-morbidities, which may lead to more aggressive disease progression. Hence, careful attention to assessing for and optimizing management of metabolic co-morbidities is also critically important.
- Young adults, women, and ethnic minority populations have been particularly affected by increasing ALD prevalence and ALD-related morbidity and mortality.

DISCLOSURES

W. Zhang has no disclosures. R.J. Wong has received funding (to his institution) from Gilead Sciences, Exact Sciences, Thera Technologies, and Durect Corporation, and has served as a consultant (without compensation) for Gilead Sciences.

REFERENCES

1. Singal AK, Mathurin P. Diagnosis and treatment of alcohol-associated liver disease: a review. JAMA 2021;326:165–76.
2. GBDCoD Collaborators. Global, regional, and national age-sex specific mortality for 264 causes of death, 1980-2016: a systematic analysis for the Global Burden of Disease Study 2016. Lancet 2017;390:1151–210.
3. Dang K, Hirode G, Singal AK, et al. Alcoholic liver disease epidemiology in the United States: a retrospective analysis of 3 us databases. Am J Gastroenterol 2020;115:96–104.
4. Kwong AJ, Ebel NH, Kim WR, et al. OPTN/SRTR 2021 annual data report: liver. Am J Transplant 2023;23:S178–263.
5. Asrani SK, Mellinger J, Arab JP, et al. Reducing the global burden of alcohol-associated liver disease: a blueprint for action. Hepatology 2021;73:2039–50.
6. Deutsch-Link S, Jiang Y, Peery AF, et al. Alcohol-associated liver disease mortality increased from 2017 to 2020 and accelerated during the COVID-19 pandemic. Clin Gastroenterol Hepatol 2022;20:2142–2144 e2.
7. Kulkarni NS, Wadhwa DK, Kanwal F, et al. Alcohol-associated liver disease mortality rates by race before and during the COVID-19 pandemic in the US. JAMA Health Forum 2023;4:e230527.
8. Julien J, Ayer T, Bethea ED, et al. Projected prevalence and mortality associated with alcohol-related liver disease in the USA, 2019-40: a modelling study. Lancet Public Health 2020;5:e316–23.
9. Anouti A, Mellinger JL. The changing epidemiology of alcohol-associated liver disease: gender, race, and risk factors. Semin Liver Dis 2023;43:50–9.
10. Diaz LA, Arab JP, Louvet A, et al. The intersection between alcohol-related liver disease and nonalcoholic fatty liver disease. Nat Rev Gastroenterol Hepatol 2023;20(12):764–83.
11. Rinella ME, Lazarus JV, Ratziu V, et al. A multisociety Delphi consensus statement on new fatty liver disease nomenclature. Hepatology 2023. https://doi.org/10.1097/HEP.0000000000000520.

12. Israelsen M, Torp N, Johansen S, et al. MetALD: new opportunities to understand the role of alcohol in steatotic liver disease. Lancet Gastroenterol Hepatol 2023;8: 866–8.

13. Crabb DW, Im GY, Szabo G, et al. Diagnosis and treatment of alcohol-associated liver diseases: 2019 practice guidance from the American Association for the Study of Liver Diseases. Hepatology 2020;71:306–33.

14. Singal AK, Bataller R, Ahn J, et al. ACG clinical guideline: alcoholic liver disease. Am J Gastroenterol 2018;113:175–94.

15. Wong T, Dang K, Ladhani S, et al. Prevalence of alcoholic fatty liver disease among adults in the United States, 2001-2016. JAMA 2019;321:1723–5.

16. Aslam A, Kwo PY. Epidemiology and disease burden of alcohol associated liver disease. J Clin Exp Hepatol 2023;13:88–102.

17. Parker R, Aithal GP, Becker U, et al. Natural history of histologically proven alcohol-related liver disease: a systematic review. J Hepatol 2019;71:586–93.

18. Hagstrom H, Thiele M, Sharma R, et al. Cardiovascular outcomes in patients with biopsy-proven alcohol-related liver disease. Clin Gastroenterol Hepatol 2023;21: 1841–1853 e12.

19. Aryan M, Qian S, Chen Z, et al. Patients with early-stage alcohol-associated liver disease are at increased risk of hospital readmission and death. Eur J Gastroenterol Hepatol 2023. https://doi.org/10.1097/MEG.0000000000002701.

20. Bataller R, Arab JP, Shah VB. 2022 #23}. H. alcohol-associated hepatitis. N Engl J Med 2022;387:2436–48.

21. Clemente-Sanchez A, Oliveira-Mello A, Bataller R. Moderate alcoholic hepatitis. Clin Liver Dis 2021;25:537–55.

22. Seitz HK, Bataller R, Cortez-Pinto H, et al. Alcoholic liver disease. Nat Rev Dis Prim 2018;4:16.

23. Singal AK, Arora S, Wong RJ, et al. Increasing burden of acute-on-chronic liver failure among alcohol-associated liver disease in the young population in the United States. Am J Gastroenterol 2020;115:88–95.

24. Garg SK, Sarvepalli S, Singh D, et al. Incidence and risk factors associated with 30-day readmission for alcoholic hepatitis. J Clin Gastroenterol 2019;53:759–64.

25. Arab JP, Diaz LA, Baeza N, et al. Identification of optimal therapeutic window for steroid use in severe alcohol-associated hepatitis: a worldwide study. J Hepatol 2021;75:1026–33.

26. Mookerjee RP, Lackner C, Stauber R, et al. The role of liver biopsy in the diagnosis and prognosis of patients with acute deterioration of alcoholic cirrhosis. J Hepatol 2011;55:1103–11.

27. Mathurin P, Duchatelle V, Ramond MJ, et al. Survival and prognostic factors in patients with severe alcoholic hepatitis treated with prednisolone. Gastroenterology 1996;110:1847–53.

28. Dominguez M, Rincon D, Abraldes JG, et al. A new scoring system for prognostic stratification of patients with alcoholic hepatitis. Am J Gastroenterol 2008;103: 2747–56.

29. Collaborators GBDC. The global, regional, and national burden of cirrhosis by cause in 195 countries and territories, 1990-2017: a systematic analysis for the Global Burden of Disease Study 2017. Lancet Gastroenterol Hepatol 2020;5: 245–66.

30. Diseases GBD, Injuries C. Global burden of 369 diseases and injuries in 204 countries and territories, 1990-2019: a systematic analysis for the Global Burden of Disease Study 2019. Lancet 2020;396:1204–22.

31. Barbosa C, Cowell AJ, Dowd WN. Alcohol consumption in response to the COVID-19 pandemic in the United States. J Addiction Med 2021;15:341–4.
32. Lee BP, Dodge JL, Leventhal A, et al. Retail alcohol and tobacco sales during COVID-19. Ann Intern Med 2021;174:1027–9.
33. Acuff SF, Strickland JC, Tucker JA, et al. Changes in alcohol use during COVID-19 and associations with contextual and individual difference variables: a systematic review and meta-analysis. Psychol Addict Behav 2022;36:1–19.
34. Sohal A, Khalid S, Green V, et al. The pandemic within the pandemic: unprecedented rise in alcohol-related hepatitis during the COVID-19 pandemic. J Clin Gastroenterol 2022;56:e171–5.
35. Deutsch-Link S, Curtis B, Singal AK. Covid-19 and alcohol associated liver disease. Dig Liver Dis 2022;54:1459–68.
36. Gao X, Lv F, He X, et al. Impact of the COVID-19 pandemic on liver disease-related mortality rates in the United States. J Hepatol 2023;78:16–27.
37. Hagstrom H, Thiele M, Roelstraete B, et al. Mortality in biopsy-proven alcohol-related liver disease: a population-based nationwide cohort study of 3453 patients. Gut 2021;70:170–9.
38. Stein E, Cruz-Lemini M, Altamirano J, et al. Heavy daily alcohol intake at the population level predicts the weight of alcohol in cirrhosis burden worldwide. J Hepatol 2016;65:998–1005.
39. Roerecke M, Vafaei A, Hasan OSM, et al. Alcohol consumption and risk of liver cirrhosis: a systematic review and meta-analysis. Am J Gastroenterol 2019;114:1574–86.
40. Askgaard G, Gronbaek M, Kjaer MS, et al. Alcohol drinking pattern and risk of alcoholic liver cirrhosis: a prospective cohort study. J Hepatol 2015;62:1061–7.
41. Delacote C, Bauvin P, Louvet A, et al. A model to identify heavy drinkers at high risk for liver disease progression. Clin Gastroenterol Hepatol 2020;18:2315–2323 e6.
42. Masson S, Emmerson I, Henderson E, et al. Clinical but not histological factors predict long-term prognosis in patients with histologically advanced non-decompensated alcoholic liver disease. Liver Int 2014;34:235–42.
43. Tapper EB, Parikh ND. Mortality due to cirrhosis and liver cancer in the United States, 1999-2016: observational study. BMJ 2018;362:k2817.
44. Singal AK, Arsalan A, Dunn W, et al. Alcohol-associated liver disease in the United States is associated with severe forms of disease among young, females and Hispanics. Aliment Pharmacol Ther 2021;54:451–61.
45. Becker U, Deis A, Sorensen TI, et al. Prediction of risk of liver disease by alcohol intake, sex, and age: a prospective population study. Hepatology 1996;23:1025–9.
46. Osna NA, Donohue TM Jr, Kharbanda KK. Alcoholic liver disease: pathogenesis and current management. Alcohol Res 2017;38:147–61.
47. Grant BF, Chou SP, Saha TD, et al. Prevalence of 12-month alcohol use, high-risk drinking, and DSM-IV alcohol use disorder in the United States, 2001-2002 to 2012-2013: results from the National epidemiologic Survey on alcohol and related conditions. JAMA Psychiatr 2017;74:911–23.
48. Stickel F, Hampe J. Genetic determinants of alcoholic liver disease. Gut 2012;61:150–9.
49. Norden-Krichmar TM, Rotroff D, Schwantes-An TH, et al. Genomic approaches to explore susceptibility and pathogenesis of alcohol use disorder and alcohol-associated liver disease. Hepatology 2023. https://doi.org/10.1097/HEP.0000000000000617.

50. Zaso MJ, Goodhines PA, Wall TL, et al. Meta-analysis on associations of alcohol metabolism genes with alcohol use disorder in East Asians. Alcohol Alcohol 2019; 54:216–24.
51. Stickel F, Moreno C, Hampe J, et al. The genetics of alcohol dependence and alcohol-related liver disease. J Hepatol 2017;66:195–211.
52. Whitfield JB, Schwantes-An TH, Darlay R, et al. A genetic risk score and diabetes predict development of alcohol-related cirrhosis in drinkers. J Hepatol 2022;76: 275–82.
53. Aberg F, Puukka P, Salomaa V, et al. Combined effects of alcohol and metabolic disorders in patients with chronic liver disease. Clin Gastroenterol Hepatol 2020; 18:995–997 e2.
54. Mallet V, Parlati L, Martinino A, et al. Burden of liver disease progression in hospitalized patients with type 2 diabetes mellitus. J Hepatol 2022;76:265–74.
55. Innes H, Crooks CJ, Aspinall E, et al. Characterizing the risk interplay between alcohol intake and body mass index on cirrhosis morbidity. Hepatology 2022; 75:369–78.
56. Blomdahl J, Nasr P, Ekstedt M, et al. Moderate alcohol consumption is associated with significant fibrosis progression in NAFLD. Hepatol Commun 2023;7:e0003.
57. Aberg F, Puukka P, Salomaa V, et al. Risks of light and moderate alcohol use in fatty liver disease: follow-up of population cohorts. Hepatology 2020;71:835–48.
58. Levy R, Catana AM, Durbin-Johnson B, et al. Ethnic differences in presentation and severity of alcoholic liver disease. Alcohol Clin Exp Res 2015;39:566–74.
59. Nguyen GC, Thuluvath PJ. Racial disparity in liver disease: biological, cultural, or socioeconomic factors. Hepatology 2008;47:1058–66.
60. Damjanovska S, Karb DB, Cohen SM. Increasing prevalence and racial disparity of alcohol-related gastrointestinal and liver disease during the COVID-19 pandemic: a population-based national study. J Clin Gastroenterol 2023;57: 185–8.
61. Mathurin P, Moreno C, Samuel D, et al. Early liver transplantation for severe alcoholic hepatitis. N Engl J Med 2011;365:1790–800.
62. Louvet A, Labreuche J, Moreno C, et al. Early liver transplantation for severe alcohol-related hepatitis not responding to medical treatment: a prospective controlled study. Lancet Gastroenterol Hepatol 2022;7:416–25.
63. Herrick-Reynolds KM, Punchhi G, Greenberg RS, et al. Evaluation of early vs standard liver transplant for alcohol-associated liver disease. JAMA Surg 2021; 156:1026–34.
64. Lee BP, Vittinghoff E, Dodge JL, et al. National trends and long-term outcomes of liver transplant for alcohol-associated liver disease in the United States. JAMA Intern Med 2019;179:340–8.
65. Cholankeril G, Goli K, Rana A, et al. Impact of COVID-19 pandemic on liver transplantation and alcohol-associated liver disease in the USA. Hepatology 2021;74: 3316–29.
66. Chen PH, Ting PS, Almazan E, et al. Inter-hospital escalation-of-care referrals for severe alcohol-related liver disease with recent drinking during the COVID-19 pandemic. Alcohol Alcohol 2022;57:185–9.
67. Cotter TG, Sandikci B, Paul S, et al. Liver transplantation for alcoholic hepatitis in the United States: excellent outcomes with profound temporal and geographic variation in frequency. Am J Transplant 2021;21:1039–55.
68. Bittermann T, Mahmud N, Abt P. Trends in liver transplantation for acute alcohol-associated hepatitis during the COVID-19 pandemic in the US. JAMA Netw Open 2021;4:e2118713.

Alcohol and Metabolic Syndrome Interaction

Ryuki Hashida, MD, PhD[a,b,c], Pegah Golabi, MD[a,d],
Janus Ong, MD, MPH[e,d], Takumi Kawaguchi, MD, PhD[b,f],
Zobair M. Younossi, MD, MPH[a,d],*

KEYWORDS

- Alcohol • Metabolic syndrome • Steatosis • Fibrosis • Mortality

KEY POINTS

- Metabolic syndrome and alcohol use are both associated with hepatic steatosis.
- Alcohol and metabolic syndrome both can cause hepatic steatosis, fibrosis, cirrhosis, hepatocellular carcinoma, and liver mortality.
- The term "non-alcoholic fatty liver disease" has been replaced with "metabolic dysfunction associated steatotic liver disease (MASLD)" to reflect the association of this liver disease with its root cause associated with metabolic abnormalities. In this context, MASLD, Met-alcohol related liver disease (ALD), and ALD are now part of the spectrum of steatoic liver diseases. Therefore, understanding the interaction between alcohol and metabolic dysfunction in promoting liver disease is very important and is being highlighted.

SUMMARY

Alcohol-related liver disease (ALD) and metabolic dysfunction associated steatotic liver disease (MASLD) are the most common causes of chronic liver disease (CLD). Globally, excessive alcohol intake, and metabolic syndrome driven by excessive caloric intake and sedentary lifestyle have steadily increased over the past decades. *Given the high prevalence of both excessive alcohol consumption and components of metabolic syndrome, both conditions frequently coexist in the same individuals causing liver disease and its associated complications.* In this article, we review the interaction of alcohol and metabolic syndrome on liver-related outcomes. *In this*

Funding: None.
[a] Beatty Liver and Obesity Research Program, Inova Health System, 3300 Gallows Road, Falls Church, VA, USA; [b] Division of Rehabilitation, Kurume University Hospital, Kurume 830-0011, Japan; [c] Department of Orthopedics, Kurume University School of Medicine, Kurume 830-0011, Japan; [d] The Global NASH Council, 2411 I Street, Washington DC, USA; [e] College of Medicine, University of the Philippines, Manila, Philippines; [f] Division of Gastroenterology, Department of Medicine, Kurume University School of Medicine, Kurume 830-0011, Japan
* Corresponding author. The Global NASH Council, 2411 I street, Washington DC 20037
E-mail address: zobair.younossi@cldq.org

Clin Liver Dis 28 (2024) 601–620
https://doi.org/10.1016/j.cld.2024.06.002
1089-3261/24/© 2024 Elsevier Inc. All rights reserved, including those for text and data mining, AI training, and similar technologies.

context, heavy alcohol consumption and metabolic syndrome can affect the liver independently or synergistically to cause hepatic fibrosis, cirrhosis, hepatocellular carcinoma (HCC), and liver mortality.

Although heavy consumption of alcohol has been shown to cause liver disease, even smaller amounts of alcohol intake may also have a negative impact on patients with existing CLD, especially those associated with concurrent metabolic liver disease such as MASLD.

BACKGROUND

CLD is one of the important causes of death worldwide.[1] Furthermore, ALD and MASLD or non-alcoholic fatty liver disease (NAFLD) are among the top leading causes of death among patients with CLD. *Histologically,* ALD and MASLD/NAFLD have similar features, which *include hepatic steatosis (triglyceride content of hepatocytes> 5%), steatohepatitis (steatosis with liver cell injury), and cirrhosis. Furthermore,* ALD and MASLD/NAFLD share pathophysiologic mechanisms, and genetic and epigenetic factors.[2] In fact, ALD and MASLD/NAFLD *can only be* distinguished clinically mainly by the amount of alcohol consumed. The cut-off value for alcohol intake for studies of MASLD/NAFLD considered alcohol consumption of 30 g/day (210 g/week) for men and 20 g/day (140 g/week) for women. On the other hand, the diagnostic cut-off value for ALD is 60 g/day (420 g/week) for men and 50 g/day (350 g/week) for women.

Alcohol use has remained a global public health problem with alcohol consumption steadily increasing in the past 2 decades in almost all regions of the world.[3,4] In 2018, the average global alcohol consumption was 6.2 L of pure ethanol per person older than 15.[5] The World Health Organization (WHO) recommends that men and women consume no more than 20 g (2 standard drinks) of pure ethanol daily.[6] Excessive alcohol consumption causes various diseases including but not limited to liver disease, pancreatitis, injury to the central nervous system, alcoholic psychosis, and cancer.[7–9] In this context, ALD is now the most common cause of liver disease and indication for liver transplantation in the United States (US).[10]

In addition to alcohol consumption, metabolic syndrome has become a worldwide problem due to excessive calorie intake, consumption of poor quality nutrition/ultra-processed foods and inactivity.[11] *Although still being debated, metabolic syndrome has been defined as having visceral obesity, hypertension, glucose intolerance, hyperinsulinemia, and dyslipidemia.*[12] Recent data suggest that the prevalence of metabolic syndrome has increased from 36.2% (1999–2000) to 47.3% (2017–2018).[13] It is well known that metabolic syndrome is associated with cardiovascular disease, liver disease, cancer, diabetes, and stroke.[11,14,15] Given the high prevalence of both metabolic syndrome or alcohol use in the general population, they can often coexist in many individuals and can drive adverse outcomes in these patients. In this context, metabolic syndrome and its components are independent drivers of liver fibrosis and liver-related outcomes.[16] Similarly, excessive alcohol consumption is *another major driver of these adverse liver-related* outcomes.[17] Therefore, presence of *metabolic syndrome and excessive alcohol consumption in the same individual* can independently and synergistically drive adverse liver-related outcomes. For example, *a recent study among US Veterans demonstrated that 1 of 9 patients with steatotic liver disease (SLD) reported concurrent high risk alcohol intake, which was associated with greater than 40% increased risk of cirrhosis development.*[18]

Interestingly, increased alcohol intake can also exacerbate components of metabolic syndrome. Recent research reported an association of excessive alcohol intake with obesity.[19,20] A Finnish study reported that ALD patients with alcohol intake higher than the threshold used for MASLD had higher rates of metabolic complications.[21]

These data demonstrate the possibility that heavy alcohol intake and metabolic syndrome can interact synergistically. In fact, the recent effort to change the term NAFLD to MASLD was partially undertaken to emphasize the role of metabolic *abnormality* as the culprit causing NAFLD/MASLD. In this context, MASLD is a part of SLD, which also contains the new category of Met-ALD, further describing the interaction between MASLD and ALD.[22] In this review, we summarize the interaction of alcohol consumption and metabolic syndrome and discuss their independent and combined impacts, particularly on liver-related clinical outcomes.

Alcohol, Metabolic Syndrome, and Mortality in Patients with Chronic Liver Disease

Table 1 depicts the summary of some studies regarding mortality in subjects with MASLD and alcohol consumption. As summarized, alcohol consumption and obesity have been associated with mortality. *In these cohort (N = 4) and retrospective (N = 2) studies, different cut-offs for alcohol consumption with only 4 studies specified the amount of alcohol consumed. This heterogeneity of the study design makes drawing conclusions more difficult. Nevertheless, we will address the interaction by assessing the literature using separate type of liver disease (ALD and MASLD).*

Alcohol, metabolic syndrome, and mortality in patients with metabolic dysfunction associated steatotic liver disease

In one study, using the National Health and Nutrition Examination Survey (NHANES) data, the long-term outcomes of those classified as NAFLD was compared to those classified as metabolic-associated fatty liver disease (MAFLD).[23] In this study, MAFLD was defined as fatty liver disease (FLD) and metabolic dysfunction but with expanded use of alcohol consumption. The results of the study found that insulin resistance was associated with liver-related mortality among NAFLD patients while excessive alcohol drinking was independently associated with increasing liver-related mortality among MAFLD patients.[23] Decraeker and colleagues reported that patients with NAFLD/MASLD had an increased overall mortality rate (heart rate [HR]: 1.9) for each unit per week increase in alcohol intake.[24] On the other hand, Pearson and colleagues investigated the effect of alcohol on mortality in patients with cirrhosis of NAFLD/MASLD, Hepatitis C virus (HCV), and ALD. The author demonstrated that alcohol use was not associated with decompensation and low-level alcohol use was associated with a decreased risk of mortality in patients with NAFLD/MASLD cirrhosis.[25] However, a more recent study (2019) utilizing a large, population-based database focused on the effects of alcohol and metabolic syndrome on mortality among patients with fatty liver.[26] This study demonstrated that compared to patients with non-excessive alcohol intake, overall mortality was significantly higher in patients with excessive alcohol intake. Furthermore, both presence of metabolic syndrome and excessive alcohol consumption were independently associated with an increased risk of death in patients with fatty liver. Finally, it was also reported that the association of excessive alcohol use with mortality was significant in patients with metabolic syndrome but not without it.[26] *Another study evaluated the histologic and biochemical effects of alcohol use among patients with NAFLD[27]. It was reported that among patients with NAFLD, modest alcohol consumption was not only associated with less improvement in steatosis and asparate aminotransferase (AST) level, but also lower odds of nonalchoholic steatohepatitis (NASH) resolution, compared to NAFLD patients without alcohol use.[27]* Although these studies suggest deleterious effects of excessive alcohol use and metabolic abnormality, the impact of smaller amounts of alcohol consumption and the long-term outcomes of these patients remain controversial and more research is needed.

Table 1
Interaction between alcohol and metabolic syndrome on mortality in patients with chronic liver disease

Author Name	Country	Study Design	Subject number Population Sample	Diagnosis NAFLD	Alcohol Consumption Definition	Main Outcome	Conclusion
Zobair M Younossi	USA	Cohort study NHANES III (1988–1994) And NHANES 2017–2018	NHANES III participants (n = 12,878) NHANES 2017–2018 participants (n = 4328)	VCTE (Fibro Scan)	Excessive alcohol consumption (alcoholconsumption < 20 g/day for males and 10 g/day for females).	Over 40% of the study population died during the follow-up period of 27 y. Again, there were no differences in the cumulative mortality among MAFLD + or among NAFLD+. In addition, among MAFLD+, it was the presence of excess alcohol use and/or ALD that increased the risk of liver-specific mortality over 4 times.	MAFLD and NAFLD have similar clinical profiles and long-term outcomes. The increased liver-related mortality among NAFLD is driven by insulin resistance, and among MAFLD is primarily driven by ALD.
Marie Decraecker	France	Cohort study January 2003 to December 2016	3365 patients (1667 with ALD and 1698 with NAFLD)	Presence of steatosis assessed by ultrasound	Alcohol consumption thresholds: 14 units/week for women or 21 units/week for men	In the NAFLD group, weekly alcohol consumption >1 unit was associated with higher overall mortality (HR: 1.9 [1.1–3.4]). In the ALD group, the presence of metabolic syndrome was associated with higher overall mortality (HR:1.27 [1.02–1.57]).	In fatty liver diseases, light alcohol consumption and metabolic syndrome are prognosis cofactors.

Meredith M. Pearson	USA	Retrospective study the VAHS is the largest integrated health care system	44,349 patients with cirrhosis	Patients with ICD-9 codes for diabetes mellitus, recorded at least twice, or body mass index ≥30 kg/m2 before the diagnosis of cirrhosis were categorized as NAFLD.	AUDIT-C Questions and Scoring System	Among patients with NAFLD-cirrhosis, the association between unhealthy drinking (vs. no drinking)was not statistically significantly associated with mortality (aHR = 0.95, 95% CI = 0.77–1.18), cirrhosis decompensation (aHR = 0.91, 95% CI = 0.63–1.32),or HCC (aHR = 0.86, 95% CI = 0.42–1.75).	Unhealthy alcohol use was common in patients with cirrhosis and was associated with higher risks of mortality and cirrhosis decompensation in patients with HCV-cirrhosis and ALD-cirrhosis. Therefore, healthcare providers should make every effort to help patients achieve abstinence.
Orly Termeie	USA	Retrospective studycompare between 1999 and 2019	6007 deaths from alcoholic cirrhosis among a total US population of 180,408,769 in 1999 23,780 deaths from alcoholic cirrhosis among a total US population of 224,981,167 in 2019	Not evaluated	The International Classification of Diseases code K70.3 (alcoholic cirrhosis of liver).	In 1999, there were 6007 deaths from alcoholic cirrhosis among a total US population of 180,408,769 aged 25–85+ years yielding a mortality rate of 3.3 per 100,000. In 2019 there were 23,780 deaths from alcoholic cirrhosis among a total US population of 224,981,167 aged 25–85+ years, yielding a mortality rate of 10.6 per 100,000.	Clinical and public health efforts are necessary to curb the epidemic of heavy alcohol consumption, the epidemic of overweight and obesity.

(continued on next page)

Table 1
(continued)

Author Name	Country	Study Design	Subject number Population Sample	Diagnosis NAFLD	Alcohol Consumption Definition	Main Outcome	Conclusion
						The overall mortality rate ratio of 3.2 was statistically significant. ($P<.001$) and was apparent in each 10-y age group.	
Richard Parker	UK and USA	Cohort study	233 patients with alcoholic hepatitis	Not evaluated	Standard definitions of AH were used to identify or exclude patients: alcohol use of at least 60 g/d in men and > 40 g/d in women for > 5 y, hazardous drinking until at least 6 weeks before admission.	Obesity was common amongst patients with AH, seen in 19% of individuals. Obesity (HR 2.22, 95%CI1.1–4.3, P = .022) and underweight (HR 2.38, 1.00–5.6, P = .049) were independently associated with mortality at 3 mo.	Obesity is common in AH and associated with a greater than two-fold increase in short-term mortality.

| Huang Y | Australia | Cohort study | 10,933 patients with CLD | Hospital medical records and/or ICD-10 code of K75.8 or K76.0 in WADLU databases. | Hospital medical records and/or ICD-10 code of K70 in WADLU databases. | Patients with AALD had the highest 5-y cumulative risk of liver-related death (17.1%). Multivariate analysis found patients with AALD had significantly higher risks of liver-related death and decompensation than patients with HCV infection with hazard ratios (HRs) of 2.39 (95% CI, 1.88–3.03) and 3.42 (95% CI, 2.74–4.27), respectively. Patients with NAFLD had a significantly lower risk of liver-related death than patients with HCV infection, with HRs of 0.67 (95% CI, 0.48–0.95). | Patients with AALD have a significantly higher risk of decompensation and liver-related death than patients with HCV infection, whereas patients with NAFLD have significantly lower risks of either outcome. |

Abbreviations: AALD, Alcohol-associated liver disease; ACLF, acute-on-chronic liver failure; AH, alcoholic hepatitis; ALD, alcohol-related liver disease; AUDIT-C, alcohol use disorders identification test consumption; CLD, chronic liver disease; HCV, hepatitis C virus; MAFLD, metabolic fatty liver disease; NAFLD, non-alcohol fatty liver disease; NHANES, nutritional health and nutritional examination survey.

Alcohol, metabolic syndrome and mortality in patients with alcohol-related liver disease

Termeie and colleagues reported that the number of deaths due to alcoholic cirrhosis in the USA increased in 2019 as compared to 1999.[28] Among the total USA population aged 25 to 85 years old, the number of deaths due to alcoholic cirrhosis increased. The number of deaths was 23780, and the mortality rate was 10.6 per 100000 people. Authors stressed the impacts of increased alcohol consumption, as well as contribution of overweight and obesity status, to the observed increases in mortality from alcoholic cirrhosis. According to a report on alcoholic hepatitis from the United Kingdom (UK) and USA, alcohol-related hospitalizations are rapidly increasing, especially in patients under 35 years of age.[29] In this context, obesity was observed in 19% of ALD patients. Furthermore, obesity was associated with short-term mortality at 3 months (HR 2.22). Decreaker and colleagues reported that the presence of metabolic syndrome was associated with higher overall mortality (HR:1.2) in patients with ALD.[30]

In another study, Huang and colleagues compared the long-term liver-related outcomes of CLD in Australia.[30] Multivariate analysis found patients with alcohol-associated liver disease had significantly higher risks of liver-related death than patients with HCV infection with hazard ratios (HRs) of 2.39. Patients with NAFLD had a significantly lower risk of liver-related death than patients with HCV infection, with HRs of 0.67. On the other hand, alcohol-associated liver disease and metabolic risk factors had intermediate risk compared to ALD or NAFLD (HR 1.55). The authors pointed out that the study used a hospital medical code, and there could be potential biases due to alcohol consumption, metabolic syndrome, etc. *On the other hand, a recent study from the UK demonstrated some interesting findings[31]. In that study, authors defined first-time hospitalization for cirrhosis as cirrhosis morbidity and investigated the cumulative incidence of this outcome over a 10-year period, categorized by body mass index (BMI) levels and drinking habits. The authors reported that compared to safe drinkers, 10-year cumulative incidence was 8.6 times higher among harmful drinkers, (1.38% vs 0.16%) if BMI was healthy; however, it was only 3.6 times higher for obese participants. They concluded that even though alcohol use and obesity are independent risk factors for cirrhosis morbidity, they may not need to interact supra-additively to modulate this effect[31].*

The Impact of Alcohol and Metabolic Syndrome on Liver-related Outcome

Most studies (N = 5) assessing the association of alcohol, and metabolic syndrome with liver-related outcomes (liver fibrosis, FLD, and HCC) were of retrospective design (**Table 2**).

In a population-based study from Spain, the relationship between liver fibrosis/stiffness (LS) using vibration controlled transient elastography , metabolic syndrome and alcohol consumption was investigated.[32] In subjects with alcohol consumption, LS was associated with male gender, AST, ALT, years of alcohol use, and metabolic syndrome. In high-risk drinkers, both metabolic syndrome and alcohol consumption were associated with significantly higher LS. In another study, Mallet and colleagues investigated the factors related to the exacerbation of liver-related diseases in approximately 50000 patients with type 2 diabetes (T2D) in France.[33] Regarding the factors associated with liver disease progression, alcohol use disorder had a more significant influence than metabolic syndrome and obesity. The study concluded the importance of counseling regarding alcohol consumption in patients with T2D to prevent the progression of liver disease. Furthermore, patients with T2D and alcohol use disorders should be prioritized in managing the risk of liver fibrosis.

Table 2
Interaction between alcohol and metabolic syndrome on liver-related outcomes in patients with chronic liver disease

Author Name	Country	Study Design	Subject	Subject Number Population Sample	Diagnosis NAFLD	Alcohol Consumption Definition	Main Outcome	Conclusion
Elisa Pose	Spain	Population-based study	Liver fibrosis	2980 patients who had information about alcohol consumption	VCTE (Fibro scan)	Patients who drank (>21 units/week men, >14 units/week women) were defined as high-risk drinkers	LS was associated with male gender, AST, ALT, years of consumption, and metabolic syndrome. In high-risk drinkers, metabolic syndrome and intensity of consumption were the only factors associated with significant LS (OR 3.7 and 4.6 for LS $\geq$ 8 kPa and 3.9 and 9.2 kPa for LS $\geq$ 9.1 kPa, respectively).	This observation should be taken into account for the management of subjects with ALD and underlines the need for strict control of metabolic risk factors especially in high-risk drinkers.

(continued on next page)

Table 2
(continued)

Author Name	Country	Study Design	Subject	Subject Number Population Sample	Diagnosis NAFLD	Alcohol Consumption Definition	Main Outcome	Conclusion
Vincent Mallet	France	Retrospective, longitudinal study in a large, multicenter cohort	Liver disease progression	52,066 hospitalized patients with T2D	Not evaluated	Alcohol use disorders were identified by 3 categories of discharge diagnosis codes: (ICD-10: K70), (ICD-10: K86.0), (ICD-10: F10.1-F10.9, Z50.2).	Alcohol use disorders contributed to more than half (55%) of the liver disease progression in patients with diabetes. Obesity accounted for 6% of the liver disease progression.	Alcohol use disorders account for more than half of the liver disease burden of patients with T2D and correlate with all other risk factors of liver disease progression. The contribution of metabolic syndrome and obesity was lower (<10%) than previous estimations. Based on these study findings, patients with T2D and alcohol use should be prioritized for case-finding of advanced fibrosis.

| Yuta Yoshimura | Japan | Retrospective cohort study The NAGALA study database consists of the results of health check-up programs. | The risk factor for alcoholic fatty liver disease | 640 participants (men) | Not evaluated | Subjects with an ethanol intake $\geq$ 420 g/week at baseline were defined as subjects who consume alcohol habitually. | The hazard ratio for a 1 kg/m2 increase in body mass index was 1.2 (1.12–1.28). The hazard ratio of subjects with high triglyceride and low high-density lipoprotein-cholesterol levels were 1.56 (1.12–2.18) and 1.52 (1.03–2.25), respectively. | Obesity, high triglyceridemia, and low HDL-cholesterolemia were independent risk factors for alcoholic fatty liver disease. |
| Charlotte E Costentin | France | Retrospective study compare between 2007 and 2013 | HCC | 11,363 patients with alcohol-associated hepatocellular carcinoma | Not evaluated | Alcohol use disorders (any combination of K700, K701, K702 K703, K704, K709, F100–109, Z502) | Patients with alcohol-associated hepatocellular carcinoma, of which 71.2% had at least one metabolic comorbidity. | A majority of patients with alcohol-associated HCC combine risk factors for metabolic-associated fatty liver disease. |

(continued on next page)

Table 2
(continued)

Author Name	Country	Study Design	Subject	Subject Number Population Sample	Diagnosis NAFLD	Alcohol Consumption Definition	Main Outcome	Conclusion
Philippe Mathurin	France	Retrospective cohort study	HCC	10,193 patients with alcohol-related disease 4016 patients with viral hepatitis 8930 patients with NAFLD, NASH	NASH and NAFLD were identified by the codes K758, and K760	ALD were identified by using ICD-10 code K70	The highest rates of curative treatments were found in patients with viral hepatitis. Median survival time months ALD 12.1[11.3–12.9] Viral hepatitis-related liver disease 27.5[23.9–34.5] Metabolic risk factor (NASH, NAFLD) 8.4 [7.6–9.7]	Alcohol and metabolic factors are the two main risk factors of HCC in France. Viral etiology was associated with the best survival.

Abbreviations: AALD, Alcohol-associated liver disease; ACLF, acute-on-chronic liver failure; ALD, alcohol-related liver disease; ALT, alanine aminotransferase; AST, aspartate aminotransferase; HCC, hepatocellular carcinoma; HDL, high density lipoprotein; LS, liver stiffness; NAFLD, non-alcoholic fatty liver diseaseNASH, non-alcoholic steatohepatitis; T2DM, type 2 diabetes mellitus.

Yoshimura and colleagues reported a retrospective cohort study in Japan using the Japanese health check-up data.[34] Six hundred forty men who consumed alcohol over 420g per week were included in this study. The author investigated the factors associated with alcohol-related liver steatosis and reported that obesity was an independent factor for alcohol-related liver steatosis. *In fact, combination of obesity and alcohol use leads to adverse liver-related outcomes, such as HCC, not only in patients with MASLD, but also with other CLDs. In this context, it was previously shown that among hepatitis B surface antigen positive men, synergistic effects of obesity and alcohol use increased the risk of incident HCC cases over 14 years of follow-up.*[35]

In a retrospective study from France, investigators assessed the incidence of alcohol-related HCC using the French nationwide administrative hospital database.[36] The author included 11363 patients with alcohol-associated HCC and investigated metabolic comorbidities. Seventy-one percent of patients with alcohol-associated HCC had at least 1 component of metabolic comorbidities, including T2D, obesity, dyslipidemia, and hypertension. The study suggested that alcohol-associated HCC cases are, in fact, most frequently related to both alcohol- and metabolic conditions.

In another retrospective study, Mathurin and colleagues investigated HCC cases in France from 2015 to 2017.[37] In this context, the most common etiologies were ALD, which was seen in 50.8% of patients. NAFLD/MASLD was the next most frequent risk factor, which was present in 44.5% of patients. Viral hepatitis was the third most frequent risk factor in 20% of patients. Patients with alcohol or metabolic disease-related HCC frequently received best supportive care and palliative care as the only treatment option. This may be due to late presentation and advanced stage of HCC. In fact, this was also shown by a retrospective analysis of SEERs database.[38] In this study, NAFLD/MASLD-HCC patients were older, had shorter survival time, more heart disease, and were more likely to die from their primary liver cancer. In fact, NAFLD independently increased the risk of 1-year mortality suggesting the possibility of presenting late with HCC that is not potentially treatable with curative treatment such as liver transplantation. Nevertheless, the number of cases of NAFLD/MASLD-related HCC and ALD-related HCC is increasing. In a study of the US transplant database, NAFLD/MASLD was the most common indication for liver transplantation (LT) in those listed for HCC in 2022.[39] Although ALD is the third common indication for HCC-LT listing, it is rapidly overtaking HCV to become the second indication for HCC-LT.[39] These data suggest that the liver-related outcomes of mortality, HCC and liver transplantation are increasingly being driven by NAFLD/MASLD and ALD. In this context, the combination of both ALD and metabolic syndrome and associated liver disease can be a major culprit in promoting liver disease burden.

Weight Loss Surgery and Its Association with Alcohol Use Disorder

Bariatric surgery is an effective treatment for severe obesity leading to significant weight loss and reduction in complications of obesity, including cardiovascular disease, hypertension, T2D, and MASLD. The number of patients undergoing bariatric surgery has been rapidly increasing as the prevalence of obesity is rising. Interestingly, bariatric surgeries, especially those related the Roux-en-Y gastric bypass (RYGB), has been associated with alcohol use disorder and ALD. Although a number of reasons for alcohol use disorder have been proposed, the damaging impact of alcohol could also be explained by anatomic changes that happen post-surgery. In this context, due to anatomic changes, patients with RYGB who ingest alcohol have higher peak blood alcohol concentrations compared to patients with normal stomach anatomy, which is more directly toxic to the liver and accelerates the development of ALD. In a retrospective study, Anugwom and colleagues reported the relationship between RYGB and overall mortality, readmissions, and cirrhosis.[40] The author enrolled 2634 patients with alcoholic hepatitis who met the inclusion criteria. Among them, 153 patients had undergone RYGB. The patients, who underwent RYGB with alcoholic hepatitis compared to patients with hepatitis, had significantly increased.[41] Thirty-day readmission (20.3% vs11.7%, P<.01), development of cirrhosis (37.5% vs 20.9%, P<.01), and overall mortality (31.4% vs 24%, P = .03). Hannah and colleagues investigated the impact of different types of bariatric surgery (RYGB; adjustable gastric band, AGB; sleeve gastrectomy, SG) on ALD. RYGB was significantly associated with an increased hazard of ALD (HR 1.51). On the other hand, AGB (HR 0.55) and SG (HR 0.77) had decreased hazards for ALD. *Mellinger and colleagues reported similar findings in a retrospective analysis of almost 400.000 patients. It was shown that overall risk of alcoholic cirrhosis was lower for patients that had undergone sleeve gastrectomy and laparoscopic banding, and alcohol misuse was higher in RYGB recipients*[42]. *A retrospective study from the US evaluated the impact of RYGB in patients with alcoholic liver disease and reported that among patients with alcoholic cirrhosis, previous RYGB was associated with increased risk of alcoholic hepatitis, hepatic encephalopathy and infection, but similar in-hospital mortality rates.*[43] These results suggest long-term follow-up is needed for patients who underwent bariatric surgery, and continued engagement in alcohol use.

Evaluation of Fatty Liver Disease and Alcohol Consumption

Given the definition of NAFLD/MASLD, excessive alcohol use must be excluded. In one study, Oscar and colleagues investigated the effect of alcohol on diagnosing FLD.[44] The author investigated the relationship between alcohol consumption and Fatty Liver Index, Hepatic Steatosis Index, Lipid Accumulation Product, and Dallas Steatosis Index. The author defined heavy drinkers as alcohol consumption greater than 50 g per day. When alcohol intake was less than 50 g per day, all indexes identified FLD, with the area under the receiver operating characteristic (AUROC) ranging from 0.82 to 0.88. AUROC for heavy drinkers (>50 g/day) was 0.61 to 0.66. In the highest binge drinking category (more than twice a week), AUROC ranged between 0.74 and 0.80. Heavy alcohol consumption reduces the ability to diagnose the index for FLD.

Thus, there is a need for a biomarker for evaluating alcohol intake that is not affected by liver dysfunction or metabolic syndrome. Morinaga and colleagues investigated the usefulness of the ratio of carbohydrate-deficient transferrin to total transferrin (%CDT) as a biomarker for alcohol consumption.[45] The %CDT is associated with the consumption of alcohol intake, an independent biomarker for alcohol consumption. Morinaga showed that the cut-off to identify nondrinkers to low-intake drinkers was 1.78% (AUROC: 0.851), and the cut-off for high-intake drinkers was 2.08% (AUROC: 0.815).

Katharina and colleagues evaluated ethyl glucuronide in hair (hEtG) and urine (uEtG) as a biomarker for the consumption of alcohol.[46] The uEtG is a valuable marker for binary screening of recent alcohol intake in patients with liver disease. On the other hand, hEtG is a long-term EtOH marker that reflects the past 3 to 6 months of alcohol consumption. The author concluded that the evaluation of alcohol intake using hEtG and uEtG is useful for screening fatty liver patients. Using %CDT, hEtG, and uEtG is useful to confirm accurate alcohol intake.

Mechanism of Liver Injury Caused by Co-existence of Alcohol and Metabolic Syndrome

As previously noted, alcohol and metabolic syndrome can negatively influence mortality,[24] liver fibrosis,[32] and HCC.[36] In this context, alcohol and metabolic syndrome can independently and synergistically cause liver disease. Several mice and human experimental studies have reported the mechanisms by which alcohol and metabolic syndrome can affect liver disease.

There is experimental evidence regarding the mechanism of synergically liver injury caused by alcohol and obesity as follows. Jun and colleagues investigated the synergic mechanism of alcohol and obesity in mice.[47] Obese mice had steatohepatitis depending on alcohol volume. Obese mice that took a high alcohol dose (32 g/kg/d) were observed, for severe steatohepatitis with pericellular fibrosis, marked M1 macrophage activation, a 40-fold induction of iNos, and intensified nitrosative stress in the liver. Nitrosative stress mediated by M1 macrophage activation is one of the mechanisms for synergistic steatohepatitis caused by metabolic syndrome and alcohol. In addition, Binxia and colleagues showed that acute ethanol binge induces hepatic or serum FFAs elevation in HFD-fed mice, up-regulating hepatic chemokine CXCL1 production.[48] Hepatic Cxcl1 mRNA was up-regulated by more than 35-fold in the HFD-plus-ethanol groups, respectively, compared to control groups. CXCL1 induces neutrophil infiltration and causes acute liver injury in those mice.

In addition to animal studies, there are a number of studies addressing this issue in humans. A recent study suggests that lipid metabolism may be different between patients with NAFLD/MASLD and ALD during acute alcohol intoxication.[49] Israelsen and colleagues found that patients with NAFLD/MASLD have reduced lipid turnover during alcohol intoxication compared with people with alcohol-related FLD.[49] The author showed a decrease in circulating lysophosphatidylcholine (LPC) alcohol after alcohol intake in NAFLD patients. On the other hand, alcohol intake increases hepatic LPC uptake, which leads to caspase activation and the generation of oxidative stress, resulting in lipoapoptosis of hepatocytes and steatohepatitis. Therefore, metabolic syndrome and alcohol cause liver damage through activation of M1 macrophages, activation of the chemokine CXCL1, and changes in lipid metabolism.

Binge Drinking

In addition to excessive daily use of alcohol, binge drinking seems to have detrimental impact on health. Binge drinking is defined as 5 or more drinks on at least 1 occasion for men or 4 or more drinks for women. According to a report in 2018 in the US, 1 in 6 adults reported binge drinking in the previous month. Among them, 25% reported binge drinking at least weekly.[50] Claudia and colleagues reported that binge drinking is the cause of insulin resistance and insulin resistance persists days after all ethanol has been metabolized. It implies that binge drinking induces metabolic syndrome and type 2 diabetes.[51] Chronic binge drinking induces higher levels of steatosis, serum alanine transaminase, and liver inflammation.[52] Younossi and colleagues reported that more than 13 days of binge drinking per year increases the risk of mortality (HR; 1.49) after adjusting for the presence of metabolic syndrome and the average amount of daily alcohol use.[26] There are still not many studies evaluating the effects of binge drinking. However, there is a possibility that some cross-sectional studies have not been able to assess past drinking habits or binge drinking accurately. For example, a participant who reported heavy drinking every weekend and an average of 2 drinks on weekdays may have reported drinking the same amount as a participant who reported an average of 2 drinks on weekdays. Therefore, in patients with liver disease, in addition to average daily alcohol intake, binge drinking must also be considered in future studies.

The Impact of Light to Moderate Alcohol Ingestion on Liver Disease

As previously noted, the fact that excessive alcohol intake is harmful is the consensus among experts. However, some reports suggest that light to moderate alcohol intake may have beneficial metabolic impact. In one study, Dunn and colleagues assessed the effect of alcohol on 251 lifetime non-drinkers and 331 modest drinkers.[53] Modest drinkers, compared to non-drinkers, had lower odds of having a diagnosis of NASH/MASH (odds 0.56). Furthermore, modest drinkers also had significantly lower odds for fibrosis (OR 0.56) and ballooning hepatocellular injury (OR 0.66) than lifetime non-drinkers. In another study, Wasit and colleagues performed a meta-analysis of 11435 patients with NAFLD, which includes 14 cohorts and cross-sectional studies.[54] In this study, moderate alcohol intake decreased risks for steatohepatitis (OR 0.59), and advanced liver fibrosis (OR 0.59). Moreover, NAFLD/MASLD patients with modest alcohol intake had a lower mortality risk than lifelong abstainers (HR 0.85). Therefore, these studies suggest that light to moderate amounts of alcohol do not worsen liver disease in NAFLD/MASLD patients. On the other hand, it is important to recognize that studies showing beneficial impact of light to moderate alcohol intake may be flawed with potential biases. One important flaw may be related to their study design. Most studies that evaluated the impact of alcohol on liver disease were cross-sectional studies. Some studies assess only diagnosis codes, and some studies do not evaluate alcohol intake. Even if the studies evaluated alcohol intake, there is a possibility that patients report a lower alcohol intake than actual intake because alcohol is a stigma for patients.[46] In contrast to these studies, Helen and colleagues demonstrated that even small amounts of alcohol intake can worsen liver outcomes in patients with NAFLD/MASLD.[55] Furthermore, Kimura and colleagues reported the impact of small amounts of drinking habits (less than 20 g/d of ethanol) on the clinical course of NAFLD/MASLD.[56] They enrolled 301 patients with NAFLD/MASLD who were divided into a small amount drinking group and a non-drinking group. The HCC appearance rate was significantly higher in the small amount drinking group. Especially in patients with advanced fibrosis (F3-4), drinking habit was a significant factor for HCC. Moreover, another study reported that a small amount of alcohol increases the risk of breast cancer and colon cancer.[57] Thus, a small amount of alcohol can be harmful to other organs and tissues. Clinicians need to be careful about the amount of alcohol and drinking habits of patients with liver disease.

The New Term for a Subtype of Steatotic Liver Disease, Met-ALD

In addition to MASLD, a new term MetALD has been selected for patients with SLD who consume alcohol per week (140–350 g/week and 210–420 g/week, respectively, for females and males). According to the new classification, MASLD, MetALD, and ALD are included under the umbrella term of SLD. This new nomenclature is expected to reveal the impact of alcohol on steatosis and the interaction between alcohol and metabolic abnormalities in patients with SLD.[58,59]

Lii and colleagues investigated all-cause mortality of MASLD, MetALD, and ALD with metabolic dysfunction using the data from NHANES III.[60] Patients with MetALD and ALD with metabolic dysfunction had a higher all-cause mortality compared to patients without liver steatosis (Patients with MetALD; HR 1.368, ALD patient with metabolic dysfunction; HR 1.774). Patients with MASLD were not associated with a significant increase in all-cause mortality compared to patients without hepatic steatosis. The findings indicated that patients with MetALD and ALD with metabolic dysfunction had a poorer prognosis and harmful impact of alcohol consumption. With the creation of a new diagnostic concept, further research on the interaction between alcohol and metabolic syndrome is desired.

SUMMARY

In summary, MASLD/NAFLD and ALD are common causes of liver disease and can co-exist in the same patient. In this context, alcohol and metabolic syndrome can negatively influence mortality, liver fibrosis, and HCC. However, the design of studies reviewed was cross-over or retrospective in which the accuracy of assessments of alcohol consumption remains questionable. Thus, evidence generated thus far may not be sufficient to completely understand the interaction of metabolic components and alcohol ingestion with liver related outcome which warrants further research. In this context, the new nomenclature of MASLD and MetALD may better clarify the inter-relationship between alcohol and metabolic syndrome and help with the development of new diagnostic biomarkers and treatments.

CLINICS CARE POINTS

- ALD and MASLD are common causes of liver disease that can individually and synergistically affect a large number of people.
- Given the rising trends of alcohol consumption as well as rates of obesity and type 2 diabetes, the clinical and economic burden of these liver diseases are expected to increase.

DISCLOSURE

Dr Z. M. Younossi is a consultant to BMS, GSK, Cymabay, Ipsen, Abbott, Novo Nordisk, Madrigal, Merck, Siemens, and Intercept. Other authors have no conflict of interest to disclose.

REFERENCES

1. Åberg F, Helenius-Hietala J, Puukka P, et al. Interaction between alcohol consumption and metabolic syndrome in predicting severe liver disease in the general population. Hepatology 2018;67(6):2141–9.
2. Anstee QM, Seth D, Day CP. Genetic factors that affect risk of alcoholic and nonalcoholic fatty liver disease. Gastroenterology 2016;150(8):1728–44.e7.
3. Alcohol consumption per capita from all beverages in the U.S. from 1850 to 2021. Statista; 2023. Available at: https://www.statista.com/statistics/442818/per-capita-alcohol-consumption-of-all-beverages-in-the-us/. [Accessed 10 January 2024].
4. Åberg F, Byrne CD, Pirola CJ, et al. Alcohol consumption and metabolic syndrome: clinical and epidemiological impact on liver disease. J Hepatol 2023;78(1):191–206.
5. Åberg F, Färkkilä M. Drinking and obesity: alcoholic liver disease/nonalcoholic fatty liver disease interactions. Semin Liver Dis 2020;40(2):154–62.
6. Babor TF, Higgins-Biddle JC. Brief intervention for hazardous and harmful drinking: a manual for use in primary care. World Health Organizaton Department of Mental Health and Substance Abuse 2001. Available at: https://www.drugsandalcohol.ie/14105/. [Accessed 10 January 2023].
7. Esser MB, Sherk A, Liu Y, et al. Deaths and years of potential life lost from excessive alcohol use - United States, 2011-2015. MMWR Morb Mortal Wkly Rep 2020;69(39):1428–33.
8. Rehm J, Taylor B, Mohapatra S, et al. Alcohol as a risk factor for liver cirrhosis: a systematic review and meta-analysis. Drug Alcohol Rev 2010;29(4):437–45.
9. Abeysekera KWM, Fernandes GS, Hammerton G, et al. Prevalence of steatosis and fibrosis in young adults in the UK: a population-based study. Lancet Gastroenterol Hepatol 2020;5(3):295–305.

10. Philip G, Hookey L, Richardson H, et al. Alcohol-associated liver disease is now the most common indication for liver transplant waitlisting among young American adults. Transplantation 2022;106(10):2000–5.
11. Saklayen MG. The global epidemic of the metabolic syndrome. Curr Hypertens Rep 2018;20(2):12.
12. Cornier MA, Dabelea D, Hernandez TL, et al. The metabolic syndrome. Endocr Rev 2008;29(7):777–822.
13. O'Hearn M, Lauren BN, Wong JB, et al. Trends and disparities in cardiometabolic health among U.S. Adults, 1999-2018. J Am Coll Cardiol 2022;80(2):138–51.
14. Kurl S, Laaksonen DE, Jae SY, et al. Metabolic syndrome and the risk of sudden cardiac death in middle-aged men. Int J Cardiol 2016;203:792–7.
15. Son DH, Ha HS, Park HM, et al. New markers in metabolic syndrome. Adv Clin Chem 2022;110:37–71.
16. Ren H, Wang J, Gao Y, et al. Metabolic syndrome and liver-related events: a systematic review and meta-analysis. BMC Endocr Disord 2019;19(1):40.
17. Ramkissoon R, Shah VH. Alcohol use disorder and alcohol-associated liver disease. Alcohol Res 2022;42(1):13.
18. Wong RJ, Yang Z, Cheung R, et al. Impact of longitudinal alcohol use patterns on long-term risk of cirrhosis among U.S. Veterans with steatotic liver disease. Gastroenterology 2024. https://doi.org/10.1053/j.gastro.2024.02.032.
19. Traversy G, Chaput JP. Alcohol consumption and obesity: an update. Curr Obes Rep 2015;4(1):122–30.
20. Fazzino TL, Fleming K, Sher KJ, et al. Heavy drinking in young adulthood increases risk of transitioning to obesity. Am J Prev Med 2017;53(2):169–75.
21. Kotronen A, Yki-Järvinen H, Männistö S, et al. Non-alcoholic and alcoholic fatty liver disease - two diseases of affluence associated with the metabolic syndrome and type 2 diabetes: the FIN-D2D survey. BMC Publ Health 2010;10:237.
22. Rinella ME, Lazarus JV, Ratziu V, et al. A multisociety Delphi consensus statement on new fatty liver disease nomenclature. Hepatology 2023;78(6):1966–86.
23. Younossi ZM, Paik JM, Al Shabeeb R, et al. Are there outcome differences between NAFLD and metabolic-associated fatty liver disease? Hepatology 2022;76(5):1423–37.
24. Decraecker M, Dutartre D, Hiriart JB, et al. Long-term prognosis of patients with alcohol-related liver disease or non-alcoholic fatty liver disease according to metabolic syndrome or alcohol use. Liver Int 2022;42(2):350–62.
25. Pearson MM, Kim NJ, Berry K, et al. Associations between alcohol use and liver-related outcomes in a large national cohort of patients with cirrhosis. Hepatol Commun 2021;5(12):2080–95.
26. Younossi ZM, Stepanova M, Ong J, et al. Effects of alcohol consumption and metabolic syndrome on mortality in patients with nonalcoholic and alcohol-related fatty liver disease. Clin Gastroenterol Hepatol 2019;17(8):1625–33.e1.
27. Ajmera V, Belt P, Wilson LA, et al. Among patients with nonalcoholic fatty liver disease, modest alcohol use is associated with less improvement in histologic steatosis and steatohepatitis. Clin Gastroenterol Hepatol 2018;16(9):1511–20.e5.
28. Termeie O, Fiedler L, Martinez L, et al. Alarming trends: mortality from alcoholic cirrhosis in the United States. Am J Med 2022;135(10):1263–6.
29. Parker R, Kim SJ, Im GY, et al. Obesity in acute alcoholic hepatitis increases morbidity and mortality. EBioMedicine 2019;45:511–8.
30. Huang Y, Joseph J, de Boer WB, et al. Long-term liver-related outcomes of patients with chronic liver diseases in Australia. Clin Gastroenterol Hepatol 2020;18(2):496–504.e3.

31. Innes H, Crooks CJ, Aspinall E, et al. Characterizing the risk interplay between alcohol intake and body mass index on cirrhosis morbidity. Hepatology 2022; 75(2):369–78.

32. Pose E, Pera G, Torán P, et al. Interaction between metabolic syndrome and alcohol consumption, risk factors of liver fibrosis: a population-based study. Liver Int 2021;41(7):1556–64.

33. Mallet V, Parlati L, Martinino A, et al. Burden of liver disease progression in hospitalized patients with type 2 diabetes mellitus. J Hepatol 2022;76(2):265–74.

34. Yoshimura Y, Hamaguchi M, Hashimoto Y, et al. Obesity and metabolic abnormalities as risks of alcoholic fatty liver in men: NAGALA study. BMC Gastroenterol 2021;21(1):321.

35. Loomba R, Yang HI, Su J, et al. Obesity and alcohol synergize to increase the risk of incident hepatocellular carcinoma in men. Clin Gastroenterol Hepatol 2010; 8(10):891–8.

36. Costentin CE, Minoves M, Kotzki S, et al. Alcohol-related hepatocellular carcinoma is a heterogenous condition: lessons from a latent class analysis. Liver Int 2022;42(7):1638–47.

37. Mathurin P, de Zélicourt M, Laurendeau C, et al. Treatment patterns, risk factors and outcomes for patients with newly diagnosed hepatocellular carcinoma in France: a retrospective database analysis. Clin Res Hepatol Gastroenterol 2023;47(5): 102124.

38. Younossi ZM, Otgonsuren M, Henry L, et al. Association of nonalcoholic fatty liver disease (NAFLD) with hepatocellular carcinoma (HCC) in the United States from 2004 to 2009. Hepatology 2015;62(6):1723–30.

39. Younossi ZM, Stepanova M, Al Shabeeb R, et al. The changing epidemiology of adult liver transplantation in the United States in 2013-2022: the dominance of metabolic dysfunction-associated steatotic liver disease and alcohol-associated liver disease. Hepatol Commun 2024;8(1).

40. Anugwom C, Thomson M, Freese RL, et al. Lower survival and higher rates of cirrhosis in patients with ROUX-EN-Y gastric bypass hospitalised with alcohol-associated hepatitis. BMJ Open Gastroenterol 2023;10(1).

41. Kim HP, Jiang Y, Farrell TM, et al. Barritt AS 4th. Roux-en-Y gastric bypass is associated with increased hazard for de Novo alcohol-related complications and liver disease. J Clin Gastroenterol 2022;56(2):181–5.

42. Mellinger JL, Shedden K, Winder GS, et al. Bariatric surgery and the risk of alcohol-related cirrhosis and alcohol misuse. Liver Int 2021;41(5):1012–9.

43. Yarra P, Dunn W, Younossi Z, et al. Association of previous gastric bypass surgery and patient outcomes in alcohol-associated cirrhosis hospitalizations. Dig Dis Sci 2023;68(3):1026–34.

44. Danielsson O, Nano J, Pahkala K, et al. Validity of fatty liver disease indices in the presence of alcohol consumption. Scand J Gastroenterol 2022;57(11):1349–60.

45. Morinaga M, Kon K, Uchiyama A, et al. Carbohydrate-deficient transferrin is a sensitive marker of alcohol consumption in fatty liver disease. Hepatol Int 2022; 16(2):348–58.

46. Staufer K, Huber-Schönauer U, Strebinger G, et al. Ethyl glucuronide in hair detects a high rate of harmful alcohol consumption in presumed non-alcoholic fatty liver disease. J Hepatol 2022;77(4):918–30.

47. Xu J, Lai KKY, Verlinsky A, et al. Synergistic steatohepatitis by moderate obesity and alcohol in mice despite increased adiponectin and p-AMPK. J Hepatol 2011; 55(3):673–82.

48. Chang B, Xu MJ, Zhou Z, et al. Short- or long-term high-fat diet feeding plus acute ethanol binge synergistically induce acute liver injury in mice: an important role for CXCL1. Hepatology 2015;62(4):1070–85.
49. Israelsen M, Kim M, Suvitaival T, et al. Comprehensive lipidomics reveals phenotypic differences in hepatic lipid turnover in ALD and NAFLD during alcohol intoxication. JHEP Rep 2021;3(5):100325.
50. Bohm MK, Liu Y, Esser MB, et al. Binge drinking among adults, by select characteristics and state - United States, 2018. MMWR Morb Mortal Wkly Rep 2021;70(41):1441–6.
51. Lindtner C, Scherer T, Zielinski E, et al. Binge drinking induces whole-body insulin resistance by impairing hypothalamic insulin action. Sci Transl Med 2013;5(170):170ra14.
52. Llerena S, Arias-Loste MT, Puente A, et al. Binge drinking: burden of liver disease and beyond. World J Hepatol 2015;7(27):2703–15.
53. Dunn W, Sanyal AJ, Brunt EM, et al. Modest alcohol consumption is associated with decreased prevalence of steatohepatitis in patients with non-alcoholic fatty liver disease (NAFLD). J Hepatol 2012;57(2):384–91.
54. Wongtrakul W, Niltwat S, Charatcharoenwitthaya P. The effects of modest alcohol consumption on non-alcoholic fatty liver disease: a systematic review and meta-analysis. Front Med 2021;8:744713.
55. Jarvis H, O'Keefe H, Craig D, et al. Does moderate alcohol consumption accelerate the progression of liver disease in NAFLD? A systematic review and narrative synthesis. BMJ Open 2022;12(1):e049767.
56. Kimura T, Tanaka N, Fujimori N, et al. Mild drinking habit is a risk factor for hepatocarcinogenesis in non-alcoholic fatty liver disease with advanced fibrosis. World J Gastroenterol 2018;24(13):1440–50.
57. Seitz HK, Mueller S, Hellerbrand C, et al. Effect of chronic alcohol consumption on the development and progression of non-alcoholic fatty liver disease (NAFLD). Hepatobiliary Surg Nutr 2015;4(3):147–51.
58. Younossi ZM, AlQahtani SA, Alswat K, et al. Global survey of stigma among physicians and patients with nonalcoholic fatty liver disease. J Hepatol 2023. https://doi.org/10.1016/j.jhep.2023.11.004.
59. Moreno C, Sheron N, Tiniakos D, et al, EASL Consortium for the Study of Alcohol-related LiVer disease in Europe (SALVE). "Dual aetiology fatty liver disease": a recently proposed term associated with potential pitfalls. J Hepatol 2021;74(4):979–82.
60. Li M, Xie W. Are there all-cause mortality differences between metabolic dysfunction-associated steatotic liver disease subtypes? J Hepatol 2024;80(2):e53–4.

Alcohol-Associated Liver Diseases
Spectrum, Nomenclature, and Definitions

Saggere Muralikrishna Shasthry, MD, DM,
Shiv Kumar Sarin, MD, DM, DSc*

KEYWORDS

- Alcohol-associated liver disease • Alcoholic hepatitis • Alcohol use disorder

KEY POINTS

- Alcohol-associated liver disease (AALD) is a nonmutually exclusive spectrum ranging from steatosis, alcoholic hepatitis to cirrhosis.
- There is a need for having universally acceptable definitions of individual stages for clinical and research utility.
- Noninvasive tests (NITs) like enhanced liver fibrosis score, fibrosis-4, and transient elastography with specific cutoffs are useful in identifying early disease especially in high-risk populations (alcohol-use disorder [AUD]).
- Alcoholic hepatitis (AH) should be defined as per National Institute on Alcohol Abuse and Alcoholism and stratified as definite, probable, and possible.
- Many areas still need granularity—defining AH in cirrhosis and cirrhosis without AH, AUD in patients with cirrhosis, stratifying AALD in the presence of cardiometabolic risk factors, identifying best cutoffs for NITs especially in the presence of inflammation, and so forth.

Alcohol-associated liver disease (AALD) is an increasingly reported cause for liver diseases with high mortality.[1,2] Chronic and hazardous alcohol consumption is a risk factor for the development of a spectrum of liver injuries—ranging from steatosis, alcohol-associated steatohepatitis, alcohol-associated fibrosis to cirrhosis. Clinically, alcohol-associated hepatitis is the most severe form of AALD and carries a high mortality and rapid progression of cirrhosis and its complications. So, defining the patient population and its spectrum is imperative in bringing out uniformity in clinical trials and optimizing the patient care. Using consistent definitions will also provide reliable and reproducible results from clinical trials, and bring out a change in clinical approach and rationalize resource allocation.

Funding sources: None.
Department of Hepatology, Institute of Liver and Biliary Sciences, Sector D1, Vasantkunj, New Delhi 110070, India
* Corresponding author.
E-mail addresses: shivsarin@gmail.com; sksarin@ilbs.in

In its broad sense AALD is a sequel to alcohol use disorder (AUD), encompassing pathologic and clinical spectrum ranging from asymptomatic steatosis to alcoholic hepatitis (AH) to alcohol-associated cirrhosis (compensated/decompensated), which further can progress to hepatocellular carcinoma (HCC). Volunteers consuming approximately 10 drinks per day (one standard US drink = 14 g of alcohol) for 2 to 3 weeks consistently develop steatosis.[3] Such a level of consumption remains for years in patients developing alcohol-associated hepatitis,[4] with only a minority of them developing the severe alcoholic hepatitis (SAH). Although, prior to National Institute on Alcohol Abuse and Alcoholism definition of AH[5] the publications were heterogenous, even today AH is variably defined, and the definition needs to be made more robust and inclusive. Presence of cardiometabolic risk factors and hepatitis B virus and hepatitis C virus infections complicates the issue further. There are challenges for physicians in understanding and appropriately using AUD, alcohol-associated hepatitis, AH, SAH, alcohol-associated cirrhosis, and similar terminologies. We, therefore, need serious efforts to list out the knowledge gaps, different facets of AUD in the context of hepatitis or cirrhosis condition, nature and period of last drinking, diagnostic and treatment needs, and then undertake global efforts through multinational societies for standardization of the definition. We are using the term AALD in this review knowing fully well the reservations and limitations of the term. With this background heterogeneity and knowledge gaps, we provide a narrative, which summarizes the current scenario and future needs in the context of AALD spectrum, nomenclature, and definitions. We also provide action points for investigators to ponder and resolve.

IDENTIFYING AND DEFINING ALCOHOL USE DISORDER

The diagnosis of AALD becomes complete with concomitant identification of AUD. The AUD depends on identifying problem drinking for which we need to quantify the amount of alcohol consumed. It is cumbersome to quantify alcohol consumption in clinical practice. Quantifying in grams per day or per week is the more precise way to do so. At times, it will be difficult to recall the history of the types and quantity of alcoholic beverages consumed by the patients. There is also a lot of discrepancy in defining what constitutes one "drink." In United States, one "standard" drink (or one alcoholic drink equivalent) contains roughly 14 g of pure alcohol.[6] European association for the study of the liver (EASL) and the World Health Organization define one drink as 10 g of pure alcohol while in some countries "one drink" consists of 8 to 16 g of alcohol.[7]

Point 1: A uniform definition of "one drink" by all the leading global societies will help not only future studies but may simplify commercial usages and warnings.

Patients with AALD suffer from at least 2 disorders: one affecting the liver and the other, AUD. AUD, according to Diagnostic and statistical manual of mental disorders, fifth edition (DSM-V), is defined as "a problematic pattern of alcohol use leading to clinically significant impairment or distress, as manifested by [two or more symptoms out of a total of 11], occurring within a 12-month period" and graded as mild, moderate, or severe. Even a mild disorder can lead to problems, so treatment is important.[8] Alcohol use disorders identification test (AUDIT) with 10 questions (that explore consumption [1–3], dependence [4–6], and alcohol-related problems [7–10]) remains the gold standard screening tool for diagnosis of AUD. A concise form AUDIT-C[9] with only 3 questions (scored 0–4, maximum score 12) can also be used to identify problem drinking. Alternatively, a simple, single initial screening question[10] asking about the number of times the person has exceeded the daily drinking recommendations[11] (2 drinks for men and one for women) in the previous 1 year, would be an easy way to identify a person needing a detailed specialist assessment, even if there is a single occurrence of such an episode. AUD, its definitions and diagnosis in difficult populations like liver diseases and post liver transplantation and so forth, is discussed in detail in a separate article in this journal. It is important to identify AUD in a health care setting as an integral part of AALD diagnosis and vice versa.[12]

Point 2: We need to define and list the facets of AUD to be assessed in patients with AALD. There is a need to standardize the duration of continued/intermittent/binge drinking and the period of abstinence for patients with AALD.

ALCOHOL-ASSOCIATED LIVER DISEASES: SPECTRUM AND DEFINITIONS

ALD carries a significant stigma in society. It is increasingly recognized to use the term "alcohol associated" in place of "alcoholic" to alleviate social stigma; thus, alcohol-associated liver disease, alcohol-associated steatohepatitis, and alcohol-associated cirrhosis are preferred, retaining the familiar abbreviations (alcoholic liver disease [ALD] or AALD, alcoholic steato hepatitis [ASH], and alcoholic cirrhosis [AC], respectively).[13] AALD encompasses overlapping clinical spectrum of alcohol-associated fatty liver, hepatitis, cirrhosis (compensated/decompensated), alcohol-associated acute-on-chronic liver failure (ACLF), and HCC. Histologically, the spectrum of AALD includes alcohol-associated steatosis, steatohepatitis, sclerosing hyaline necrosis, alcohol-associated fibrosis, and alcohol-associated cirrhosis. About 90% to 95% of the harmful alcoholic consumers have steatosis, of which around 20% to 40% develop some amount of fibrosis. Nearly half of those developing the fibrosis (8%–20%) will further progress to the stage of cirrhosis.[12]

Alcohol-Associated Fatty Liver/Steatosis

There is no unique presentation of AALD to confidently differentiate it from other forms of liver disease. Alcohol consumption is often not revealed, and sometimes, the history is not properly taken by the health care professional. It merits a high index of suspicion to diagnose ALD, especially in its early forms such as alcohol-associated fatty liver or steatosis. Patients with alcohol-associated steatosis are usually asymptomatic. Elevations of aspartate amino transferase and gamma-glutamyl transpeptidase (GGT) are the best indicators of significant alcohol consumption in comparison to non-alcoholic fatty liver disease (NAFLD) where alanine amino transferase levels are elevated.[14,15] Steatosis can be easily identified on ultrasonography, computed tomography (CT), or MRI of the liver. Of these modalities, MRI is the more accurate to quantify fat with added advantage of its ability to evaluate the entire liver.[16,17] Liver biopsy is rarely needed to diagnose alcohol-associated steatosis. With cessation of alcohol intake, the steatosis has a potential to resolve.

Alcohol-Associated Fibrosis/Cirrhosis

Development of alcohol-associated fibrosis and cirrhosis generally goes through multiple episodes of subclinical, biochemical, or clinical episodes of hepatitis. Progression through these various stages is dependent on continued heavy alcohol use and other risk factors, including female sex, genetic susceptibility, diet, metabolic risk factors, and comorbid liver diseases. In an earlier study, after adjustment for daily alcohol intake and total duration of alcohol abuse, body mass index, liver iron overload, and blood glucose were identified as independent risk factors for fibrosis in AALD.[18,19] The occurrence of AH hastens the progression of fibrosis and cirrhosis. There is, however, a distinct group of patients, who develop zone 3 injury, characterized as sclerosing hyaline necrosis, and develop portal hypertension and other features of

AALD, without manifesting features of AH.[20] It is to be emphasized that the stage of liver fibrosis is an important determinant of clinical outcomes in AALD. In the initial stages of fatty liver, collagen deposits around terminal hepatic veins: the perivenular fibrosis. Lobular inflammation and ballooning trigger the release of hedgehog ligands that activate hepatic stellate cells in a paracrine manner leading to deposition of matrix around hepatocytes (pericellular fibrosis) and along sinusoids (perisinusoidal fibrosis).

Individuals with early ALD (with steatosis or steatohepatitis and early stage fibrosis) may be asymptomatic with mere biochemical abnormalities of routine blood tests (reversal of aspartate aminotransferase/ alanine aminotransferase [AST/ALT] ratio, marginally low serum albumin level or low platelet count) or the presence of changes of chronic liver disease, collaterals, or splenomegaly on ultrasound/CT imaging done for other purposes. While patients in the later stages may present with complications of cirrhosis with decompensating events (ascites, hepatic encephalopathy, variceal bleeding, and HCC), or with symptomatic AH with jaundice and/or ACLF, with jaundice and ascites. At present, there are challenges in using the term SAH in the context of underlying cirrhosis and to differentiate it from ACLF and decompensation of a known alcohol-associated cirrhosis.[21]

Point 3: There is a need to put in AH and SAH in the context of underlying cirrhosis. There is also a need to define AALD and AC in the absence of AH.

Alcohol-associated hepatitis

AH is the most florid presentation of AALD. Proposed definitions have been attempted to delineate alcohol-associated hepatitis, with applicability limited to prospective clinical trials only. Among patients with suspected heavy alcohol use and new onset or worsening jaundice, clinicians should have a high suspicion for alcohol-associated hepatitis given its high short-term mortality. AH is defined as per the National Institute on Alcohol Abuse and Alcoholism (NIAAA), Alcoholic Hepatitis Consortia, to include the following[22]:

- The onset of jaundice within 60 days of heavy alcohol consumption (more than 50 g/d) for a minimum of 6 months
- Serum bilirubin more than 3 mg/dL
- Elevated AST to 50 to 400 U/L
- AST:ALT ratio of more than 1.5
- No other cause of acute hepatitis (hepatitis A virus [HAV], hepatitis E virus [HEV], drug induced liver injury [DILI], ischemic hepatitis, and so forth)
- Absence of confounding factors—possible Wilson disease or α1-antitrypsin deficiency, uncertain alcohol consumption, atypical laboratory tests (AST<50 or >400 IU/L or AST/ALT<1.5).

Once the diagnosis of AH is made, it is further stratified as *definite* AH (clinically diagnosed along with biopsy substantiated), *probable* AH (clinically diagnosed without biopsy and without confounding factors), or *possible* AH (clinically diagnosed with confounding factors[18]; **Fig. 1**). Clinical diagnosis of probable AH accurately predicted AH on 95% of the patients in the original consortia, but later some studies have shown discordance between the criteria and the explant histology—with 79% patients meeting the clinical criteria and only 59% having histologic steatohepatitis.[23] On the other hand, there are about 30% of the patients who do not meet the clinical definition of AH but have features of AH on biopsy, coexisting with presence of cirrhosis called "walking AH."[24] Some of these patients may progress to clinical AH. An important question is to how to identify such outliers so that our clinical definition of AH is very sensitive and as well as specific. Similarly, a fair proportion of patients who have

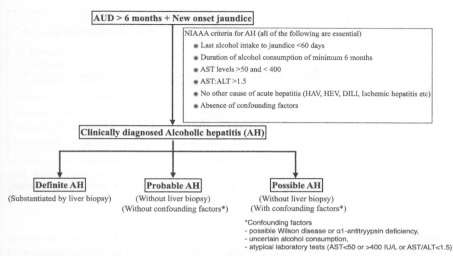

Fig. 1. Algorithm for diagnosis of symptomatic AH. *, Indicationg confounding factors.

stopped drinking for greater than 60 days continue to show clinical features of AH and the biopsy confirms the same. The current definition would exclude these patients.

Point 4: We need more studies to demonstrate clear distinction and positive predictive value of liver biopsy and definite AH over probable AH. A greater correlation between histologic and clinical criteria is also warranted.

Severity of alcohol-associated hepatitis

After diagnosing AH, the severity of the condition needs to be categorized. Severe AH is conventionally defined using the Maddrey's Discriminant Function score [4.6 (delta prothrombin time in seconds) + serum bilirubin in mg/dL], which if greater than 32, identifies patients who have low short-term survival and meet prednisolone therapy eligibility.[25] The model for end-stage liver disease (MELD) score is also frequently used to estimate disease severity and determine the eligibility for corticosteroid treatment, with scores greater than 20 indicating severe AH and 20 or less indicating moderate AH.[26,27] Recently, model for end-stage liver disease sodium (MELDNa) has also been proposed to be an accurate assessor of disease severity and eligibility for corticosteroid therapy in AH.[28] Advantages of using the MELD score in the assessment of AH severity are its better accuracy, worldwide use in organ allocation, use of International Normalized Ratio over prothrombin time, and incorporation of serum creatinine, a major determinant of outcomes in patients with AH.[12] Many other scores to identify severe AH at baseline are available (**Table 1**). Lille score helps in identifying patients with AH receiving steroids as responders (score <0.45) or nonresponders (>0.45) at day 7 and is widely accepted as a therapeutic end-point in clinical trials. Unfortunately, Lille score has limited relevance when slow-acting therapies, such as fecal microbial transplantation[29] or grannulocyte-colony stimulating factor (GCSF),[30] are employed.

Metabolic Dysfunction-Associated Fatty Liver Disease and Metabolic Dysfunction and Alcohol-Associated Liver Disease

AALD is a type of fatty liver disease caused solely by significant alcohol consumption (weekly intake 140–350 g female, 210–420 g male [average daily 20–50 g female, 30–60 g male]) in the absence of any cardiometabolic risk factors.

Table 1
Variables incorporated in the 5 prognostic scores most commonly used in alcoholic hepatitis[7]

Score	Bilirubin	PT/INR	Creatinine/Urea	Leukocytes	Age	Albumin	Change in Bilirubin by day 7
Maddrey DF	+	+	−	−	−	−	−
MELD	+	+	+	−	−	−	−
GAHS	+	+	+	+	+	−	−
ABIC	+	+	+	−	+	+	−
Lille score	+	+	+	−	+	+	+

Abbreviations: ABIC, age, serum bilirubin; GAHS, Glasgow alcoholic hepatitis score; PT/INR, prothrombin time and international normalized ratio; Maddrey DF, Maddrey discriminant function; MELD, model for end-stage liver disease.

Presence of cardiometabolic risk factors and significant alcohol consumption would make them fit into a new term called metabolic dysfunction and alcohol-associated liver disease (Met ALD). Within Met ALD, there is a continuum where, conceptually, the condition can be seen to be metabolic dysfunction-associated fatty liver disease (MAFLD) or ALD predominant based on the amount of alcohol consumed. This may vary over time within a given individual.[31] Mild, moderate alcohol consumption can be included under MAFLD based on the presence of overweight/obesity or diabetes in addition to alcohol consumption. In very early Met ALD without cirrhosis, the presence of AST greater than ALT may identify those with predominance of ALD over MAFLD. But, in patients with Met ALD and early cirrhosis of liver, it will be very difficult and important to diagnose walking AH (asymptomatic but AH on biopsy) as patients with AH on biopsy are likely to have faster progression of liver cirrhosis in comparison to those with predominant MAFLD or simple steatosis.

Point 5: There is a need for granularity in diagnosing AH in patients with mild-to-moderate drinking with metabolic dysfunctions and/or obesity and a need to add histologic features in Met ALD or MAFLD definitions distinctive from pure MAFLD or AALD.

Assessment of Fibrosis and Inflammation in Alcohol-Associated Liver Disease

Alcohol-associated cirrhosis is usually diagnosed only at the time of decompensation or uncovered incidentally during the evaluation of abnormal blood tests or physical findings. Abnormal imaging findings may include liver nodularity or presence of signs of portal hypertension and increase in transient elastography. Without a careful history of AUD and ruling out other causes, the diagnosis of AC is not easy. Fibrosis assessment is an important step in identifying asymptomatic patients with suspected high risk of fibrosis and early AALD. Very limited noninvasive studies are available in AALD with respect to identifying the fibrosis. Noninvasive blood and/or radiological tests (NITs) should be used to assess the severity of fibrosis in persons with asymptomatic AALD (**Fig 2**). Fibrosis-4 (FIB-4) score and transient elastography of liver are generally employed for fibrosis detection among persons with AALD. Persons with harmful drinking with evidence of AALD/fibrosis, detected with NITs, will need a multidisciplinary approach in managing both AUD and AALD.[8] To avoid late presentation, noninvasive tests to screen the liver disease in the harmful alcohol consumers is cost-effective, especially in those who have AUD and have a health care encounter due to any reason.

Non invasive tests (NIT) in assessing asymptomatic early AALD			

	No fibrosis	Indeterminate	Advanced fibrosis
Fib-4 score	< 1.45	>1.45 to 3.25	> 3.25
ELF score	<7.7	7.7-9.8	>9.8
TE-LSM	<8 kPa	>8 kPa- 12.2 kPa	>12.2 kPa

Red flags
1. Platelet count < 150×10^9/L
2. Serum Albumin <3.5g/dL
3. AST>ALT
4. USG or CT
    - suggestive of chronic liver disease
    - portosystemic collaterals
    - splenomegaly

Group 1 : No fibrosis and no red flags; Should be monitored annually

Group 2 : Indeterminate fibrosis and no red flags; Should be reassessed after 3 months of strict abstinence

Group 3 : Advanced fibrosis and/ or any of the red flags; Should be referred to hepatologist

Fig. 2. Algorithm on the use of NITs in identifying asymptomatic early AALD.

FIB-4 has been most studied with high sensitivity (80%–90%), but low specificity (60%–70%) in excluding advanced fibrosis (F3-4).[32,33] The enhanced liver fibrosis (ELF) score is a patented blood-based biomarkers score with higher specificity (80%–90%), but with higher cost and limited availability.[34] According to the manufacturer, ELF should be interpreted as follows: less than 7.7, no to mild fibrosis; 7.7 to less than 9.8, moderate fibrosis (F≥2); and greater than 9.8, significant fibrosis (F≥3).[35] This original ELF cohort included 64 patients with ALD and found an area under receiver operating curve (AUROC) of 0.944 (95% CI: 0.836–1.000) for diagnosis of significant fibrosis (F≥2). In another study on patients with ALD (n = 289), the utility of ELF in detecting significant and advanced fibrosis and cirrhosis was excellent, with AUROCs of 0.84 (95% CI: 0.80–0.89), 0.92 (0.89–0.96), and 0.94 (0.91–0.97), respectively, with scores greater than 11.3 indicating cirrhosis.[34] ELF score may be more reliable in patients with recent alcohol intake as the circulating markers are not affected by alcohol intake.[36] A significant correlation between ELF score and transient elastography and liver biopsy was documented in another study,[37] which also showed significantly better accuracy of ELF over FIB-4 and NFS in patients with AALD with AUROC 0.85 (95% confidence interval [CI] 0.79–0.92).

Transient elastography, a test of liver stiffness measurement (LSM), has been most extensively evaluated for fibrosis assessment in patients with AALD. Multiple meta-analyses have found acceptable sensitivity and specificity, especially for advanced fibrosis (F3–F4).[38–40] In AUD patients, an LSM on transient elastography of greater than 8 kPa is sensitive in identifying patients with grade 2 or more fibrosis. In a meta-analysis of individual patient data of 1026 patients with AALD, a cutoff LSM of 12.1 kPa was found accurate to identify advanced fibrosis with receiver operating characteristics of 0.90 (95% CI 0.86–0.94).[34] It is important to note that the underlying inflammation, elevated serum bilirubin, and recent alcohol consumption may interfere with LSM values and hence in the presence of AST greater than 100 IU/L, LSM values should be interpreted with caution as it may overestimate fibrosis. As the fibrosis stage is the strongest predictor of prognosis in liver disease,[41] individuals with advanced fibrosis and active drinking should be seen by a liver specialist.[42]

Measurement of inflammation, the hall mark of AH is a challenge. The current NITs and ELF and their cutoff values are designed to measure fibrosis at a given point and not inflammation. Serial LSM and ELF measurements after varying periods of abstinence may help in to identifying true fibrosis from inflammation and fibrosis. Hepatic

> **Box 1**
> **Requirements to be met for a new definition of alcohol-associated liver disease**
>
> Point 1: A uniform definition of "one drink" by all the leading global societies will help not only future studies but may simplify commercial usages and warnings.
>
> Point 2: We need to define and list the facets of AUD to be assessed in patients with AALD. There is a need to standardize the duration of continued/intermittent/binge drinking and the period of abstinence for patients with AALD.
>
> Point 3: There is a need to put in AH and SAH in the context of underlying cirrhosis. There is also a need to define AALD and AC in the absence of AH.
>
> Point 4: We need more studies to demonstrate clear distinction and positive predictive value of liver biopsy and definite AH over probable AH. A greater correlation between histologic and clinical criteria is also warranted.
>
> Point 5: There is a need for granularity in diagnosing AH in patients with mild-to-moderate drinking with metabolic dysfunctions/and or obesity and need to add histologic features in Met ALD or MAFLD definitions distinctive from pure MAFLD or AALD.
>
> Point 6: There is a need to identify and validate NITs to characterize and correctly classify patients with different stages of AALD and serve to assess progression or treatment response.

veinous pressure gradient (HVPG) may score above all the tests in this regard but cannot be serially done beyond clinical studies, being invasive in nature.

Point 6: There is a need to identify and validate NITs to characterize and correctly classify patients with different stages of AALD and serve to assess progression or treatment response.

The issues related to nomenclature and definitions of AALD need large data and evidence-based deliberations. While prospective large global cohort studies would be the best options, in the present, the published literature can be reanalyzed with individual case based data. Clinical and histologic data, with special attention to metabolic risk factors, age, gender, race and drinking patters, could help reduce the bias and help achieve a more homogenous and acceptable definition. We have identified 6 major issues or key points to draw attention of the investigators across the world (**Box 1**). These may help to push the agenda toward a more granular and clear definition of AALD. Our goals in considering these agenda items could be that (1) clinicians can identify the stage and clinical course of the disease and can choose the appropriate interventions and therapies, (2) clinical trials can have clear inclusion criteria and end-point for all types of therapies, and (3) policy makers can issue warnings related to harmful drinking. We need collective global efforts to achieve these goals.

CLINICS CARE POINTS

- AALD is a global health problem with increasing incidence with high morbidity and mortality.
- Identifying the disease in the initial stages of the spectrum and remaining alcohol abstinent is the key in management.
- Evaluation for AALD with proper history and non-invasive tests (ELF score, Fib-4, elastography) should be part of every enounter with health care system.
- Deliniating the spectrum of AALD with globally acceptable difinitions with possible inclusion of NITs is very much needed for uniformity in patient care and research.

DISCLOSURE

Potential conflict of interest: None.

REFERENCES

1. Mellinger JL, Shedden K, Winder GS, et al. The high burden of alcoholic cirrhosis in privately insured persons in the United States. Hepatology 2018;68:872–82.
2. Peery AF, Crockett SD, Murphy CC, et al. Burden and cost of gastrointestinal, liver, and pancreatic diseases in the United States: update 2018. Gastroenterology 2019;156:254–72.e11.
3. Rubin E, Lieber CS. Alcohol- induced hepatic injury in nonalcoholic volunteers. N Engl J Med 1968;278:869–76.
4. Mendenhall CL, Moritz TE, Roselle GA, et al. A study of oral nutritional support with oxandrolone in malnourished patients with alco- holic hepatitis: results of a Depart- ment of Veterans Affairs cooperative study. Hepatology 1993;17: 564–76.
5. Crabb DW, Bataller R, Chalasani NP, et al. Standard definitions and common data elements for clinical trials in patients with alcoholic hepatitis: recommendation from the NIAAA Alcoholic Hepatitis Consortia. Gastroenterology 2016;150: 785–90.
6. DHHS, DoA. 2015–2020 dietary guidelines for Americans. In: 8th edition. Available at: http://health.gov/dietaryguidelines/2015/guidelines/2015.
7. European Association for the Study of the Liver. Electronic address: easloffi-ceeasloffice.eu; European association for the study of the liver. EASL clinical practice guidelines: management of alcohol-related liver disease. J Hepatol 2018;69(1):154–81. Epub 2018 Apr 5. PMID: 29628280.
8. Diagnostic and statistical manual of mental disorders: DSM-5 (5th edition). Arlington, VA: American Psychiatric Association; 2013. p. 490. ISBN 978-0-89042-554-1. OCLC 830807378.
9. Bush K, Kivlahan DR, McDonell MB, et al. The AUDIT alcohol consumption questions (AUDIT-C): an effective brief screening test for problem drinking. Ambulatory Care Quality Improvement Project (ACQUIP). Alcohol Use Disorders Identification Test. Arch Intern Med 1998;158(16):1789–95.
10. Smith PC, Schmidt SM, Allensworth-Davies D, et al. Primary care validation of a single-question alcohol screening test. J Gen Intern Med 2009;24:783–8.
11. Snetselaar LG, de Jesus JM, DeSilva DM, Stoody EE. Dietary guidelines for Americans, 2020-2025: understanding the scientific process, guidelines, and key recommendations. Nutr Today 2021;56(6):287–95.
12. Jophlin LL, Singal AK, Bataller R, et al. ACG clinical guideline: alcohol-associated liver disease. Am J Gastroenterol 2024;119(1):p30–54.
13. Crabb DW, Im GY, Szabo G, et al. Diagnosis and treatment of alcohol-associated liver diseases: 2019 practice guidance from the American association for the study of liver diseases. Hepatology 2020;71(1):306–33. https://doi.org/10.1002/hep.30866.
14. Lucey MR, Connor JT, Boyer TD, et al. DIVERT Study Group. Alcohol consumption by cirrhotic subjects: patterns of use and effects on liver function. Am J Gastroenterol 2008;103:1698–706.
15. Whitfield JB, Masson S, Liangpunsakul S, et al. Evaluation of laboratory tests for cirrhosis and for alcohol use, in the context of alcoholic cirrhosis. Alcohol 2018; 66:1–7.

16. Tapper EB, Lok ASF. Use of liver imaging and biopsy in clinical practice. N Engl J Med 2017;7(377):2296–7.

17. Reeder SB, Cruite I, Hamilton G, et al. Quantitative assess- ment of liver fat with magnetic resonance imaging and spectros- copy. J Magn Reson Imaging 2011; 34:729–49.

18. Raynard B, Balian A, Fallik D, et al. Risk factors of fibrosis in alcohol-induced liver disease. Hepatology 2002;35(3):635–8.

19. Lackner C, Tiniakos D. Fibrosis and alcohol-related liver disease. J Hepatol 2019; 70(2):294–304.

20. Theise ND. Histopathology of alcoholic liver disease. Clin Liver Dis (Hoboken) 2013;2(2):64–7.

21. Maiwall R, Pasupuleti SSR, Choudhury A, et al. AARC score determines out- comes in patients with alcohol-associated hepatitis: a multinational study. Hepa- tol Int 2023;17(3):662–75.

22. Crabb DW, Bataller R, Chalasani NP, et al. Standard definitions and common data elements for clinical trials in patients with alcoholic hepatitis: recommendation from the NIAAA alcoholic hepatitis consortia. Gastroenterology 2016;150(4): 785–90.

23. Lee BP, Mehta N, Platt L, et al. Outcomes of early liver transplantation for patients with severe alcoholic hepatitis. Gastroenterology 2018;155:422–30.e1.

24. Naveau S, Montembault S, Balian A, et al. Biological diagnosis of the type of liver disease in alcoholic patients with abnormal liver function tests. Gastroenterol Clin Biol 1999;23:1215–24.

25. Maddrey WC, Boitnott JK, Bedine MS, et al. Corticosteroid therapy of alcoholic hepatitis. Gastroenterology 1978;75(2):193–9. PMID: 352788.

26. Lucey MR, Mathurin P, Morgan TR. Alcoholic hepatitis. N Engl J Med 2009;360: 2758–69.

27. Dunn W, Jamil LH, Brown LS, et al. MELD accurately predicts mortality in patients with alcoholic hepatitis. Hepatology 2005;41(2):353–8.

28. Papastergiou V, Tsochatzis EA, Pieri G, et al. Nine scoring models for short-term mortality in alcoholic hepatitis: cross-validation in a biopsy- proven cohort. Aliment Pharmacol Ther 2014;39(7):721–32.

29. Pande A, Sharma S, Khillan V, et al. Fecal microbiota transplantation compared with prednisolone in severe alcoholic hepatitis patients: a randomized trial. Hep- atol Int 2023;17(1):249–61.

30. Shasthry SM, Sharma MK, Shasthry V, et al. Efficacy of granulocyte colony-stimulating factor in the management of steroid-nonresponsive severe alcoholic hepatitis: a double-blind randomized controlled trial. Hepatology 2019;70(3): 802–11.

31. Rinella ME, Lazarus JV, Ratziu V, et al. A multisociety Delphi consensus statement on new fatty liver disease nomenclature. Hepatology 2023. https://doi.org/10.1097/HEP.0000000000000520.

32. Singal A, Mathurin P. Diagnosis and treatment of alcohol-associated liver disease: a review. JAMA 2021;326(2):165–76.

33. Moreno C, Mueller S, Szabo G. Non-invasive diagnosis and biomarkers in alcohol-related liver disease. J Hepatol 2019;70(2):273–83.

34. Thiele M, Madsen BS, Hansen JF, et al. Accuracy of the enhanced liver fibrosis test vs FibroTest, elastography, and indirect markers in detection of advanced fibrosis in patients with alcoholic liver disease. Gastroenterology 2018;154(5): 1369–79.

35. Rosenberg WM, Voelker M, Thiel R, et al. Serum markers detect the presence of liver fibrosis: a cohort study. Gastroenterology 2004;127:1704–13.
36. Ponomarenko Y, Leo MA, Kroll W, et al. Effects of alcohol consumption on eight circulating markers of liver fibrosis. Alcohol Alcohol 2002;37:252–5.
37. Kjaergaard M, Lindvig KP, Thorhauge KH, et al. Using the ELF test, FIB-4 and NAFLD fibrosis score to screen the population for liver disease. J Hepatol 2023;79(2):277–86.
38. Nguyen-Khac E, Thiele M, Voican C, et al. Non-invasive diagnosis of liver fibrosis in patients with alcohol-related liver disease by transient elastography: an individual patient data meta-analysis. Lancet Gastroenterol Hepatol 2018;3(9):614–25.
39. Cai C, Song X, Chen X, et al. Transient elastography in alcoholic liver disease and nonalcoholic fatty liver disease: a systemic review and meta- analysis. Can J Gastroenterol Hepatol 2021;2021:8859338.
40. Pavlov CS, Casazza G, Semenistaia M, et al. Ultrasonography for diagnosis of alcoholic cirrhosis in people with alcoholic liver disease. Cochrane Database Syst Rev 2016;3:CD011602.
41. Ekstedt M, Hagstrom H, Nasr P, et al. Fibrosis stage is the strongest predictor for disease-specific mortality in NAFLD after up to 33 years of follow-up. Hepatology 2015;61(5):1547–54.
42. Rasmussen DN, Thiele M, Johansen S, et al. Prognostic performance of 7 biomarkers compared to liver biopsy in early alcohol-related liver disease. J Hepatol 2021;75(5):1017–25.

Alcohol and Hepatocellular Carcinoma

Nghiem B. Ha, MD, MAS, Francis Yao, MD*

KEYWORDS

- Surgery • Cancer • Obesity • Metabolic • Viral hepatitis • Surveillance • Treatment

KEY POINTS

- Alcohol-associated liver disease (ALD) is a major contributor to chronic liver disease and primary liver cancer, responsible for nearly one-third of global hepatocellular carcinoma (HCC) cases and one-fifth of liver cancer deaths annually.
- Alcohol causes liver damage through mechanisms such as endotoxin, oxidative stress, and inflammation, which leads to a spectrum of hepatic injuries from steatosis, steatohepatitis, and fibrosis/cirrhosis. Additionally, chronic alcohol use increases conversion of procarcinogens into carcinogens and disrupts gut flora, enhancing gut permeability and inflammation, which contributes to HCC development.
- Alcohol acts a cofactor when combined with other factors including viral hepatitis and metabolic disorders, exacerbating and accelerating the progression to HCC.
- Despite high risk of HCC in patients with ALD, current surveillance strategies are not tailored specifically for this population. Improve screening and targeted-therapeutic approaches, including immunotherapy and local regional therapy, as needed to enhance outcomes for alcohol-associated HCC, given its frequent advanced-stage diagnosis and poor prognosis compared to other etiologies.

INTRODUCTION

The global incidence of alcohol-associated liver disease (ALD) has been rising in recent decades due to increased high-risk drinking, placing a significant health and economic burden on the health care system.[1,2] In the United States (US), the annual direct and indirect costs of ALD are projected to increase by 118%, from $31 billion in 2022 to $66 billion in 2040, amounting to a total of $880 billion—$355 billion in direct health care-related costs and $525 billion in lost labor and economic consumption.[3] Diminished productivity and rising health care-related costs have significant upstream impacts on public payers, programs, and policymakers, as well as downstream

Hepatology, Liver Transplant, Division of Gastroenterology and Hepatology, Department of Medicine, University of California, San Francisco, 505 Parnassus Avenue, S-357, San Francisco, CA 94112, USA
* Corresponding author.
E-mail address: francis.yao@ucsf.edu

Clin Liver Dis 28 (2024) 633–646
https://doi.org/10.1016/j.cld.2024.06.007
liver.theclinics.com
1089-3261/24/© 2024 Elsevier Inc. All rights reserved, including those for text and data mining, AI training, and similar technologies.

effects on patients and their families, who bear a substantial portion of the health-related expenses for advanced ALD care. As such, ALD remains one of the most prevalent types of chronic liver disease and accounts for nearly one-third of global incident cases of primary liver cancer, contributing to an estimated 20% of liver cancer death annually.[1,4–6] In the US, hepatocellular carcinoma (HCC) accounts for up to 75% to 85% of liver cancer cases, making it a major cause of cancer-related deaths and contributing significantly to the disease burden within the US health care system. The prevalence of alcohol-associated HCC has been steadily rising over the past 35 years, with an annual incidence ranging from 0.9% to 5.6%.[7–9] Among individuals with alcohol-associated cirrhosis, the risk of developing HCC increases over time, with a cumulative incidence of 3% at year 5% and 9% at year 10.[1] A recent population-based study estimates that the number of HCC cases in the US will surpass 56000 by 2030, largely due to a shifting etiologic landscape favoring ALD or metabolic dysfunction-associated steatotic liver disease (MASLD).[9]

The spectrum of alcohol-induced hepatic injury spans from mild or biochemical damage to more severe conditions such as alcohol-associated hepatitis, steatotic liver disease, steatohepatitis, fibrosis, and ultimately, cirrhosis.[10] Alcohol consumption damages the liver through mechanisms including endotoxins, oxidative stress, and inflammation.[11] Additionally, alcohol acts as a cofactor in the development of HCC when combined with other causative agent, such as hepatitis C virus (HCV), hepatitis B virus (HBV), steatotic liver disease, or diabetes. This interaction notably exacerbates and accelerates liver damage, partly due to alcohol's distinct disruption of several metabolic pathways including toxic reactive metabolite production, ultimately resulting in DNA damage, impaired regulation of gene expression, and enhanced tumorigenesis.

EPIDEMIOLOGY AND CO-FACTORS
Alcohol as a Carcinogen

Alcohol is recognized as a carcinogen by the International Agency for Cancer Research from the World Health Organization (WHO) and has been associated with an increased risk of several malignancies.[12] The risk of liver cancer-related mortality directly correlates with the level of alcohol consumption in a dose-dependent manner. The underlying causes of alcohol-related cancers remain unclear, although several factors have been proposed to contribute. These include the localized effects of alcohol, induction of cytochrome P450 2E1 (CYP2E1) leading to the conversion of various xenobiotics, acetaldehyde toxicity through formation of protein, and DNA adducts, increased production of reactive oxygen species (ROS), changes to lipid peroxidation and metabolism, alterations in DNA methylation, modulation of angiogenesis, malnutrition, inflammation, and impaired immune response (Fig. 1).[13,14] Alcohol is absorbed by the small intestine and metabolized by hepatocytes, where ethanol is oxidized into acetaldehyde by alcohol dehydrogenase (ADH) in the cytosol, and then further oxidized to acetate by aldehyde dehydrogenase (ALDH) in the mitochondria. Acetaldehyde, a highly reactive and directly mutagenic compound, forms diverse protein and DNA adducts, leading to DNA repair failure, lipid peroxidation, and mitochondrial damage, further contributing to tissue damage and ultimately, promoting carcinogenesis. While under normal circumstances, acetaldehyde is detoxified by mitochondrial ALDH, genetic variations in ALDH and ADH function, along with increased oxidative stress, could lower the liver's ability to control concentration of these harmful compounds.[15,16] Consequently, mitochondrial dysfunction remains a considerable factor in development of ALD-associated HCC.[15,17]

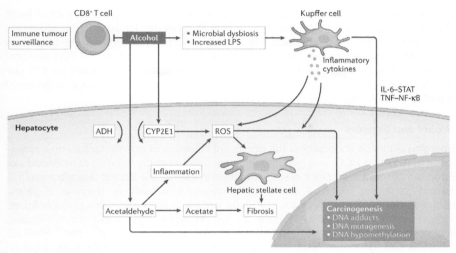

Fig. 1. Alcohol is metabolized to acetaldehyde by alcohol dehydrogenase (ADH) and cytochrome P450 2E1 (CYP2E1) within hepatocytes. This process generates reactive oxygen species (ROS), which activate hepatic stellate cells, contributing to fibrosis in conjunction with acetate. Acetaldehyde induces inflammation, forms DNA adducts, and causes DNA hypomethylation, leading to hepatocarcinogenesis. ROS formation also leads to DNA adducts via lipid peroxidation, further promoting carcinogenesis. Additionally, alcohol causes microbial dysbiosis and increases gut permeability, allowing the translocation of lipopolysaccharide (LPS) and gut bacteria to the liver. This translocation activates Kupffer cells, leading to the production of pro-inflammatory cytokines and chemokines, which promote fibrosis and activate oncogenic pathways. (Huang, D.Q., Mathurin, P., Cortez-Pinto, H. et al. Global epidemiology of alcohol-associated cirrhosis and HCC: trends, projections and risk factors. Nat Rev Gastroenterol Hepatol 20, 37-49 (2023). https://doi.org/10.1038/s41575-022-00688-6.)

Chronic alcohol consumption enhances the conversion of several procarcinogens, nitrosamines and azo compounds, into carcinogen derivatives through CYP2E1-dependent metabolism.[18–20] Additionally, ROS are generated during alcohol metabolism by CYP2E1 and through the re-oxidation of nicotinamide adenine dinucleotide within the mitochondria, further leading to ineffective electron transplant chain with downstream effects.[21,22] Furthermore, chronic alcohol use disrupts the intestinal bacterial flora, leading to increased gut permeability to lipopolysaccharides. This results in the activation of hepatic Kupffer cells, triggering the release of proinflammatory cytokines, including tumor necrosis factor-alpha, prostaglandins, and interleukins.[23–25] Genetic variations in alcohol metabolizing enzymes, influencing carcinogenic aldehyde levels, are considered potential inherited markers for HCC. Patients with ALD who are homozygous for the *ADH1C*1* allele are considered more susceptible to HCC, while the weakly active *ALDH2*2* allele is associated with HCC in moderate-to-heavy drinkers, particularly prevalent in 50% of the eastern Asian population.[26] Oxidative stress resulting from ROS generated during alcohol metabolism and inflammation remains a crucial mechanism in hepatocarcinogenesis. ROS activates hepatic stellate cells and damages cellular macromolecules, promotes lipid peroxidation, stimulates cytokine production, immune processes, and angiogenesis. Additionally, ROS accumulation affects DNA structure and function, leading to cell cycle arrest and apoptosis. The risk significantly increases after accumulating 1500 g-years of alcohol consumption, which is approximately equivalent to 60 g per day for at least 25 years.[27,28] Chronic alcohol use of more than 80 g per day for over 10 years is associated with a 5- to 7-fold increased risk of HCC, and this risk remains elevated even with lower doses of alcohol consumption, such as 25 g per day.[29–31] Furthermore, cessation of alcohol use leads to a decrease in the risk of liver cancer by 6% per year though requires an estimated 23-year period of abstinence for the risk to be equal to that of non-alcohol users.[32]

Alcohol and Genetics

Emerging evidence underscores the significant influence of genetic factors on susceptibility to ALD and HCC. In a genome-wide association study (GWAS) of individuals of European descent, new risk loci were identified in membrane-bound O-acyltransferase domain-containing protein 7 and transmembrane 6 superfamily member 2 genes, alongside the confirmation of the rs738409 variant in the patatin-like phospholipase domain-containing 3 (PNPLA3) gene as an important gene locus for developing alcohol-associated-cirrhosis.[33] Moreover, the prevalence of the PNPLA3 rs738409 GG genotype was notably higher among patients with both alcohol-associated cirrhosis and HCC.[34,35] The involvement of PNPLA3 in lipid metabolism prompts further exploration of its role in ALD and HCC pathogenesis. Contrary to PNPLA3, FAS-associated factor 2 was found to confer protection against development of alcohol-associated cirrhosis, suggesting its potential significance in lipid pathways and cirrhosis development.[36] Similarly, a case-control GWAS identified a risk locus on chromosome 1 involving WNT3A and WNT9A genes, associated with decreased risk of alcohol-associated HCC. While clinical studies have linked somatic mutations to alcohol-associated HCC, genetic data integration into risk assessment models remains limited. However, genetic risk scores hold promise in identifying high-risk patients for cirrhosis and HCC, enabling targeted screening and surveillance.[37] Further research is essential to elucidate the utility of genetic testing in HCC surveillance and screening.

Alcohol and Viral Hepatitis

Concurrent ALD and viral hepatitis independently and synergistically accelerate disease progression, increasing the risk of HCC.[30,38,39] Several studies have demonstrated significantly higher prevalence rates of HCV infection among individuals with alcohol abuse and ALD with nearly an 8-fold increase compared to the general population.[40–42] Patients with cirrhosis secondary to HCV infection and alcohol have a significantly higher risk of HCC compared to those with cirrhosis due to alcohol alone, and they may develop HCC at younger age.[43,44] Oxidative stress has been shown to increase several-fold in patients with both moderate (<50 g per day) and heavy (>50 g per day) alcohol use, further exacerbated by the combined effects of alcohol and HCV, which synergistically increase free radical formation within the liver and further diminish its antioxidant defenses.[45] Moreover, in the setting of chronic alcohol use, the expression of HCV core protein increases lipid peroxidation, hepatic tumor necrosis factor-alpha and transforming growth factor-beta, leading to the generation of ROS and development of hepatic fibrosis.[46] Additionally, HCC patients with ALD and HCV have overall reduced tumor-free survival and overall survival following hepatic resection, along with lower proportion of well-differentiated HCC, suggesting potential alteration in carcinogenesis and tumor biology.[47,48] Patients with coexisting HBV infection and ALD are also at risk for accelerated progression of liver disease and development of HCC.[49] However, the data in this area remain limited due to potential contribution of undiagnosed underlying HCV.

Alcohol and Metabolic Syndrome

With the obesity epidemic and the effectiveness of antiviral therapy for HCV and HBV, the latter including effective vaccination, MASLD and ALD have emerged as the 2 major causes of HCC (**Fig. 2**).[50] Metabolic syndrome, characterized by obesity and diabetes, in the form of MASLD, represents a significant risk factor for the development of HCC through both direct and synergistic effects.[51–55] In the US, metabolic syndrome has become the leading contributor to population-level HCC, with a population attributable fraction of 32%.[56] This contribution has steadily increased over the last decade, in contrast to alcohol-related disorders and HCV infections, which have otherwise remained stable. The accumulation of individual components of metabolic syndrome—obesity, diabetes, hypertension, and hyperlipidemia—is associated with a stepwise increase in the risk of HCC, with diabetes showing the strongest association with incident HCC.[57] Alcohol use and obesity (defined as body mass index >30 kg/m^2) have been shown to synergistically increase the risk of incident HCC.[58,59] This association was also observed among individuals with concurrent heavy alcohol use and diabetes, resulting in a substantial supra-additive effect on liver-related outcomes including HCC.[39,58] Diabetes increases the risk of cirrhosis through pro-fibrogenic properties on hepatic stellate cells, resulting in chronic inflammation. The presence of diabetes increases the risk of HCC by approximately 50% in patients with ALD-associated cirrhosis; therefore, individuals with heavy alcohol consumption should be screened for diabetes to identify those at higher risk of cirrhosis and HCC.[8,60] More specific than BMI, waist-to-hip ratio may offer a more reliable measure of visceral obesity. The degree of alcohol consumption contributes to varying risks of liver-related outcomes depending on the quartile of waist-to-hop ratio.[61] Notably, among individuals in the highest waist-to-hip ratio quartile, the intake of

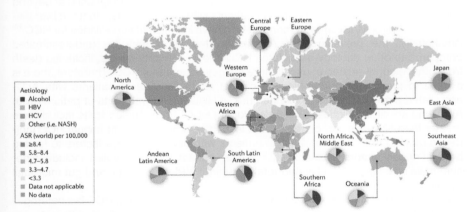

Fig. 2. Changing global landscape in age-standardized incidence rate (ASR) of hepatocellular carcinoma based on major etiologic factors involved in hepatocarcinogenesis. Hepatitis B virus remains the major etiologic factor in most parts of Asia (except Japan), South America and Africa. Hepatitis C virus is the predominant causative factor in Western Europe, North America and Japan. Alcohol intake is the etiologic factor in Central and Eastern Europe, and is expected to become one of the predominant causes of hepatocellular carcinoma in addition to metabolic dysfunction-associated steatotic liver disease. (*Figure obtained from* Llovet et al.[90])

1 unit of alcohol per day was associated with a similar risk as the intake of 4 units of alcohol per day among those in the lowest waist-to-hip ratio quartile. While the mechanisms underlying the synergistic effect between ALD and obesity and diabetes remain unclear, various pathways have been proposed to explain the development of diabetes or obesity-induced HCC in individuals with metabolic dysfunction-associated steatohepatitis (MASH).[62]

SURVEILLANCE AND MANAGEMENT
Screening and Surveillance

According to the WHO, the global prevalence of individuals meeting criteria for alcohol use disorder (AUD), defined as alcohol dependence and harmful use, is similar to that of HBV infection and nearly 4 to 5 times higher than that of HCV infection. However, there is no risk stratification to initiate surveillance for HCC in ALD patients without cirrhosis compared to available guidance for non-cirrhotic chronic HBV (eg, men age >40 years, female age >50 years, and/or family history of HCC).[63] Though alcohol consumption is recognized as a significant risk factor for HCC, quantifying the association between alcohol consumption and HCC remains challenging due to factors such as cirrhosis and other liver conditions, which often lead to a substantial decrease in alcohol consumption preceding the diagnosis of HCC. In this respect, The American Association for the Study of Liver Diseases (AASLD) and European Association for the Study of the Liver (EASL) recommend initiating surveillance for HCC in patients with Child-Pugh classification A or B cirrhosis using ultrasonography with or without alpha-fetoprotein (AFP) measurements, every 6 months, without modifying the surveillance strategy based on etiology.[63,64] Given that the annual incidence of HCC has been reported to be 1.9% to 2.9% in patients with ALD-associated cirrhosis, surveillance for HCC in this population remains cost-effective, meeting the greater than or equal to 1.5% annual prevalence threshold.[65,66] However, even with guideline-based surveillance, nearly one-third of patients with cirrhosis are diagnosed at beyond early or curable stages.[67] Compared to patients with HCV cirrhosis, steatotic liver disease (ALD and/or MASLD) were more likely to have insufficient surveillance for HCC.[68] Additionally, the prevalence of ALD-associated HCC may be underestimated compared to other etiology-associated HCC due to competing risks, including death from other alcohol-related causes before the development of HCC. Therefore, there is a need to identify demographic and clinical characteristics of patients with ALD-associated cirrhosis that increase their risk of HCC, along with traits of patients with AUD who are at the highest risk of developing HCC. Prior studied traits include age greater than 55 years and platelet count less than 125000/uL, with annual HCC incidence ranging from 0.3% to 4.8% in patients with neither of these factors to having both of these factors, respectively.[66] Other patient factors studied include older age, male sex, high AFP, elevated total bilirubin, PNPLA3 variants, and gut microbial dysbiosis.[65]

Several clinical studies have demonstrated that ALD-associated HCC is a heterogeneous condition, encompassing various phenotypes that result in different outcomes.[69] Patient demographics and tumor characteristics are notable factors contributing to why ALD is often diagnosed at a more advanced stage and is more likely to occur in the presence of cirrhosis compared to HCC from other etiologies. This is partly attributed to delayed diagnosis and limited access to appropriate screening and risk stratification for ALD.[70–73] Allocating resources to primary health care providers for screening for AUD is essential, which can further facilitate early detection and treatment of ALD before the onset of cirrhosis and HCC. Notably, modifiable risk factors, including diabetes, obesity, alcohol or tobacco use, and MASLD, contribute to 70% of HCC cases. As such, medications such as glucagon-like peptide receptor agonists (GLP-1RA) have emerged as promising interventions for improving hepatic function and reducing disease progression, particularly in patients with diabetes mellitus or obesity, potentially preventing the development of HCC. This is largely due to GLP-1RA's pleiotropic effects on reducing serum glucose, inducing weight loss, and decreasing desire for alcohol and tobacco use, while modulating immune functions to reduce chronic inflammation[74–77] GLP-1RA potentially prevent HCC development through tumor-suppression, downregulation of lipogenesis, inhibition of mammalian target of rapamycin expression, reduction inflammatory cytokines, and induction of apoptosis, while also inhibiting HCC cell proliferation.[78–80] Moreover, genetic diversity resulting from the dysregulation of specific gene clusters in ALD-associated HCC has been shown to influence the development and progression of HCC.[81] This molecular heterogeneity highlights the impracticality of a one-size-fits-all clinical approach for ALD-associated HCC. While a comprehensive comparison of molecular features among ALD-associated HCC would enhance classification and therapeutic decision-making, data in this area remain limited.

Management and Therapeutic

AASLD and EASL recommend the same therapeutic strategy for HCC regardless of etiology.[63,64] These strategies can be categorized into curative therapies that include surgical resection, orthotopic liver transplant, and thermal/radiofrequency ablation and noncurative therapies with transarterial chemoembolization, transarterial radioembolization, stereotactic body radiation therapy, and systemic chemotherapy.[63] Unfortunately, ALD-associated HCC is frequently diagnosed at an advanced stage and with concomitant cirrhosis compared to other etiologies, largely due to delayed diagnosis and insufficient screening and surveillance. This is compounded by patient-related factors such as older age and coexisting metabolic and cardiovascular comorbidities, posing significant challenges for potential curative therapies leading to suboptimal outcomes. In one large database study, ALD-associated HCC exhibited the highest 1-year mortality rate compared to other etiologies including HBV, HCV, and MASLD.[82] However, the poor survival observed among patients with ALD-associated HCC is likely due to suboptimal surveillance, resulting in the diagnosis of more advanced HCC and impaired liver function at the time of diagnosis. This was supported by 2 large-scale European studies utilizing the Barcelona Clinic Liver Cancer (BCLC) staging system. While both studies demonstrated a shorter median overall survival among patients with ALD-associated HCC compared to HCV-associated HCC, the survival difference was no longer significant when assessed at each BCLC stage, eliminating the potential influence of etiology differences.[71] Given that ALD-associated HCC tends to present at advanced stages, the potential for extrahepatic spread to other organs is a significant concern, observed in approximately 30% to 50% of cases, with the lungs, lymph nodes, and bones being common sites. Notably, one mechanistic study proposed that CYP2E1-dependent upregulation of SIRT7 plays a pivotal role in ALD-associated HCC metastasis. This mechanism impacts overall and tumor-free survival by influencing chemosensitivity through alteration of the p53-dependent pathway and promoting HCC cell migration.[20]

Compared to other etiologies, patients with ALD-associated HCC typically present with more advanced liver disease (including higher Model for End-Stage Liver Disease and Child-Pugh scores) and tumor stage (including larger tumor size, multifocality, or infiltrative HCC), limiting their options for local regional therapies or surgical resection. Therefore, systemic therapies using a combination PD-1 or programmed cell death ligand 1 (PD-L1) inhibitors with different tyrosine kinase inhibitors, vascular endothelial growth factor (VEGF), or cytotoxic T lymphocyte–associated antigen 4 (CTLA-4) inhibitors, are promising options to maintain disease within Milan criteria or achieve further downstaging. The combination of atezolizumab (anti-PD-L1) plus bevacizumab (anti-VEGF) or durvalumab (anti-PD-L1) plus tremelimumab (anti-CTLA-4) has been established as the current standard-of-care for advanced HCC.[83,84] However, recent data have shown variable responses between viral hepatitis and non-viral hepatitis-associated HCC, with immunotherapy responses favoring patients with viral hepatitis-associated HCC. Etiology-dependent mechanisms result in varied prognoses among HCC patients, influencing clinical outcomes and responses to cancer-directed therapy.[85] Compared to viral hepatitis-associated HCC, non-viral hepatitis-associated HCC demonstrated reduced responsiveness to combined immunotherapy and anti-angiogenic therapies such as atezolizumab plus bevacizumab, yielding no significant survival benefit, yet demonstrating improved response to lenvatinib.[86,87] However, it remains unclear whether patients with ALD-associated HCC have suboptimal responses to immunotherapy, as these prior studies consolidated patients with MAFLD-associated and ALD-associated HCC into 1 cohort.[88] Moreover, a multicenter study in Europe showed no significant difference in etiology and overall survival in HCC patients treated with anti-PD-L1-based immunotherapy.[89] Proposed mechanistic studies suggest that aberrant T-cell activation leading to tissue damage and impaired immune surveillance, along with decreased immune response, may occur among patients with non-viral hepatitis-associated HCC due to the accumulation of exhausted, unconventionally activated CD8+PD1+ T-cells and tumor-associated neutrophils.[88] However, due to absence of a clear definition and presence of other etiologies, ALD-associated HCC tends to be classified under non-viral hepatitis-associated HCC, or alternatively as MASLD or MASH—further complicating evaluation of ALD-associated HCC as a distinct entity in relation to HCC. Further data are needed to determine whether patients with ALD-associated HCC derive similar benefits from immunotherapy as those with viral hepatitis-associated HCC.

SUMMARY

Alcohol-associated cirrhosis is a well-established risk factor for HCC development, and when combined with other etiologies, alcohol use can increase HCC risk up to 5-fold. Alcohol remains one of the leading causes of HCC cases in the US; a trend that is expected to continue, highlighting the urgent need for public policies aimed at further reducing HCC incidence. Considering the high annual incidence of ALD-associated HCC, implementing timely and consistent screening measures would likely prove cost-effective. Such screening initiatives have the potential to decrease HCC-related morbidity and mortality and improve overall survival rates through initiating appropriate therapy, in particularly systemic therapy given controversy over varying responses to immune checkpoint inhibitors according to underlying etiology. As such, it will be important to investigate the effects of dietary factors, intestinal factors, and alcohol metabolites on development and progression of HCC in ALD with and without cirrhosis, which may aid in identifying effective prevention and management strategies of ALD-associated HCC. The future of ALD-associate HCC management lies in improved surveillance, targeted combination therapies to overcome immune evasion, and the identification of biomarkers to identify treatment responders.

CLINICS CARE POINTS

- Prevalence of alcohol-associated hepatocellular carcinoma has been rising over the past three decades, with an annual incidence ranging from 0.9% to 5.6%, and is projected to be a leading indication for liver transplantation.

- Alcohol consumption remains a significant risk factor for the development of hepatocellular carcinoma, especially in patients with cirrhosis; thus, should be advised to maintain complete abstinence from alcohol in order to improve liver function and overall prognosis.

- Alcohol-associated hepatocellular carcinoma often presents with more advanced liver disease and tumor stage compared to other liver-related etiologies, including hepatitis B and C, and metabolic dysfunction-associated steatotic liver disease.

- Implement regular surveillance with ultrasound and tumor marker alpha fetoprotein every 6 months for patients with alcohol-associated cirrhosis to detect hepatocellular carcinoma at an earlier stage.

- Major society guidelines recommend same therapeutic strategies for hepatocellular carcinoma regardless of etiology, categorized into curative therapies that include surgical resection, orthotopic liver transplant, and thermal/radiofrequency ablation and noncurative therapies with transarterial chemoembolization, transarterial radioembolization, stereotactic body radiation therapy, and systemic chemotherapy.

- Nutritional support and management of protein-caloric malnutrition are crucial to prevent frailty and sarcopenia in patients with alcohol-associated cirrhosis and hepatocellular carcinoma.

DISCLOSURE

The authors of this review were supported by the NIH, United States 5T32DK060414-18 (National Institute of Diabetes and Digestive and Kidney Diseases, United States, N.B. Ha), AASLD Anna S. Lok Advanced/Transplant Hepatology Award (AASLD Foundation, N.B. Ha). These funding agencies played no role in the analysis of the data or the preparation of this manuscript. Author contribution: N.B. Ha: Study concept and design; drafting of the manuscript; critical revision of the manuscript for important intellectual content. F. Yao: Study concept and design; drafting of the manuscript; critical revision of the manuscript for important intellectual content.

REFERENCES

1. Huang DQ, Tan DJH, Ng CH, et al. Hepatocellular carcinoma incidence in alcohol-associated cirrhosis: systematic review and meta-analysis. Clin Gastroenterol Hepatol 2023;21(5):1169–77.

2. Mellinger JL, Shedden K, Winder GS, et al. The high burden of alcoholic cirrhosis in privately insured persons in the United States. Hepatology 2018;68(3):872–82.

3. Julien J, Ayer T, Tapper EB, et al. The rising costs of alcohol-associated liver disease in the United States. Am J Gastroenterol 2024;119(2):270–7.

4. Bosch FX, Ribes J, Diaz M, et al. Primary liver cancer: worldwide incidence and trends. Gastroenterology 2004;127(5 Suppl 1):S5–16.

5. Matsushita H, Takaki A. Alcohol and hepatocellular carcinoma. BMJ Open Gastroenterol 2019;6(1):e000260.

6. Vogel A, Meyer T, Sapisochin G, et al. Hepatocellular carcinoma. Lancet 2022; 400(10360):1345–62.

7. Hagstrom H, Thiele M, Sharma R, et al. Risk of cancer in biopsy-proven alcohol-related liver disease: a population-based cohort study of 3410 persons. Clin Gastroenterol Hepatol 2022;20(4):918–929 e8.

8. N'Kontchou G, Paries J, Htar MT, et al. Risk factors for hepatocellular carcinoma in patients with alcoholic or viral C cirrhosis. Clin Gastroenterol Hepatol 2006;4(8): 1062–8.

9. Petrick JL, Kelly SP, Altekruse SF, et al. Future of hepatocellular carcinoma incidence in the United States forecast through 2030. J Clin Oncol 2016;34(15): 1787–94.

10. Crawford JM. Histologic findings in alcoholic liver disease. Clin Liver Dis 2012; 16(4):699–716.

11. Wu D, Cederbaum AI. Alcohol, oxidative stress, and free radical damage. Alcohol Res Health 2003;27(4):277–84.

12. GBDA Collaborators. Alcohol use and burden for 195 countries and territories, 1990-2016: a systematic analysis for the Global Burden of Disease Study 2016. Lancet 2018;392(10152):1015–35.

13. Fu Y, Maccioni L, Wang XW, et al. Alcohol-associated liver cancer. Hepatology 2024. https://doi.org/10.1097/HEP.0000000000000890.

14. Seitz HK, Stickel F. Molecular mechanisms of alcohol-mediated carcinogenesis. Nat Rev Cancer 2007;7(8):599–612.

15. Auger C, Alhasawi A, Contavadoo M, et al. Dysfunctional mitochondrial bioenergetics and the pathogenesis of hepatic disorders. Front Cell Dev Biol 2015;3:40.

16. Zakhari S. Overview: how is alcohol metabolized by the body? Alcohol Res Health 2006;29(4):245–54.

17. LeFort KR, Rungratanawanich W, Song BJ. Contributing roles of mitochondrial dysfunction and hepatocyte apoptosis in liver diseases through oxidative stress, post-translational modifications, inflammation, and intestinal barrier dysfunction. Cell Mol Life Sci 2024;81(1):34.

18. Cederbaum AI. CYP2E1–biochemical and toxicological aspects and role in alcohol-induced liver injury. Mt Sinai J Med 2006;73(4):657–72.

19. Tanaka E, Terada M, Misawa S. Cytochrome P450 2E1: its clinical and toxicological role. J Clin Pharm Ther 2000;25(3):165–75.

20. Zhang C, Zhao J, Zhao J, et al. CYP2E1-dependent upregulation of SIRT7 is response to alcohol mediated metastasis in hepatocellular carcinoma. Cancer Gene Ther 2022;29(12):1961–74.

21. Niemela O, Parkkila S, Pasanen M, et al. Early alcoholic liver injury: formation of protein adducts with acetaldehyde and lipid peroxidation products, and expression of CYP2E1 and CYP3A. Alcohol Clin Exp Res 1998;22(9):2118–24.

22. Yu HS, Oyama T, Isse T, et al. Formation of acetaldehyde-derived DNA adducts due to alcohol exposure. Chem Biol Interact 2010;188(3):367–75.

23. Bode C, Bode JC. Activation of the innate immune system and alcoholic liver disease: effects of ethanol per se or enhanced intestinal translocation of bacterial toxins induced by ethanol? Alcohol Clin Exp Res 2005;29(11 Suppl):166S–71S.

24. Hoek JB, Pastorino JG. Ethanol, oxidative stress, and cytokine-induced liver cell injury. Alcohol 2002;27(1):63–8.

25. Zima T, Kalousova M. Oxidative stress and signal transduction pathways in alcoholic liver disease. Alcohol Clin Exp Res 2005;29(11 Suppl):110S–5S.

26. Munaka M, Kohshi K, Kawamoto T, et al. Genetic polymorphisms of tobacco- and alcohol-related metabolizing enzymes and the risk of hepatocellular carcinoma. J Cancer Res Clin Oncol 2003;129(6):355–60.

27. Corrao G, Bagnardi V, Zambon A, et al. A meta-analysis of alcohol consumption and the risk of 15 diseases. Prev Med 2004;38(5):613–9.

28. Marrero JA, Fontana RJ, Fu S, et al. Alcohol, tobacco and obesity are synergistic risk factors for hepatocellular carcinoma. J Hepatol 2005;42(2):218–24.

29. Bagnardi V, Blangiardo M, La Vecchia C, et al. A meta-analysis of alcohol drinking and cancer risk. Br J Cancer 2001;85(11):1700–5.

30. Donato F, Tagger A, Gelatti U, et al. Alcohol and hepatocellular carcinoma: the effect of lifetime intake and hepatitis virus infections in men and women. Am J Epidemiol 2002;155(4):323–31.

31. Tagger A, Donato F, Ribero ML, et al. Case-control study on hepatitis C virus (HCV) as a risk factor for hepatocellular carcinoma: the role of HCV genotypes and the synergism with hepatitis B virus and alcohol. Brescia HCC Study. Int J Cancer 1999;81(5):695–9.

32. Heckley GA, Jarl J, Asamoah BO, et al. How the risk of liver cancer changes after alcohol cessation: a review and meta-analysis of the current literature. BMC Cancer 2011;11:446.

33. Buch S, Stickel F, Trepo E, et al. A genome-wide association study confirms PNPLA3 and identifies TM6SF2 and MBOAT7 as risk loci for alcohol-related cirrhosis. Nat Genet 2015;47(12):1443–8.

34. Romeo S, Kozlitina J, Xing C, et al. Genetic variation in PNPLA3 confers susceptibility to nonalcoholic fatty liver disease. Nat Genet 2008;40(12):1461–5.

35. Salameh H, Raff E, Erwin A, et al. PNPLA3 gene polymorphism is associated with predisposition to and severity of alcoholic liver disease. Am J Gastroenterol 2015;110(6):846–56.

36. Schwantes-An TH, Darlay R, Mathurin P, et al. Genome-wide association study and meta-analysis on alcohol-associated liver cirrhosis identifies genetic risk factors. Hepatology 2021;73(5):1920–31.

37. Schwantes-An TH, Whitfield JB, Aithal GP, et al. A polygenic risk score for alcohol-associated cirrhosis among heavy drinkers with European ancestry. Hepatol Commun 2024;8(6). https://doi.org/10.1097/HC9.0000000000000431.

38. Poynard T, Bedossa P, Opolon P. Natural history of liver fibrosis progression in patients with chronic hepatitis C. The OBSVIRC, METAVIR, CLINIVIR, and DOSVIRC groups. Lancet 1997;349(9055):825–32.

39. Yuan JM, Govindarajan S, Arakawa K, et al. Synergism of alcohol, diabetes, and viral hepatitis on the risk of hepatocellular carcinoma in blacks and whites in the U.S. Cancer 2004;101(5):1009–17.

40. Armstrong GL, Wasley A, Simard EP, et al. The prevalence of hepatitis C virus infection in the United States, 1999 through 2002. Ann Intern Med 2006;144(10):705–14.

41. Fong TL, Kanel GC, Conrad A, et al. Clinical significance of concomitant hepatitis C infection in patients with alcoholic liver disease. Hepatology 1994;19(3):554–7.

42. Hassan MM, Hwang LY, Hatten CJ, et al. Risk factors for hepatocellular carcinoma: synergism of alcohol with viral hepatitis and diabetes mellitus. Hepatology 2002;36(5):1206–13.

43. Berman K, Tandra S, Vuppalanchi R, et al. Hepatic and extrahepatic cancer in cirrhosis: a longitudinal cohort study. Am J Gastroenterol 2011;106(5):899–906.

44. Shimauchi Y, Tanaka M, Koga K, et al. Clinical characteristics of patients in their 40s with HCV antibody-positive hepatocellular carcinoma. Alcohol Clin Exp Res 2000;24(4 Suppl):64S–7S.

45. Safdar K, Schiff ER. Alcohol and hepatitis C. Semin Liver Dis 2004;24(3):305–15.

46. Perlemuter G, Letteron P, Carnot F, et al. Alcohol and hepatitis C virus core protein additively increase lipid peroxidation and synergistically trigger hepatic cytokine expression in a transgenic mouse model. J Hepatol 2003;39(6):1020–7.

47. Kubo S, Kinoshita H, Hirohashi K, et al. High malignancy of hepatocellular carcinoma in alcoholic patients with hepatitis C virus. Surgery 1997;121(4):425–9.

48. Okada S, Ishii H, Nose H, et al. Effect of heavy alcohol intake on long-term results after curative resection of hepatitis C virus-related hepatocellular carcinoma. Jpn J Cancer Res 1996;87(8):867–73.

49. Walter SR, Thein HH, Gidding HF, et al. Risk factors for hepatocellular carcinoma in a cohort infected with hepatitis B or C. J Gastroenterol Hepatol 2011;26(12): 1757–64.

50. Shah PA, Patil R, Harrison SA. NAFLD-related hepatocellular carcinoma: the growing challenge. Hepatology 2023;77(1):323–38.

51. Aberg F, Byrne CD, Pirola CJ, et al. Alcohol consumption and metabolic syndrome: clinical and epidemiological impact on liver disease. J Hepatol 2023; 78(1):191–206.

52. El-Serag HB, Hampel H, Javadi F. The association between diabetes and hepatocellular carcinoma: a systematic review of epidemiologic evidence. Clin Gastroenterol Hepatol 2006;4(3):369–80.

53. Larsson SC, Wolk A. Overweight, obesity and risk of liver cancer: a meta-analysis of cohort studies. Br J Cancer 2007;97(7):1005–8.

54. Wang P, Kang D, Cao W, et al. Diabetes mellitus and risk of hepatocellular carcinoma: a systematic review and meta-analysis. Diabetes Metab Res Rev 2012; 28(2):109–22.

55. Welzel TM, Graubard BI, Zeuzem S, et al. Metabolic syndrome increases the risk of primary liver cancer in the United States: a study in the SEER-Medicare database. Hepatology 2011;54(2):463–71.

56. Makarova-Rusher OV, Altekruse SF, McNeel TS, et al. Population attributable fractions of risk factors for hepatocellular carcinoma in the United States. Cancer 2016;122(11):1757–65.

57. Kanwal F, Kramer JR, Li L, et al. Effect of metabolic traits on the risk of cirrhosis and hepatocellular cancer in nonalcoholic fatty liver disease. Hepatology 2020; 71(3):808–19.

58. Loomba R, Yang HI, Su J, et al. Synergism between obesity and alcohol in increasing the risk of hepatocellular carcinoma: a prospective cohort study. Am J Epidemiol 2013;177(4):333–42.

59. Loomba R, Yang HI, Su J, et al. Obesity and alcohol synergize to increase the risk of incident hepatocellular carcinoma in men. Clin Gastroenterol Hepatol 2010; 8(10):891–8, 898 e1-e2.

60. Ioannou GN, Green P, Kerr KF, et al. Models estimating risk of hepatocellular carcinoma in patients with alcohol or NAFLD-related cirrhosis for risk stratification. J Hepatol 2019;71(3):523–33.

61. Sahlman P, Nissinen M, Puukka P, et al. Genetic and lifestyle risk factors for advanced liver disease among men and women. J Gastroenterol Hepatol 2020; 35(2):291–8.

62. Reeves HL, Zaki MY. Day CP. Hepatocellular carcinoma in obesity, type 2 diabetes, and NAFLD. Dig Dis Sci 2016;61(5):1234–45.

63. Singal AG, Llovet JM, Yarchoan M, et al. AASLD Practice Guidance on prevention, diagnosis, and treatment of hepatocellular carcinoma. Hepatology 2023; 78(6):1922–65.

64. European Association for the Study of the Liver. Electronic address eee, European association for the study of the L. EASL clinical practice guidelines: management of hepatocellular carcinoma. J Hepatol 2018;69(1):182–236.

65. Ganne-Carrie N, Chaffaut C, Bourcier V, et al. Estimate of hepatocellular carcinoma incidence in patients with alcoholic cirrhosis. J Hepatol 2018;69(6): 1274–83.

66. Mancebo A, Gonzalez-Dieguez ML, Cadahia V, et al. Annual incidence of hepatocellular carcinoma among patients with alcoholic cirrhosis and identification of risk groups. Clin Gastroenterol Hepatol 2013;11(1):95–101.

67. Trinchet JC, Chaffaut C, Bourcier V, et al. Ultrasonographic surveillance of hepatocellular carcinoma in cirrhosis: a randomized trial comparing 3- and 6-month periodicities. Hepatology 2011;54(6):1987–97.

68. Bucci L, Garuti F, Camelli V, et al. Comparison between alcohol- and hepatitis C virus-related hepatocellular carcinoma: clinical presentation, treatment and outcome. Aliment Pharmacol Ther 2016;43(3):385–99.

69. Costentin CE, Minoves M, Kotzki S, et al. Alcohol-related hepatocellular carcinoma is a heterogenous condition: lessons from a latent class analysis. Liver Int 2022;42(7):1638–47.

70. Avila MA, Dufour JF, Gerbes AL, et al. Recent advances in alcohol-related liver disease (ALD): summary of a Gut round table meeting. Gut 2020;69(4):764–80.

71. Costentin CE, Mourad A, Lahmek P, et al. Hepatocellular carcinoma is diagnosed at a later stage in alcoholic patients: results of a prospective, nationwide study. Cancer 2018;124(9):1964–72.

72. Costentin CE, Sogni P, Falissard B, et al. Geographical disparities of outcomes of hepatocellular carcinoma in France: the heavier burden of alcohol compared to hepatitis C. Dig Dis Sci 2020;65(1):301–11.

73. Safcak D, Drazilova S, Gazda J, et al. Alcoholic liver disease-related hepatocellular carcinoma: characteristics and comparison to general Slovak hepatocellular cancer population. Curr Oncol 2023;30(3):3557–70.

74. Wang L, Berger NA, Kaelber DC, et al. Association of GLP-1 receptor agonists and hepatocellular carcinoma incidence and hepatic decompensation in patients with type 2 diabetes. Gastroenterology 2024. https://doi.org/10.1053/j.gastro. 2024.04.029.

75. Chen J, Mei A, Wei Y, et al. GLP-1 receptor agonist as a modulator of innate immunity. Front Immunol 2022;13:997578.

76. Bendotti G, Montefusco L, Lunati ME, et al. The anti-inflammatory and immunological properties of GLP-1 Receptor Agonists. Pharmacol Res 2022;182:106320.

77. Chuong V, Farokhnia M, Khom S, et al. The glucagon-like peptide-1 (GLP-1) analogue semaglutide reduces alcohol drinking and modulates central GABA neurotransmission. JCI Insight 2023;8(12). https://doi.org/10.1172/jci.insight. 170671.

78. Chen-Liaw AY, Hammel G, Gomez G. Inhibition of exendin-4-induced steatosis by protein kinase A in cultured HepG2 human hepatoma cells. In Vitro Cell Dev Biol Anim 2017;53(8):721–7.

79. Krause GC, Lima KG, Dias HB, et al. Liraglutide, a glucagon-like peptide-1 analog, induce autophagy and senescence in HepG2 cells. Eur J Pharmacol 2017;809:32–41.

80. Zhou M, Mok MT, Sun H, et al. The anti-diabetic drug exenatide, a glucagon-like peptide-1 receptor agonist, counteracts hepatocarcinogenesis through cAMP-PKA-EGFR-STAT3 axis. Oncogene 2017;36(29):4135–49.

81. Boyault S, Rickman DS, de Reynies A, et al. Transcriptome classification of HCC is related to gene alterations and to new therapeutic targets. Hepatology 2007; 45(1):42–52.

82. Younossi ZM, Otgonsuren M, Henry L, et al. Association of nonalcoholic fatty liver disease (NAFLD) with hepatocellular carcinoma (HCC) in the United States from 2004 to 2009. Hepatology 2015;62(6):1723–30.

83. Abou-Alfa GK, Lau G, Kudo M, et al. Tremelimumab plus durvalumab in unresectable hepatocellular carcinoma. NEJM Evid 2022;1(8):EVIDoa2100070.

84. Finn RS, Qin S, Ikeda M, et al. Atezolizumab plus bevacizumab in unresectable hepatocellular carcinoma. N Engl J Med 2020;382(20):1894–905.

85. Llovet JM, Willoughby CE, Singal AG, et al. Nonalcoholic steatohepatitis-related hepatocellular carcinoma: pathogenesis and treatment. Nat Rev Gastroenterol Hepatol 2023;20(8):487–503.

86. Casadei-Gardini A, Rimini M, Tada T, et al. Atezolizumab plus bevacizumab versus lenvatinib for unresectable hepatocellular carcinoma: a large real-life worldwide population. Eur J Cancer 2023;180:9–20.

87. Rimini M, Rimassa L, Ueshima K, et al. Atezolizumab plus bevacizumab versus lenvatinib or sorafenib in non-viral unresectable hepatocellular carcinoma: an international propensity score matching analysis. ESMO Open 2022;7(6):100591.

88. Pfister D, Nunez NG, Pinyol R, et al. NASH limits anti-tumour surveillance in immunotherapy-treated HCC. Nature 2021;592(7854):450–6.

89. Scheiner B, Pomej K, Kirstein MM, et al. Prognosis of patients with hepatocellular carcinoma treated with immunotherapy - development and validation of the CRAFITY score. J Hepatol 2022;76(2):353–63.

90. Llovet JM, Kelley RK, Villanueva A, et al. Hepatocellular carcinoma. Nat Rev Dis Primers 2021;7(1):6.

Pathogenesis of Alcohol-Associated Liver Disease

Pranoti Mandrekar, PhD*, Abhishek Mandal, PhD

KEYWORDS

- Alcohol associated liver disease • Pathogenesis • Fatty liver • Inflammation
- Cytokines • Chemokines • Immune cells • Interorgan crosstalk

KEY POINTS

- The pathogenesis of alcohol-associated liver disease is complex and multifactorial, involving alcohol metabolism-mediated oxidative stress, increased triglyceride accumulation in the liver, and inflammation.
- Chronic alcohol-induced fatty liver injury is mediated by increased lipogenesis and fatty acid uptake and reduced β-oxidation of free fatty acids.
- Alcohol-associated hepatitis is triggered by various intrahepatic and extrahepatic factors resulting in activation of innate and adaptive immune cells.
- The contribution of multiple organ-organ interaction in ALD is now being recognized.

INTRODUCTION

Alcohol-associated liver disease (ALD) is one of the leading causes of deaths worldwide, accounting for 50% of cirrhosis-related deaths.[1] Recent studies reported an increase in alcohol consumption during the coronavirus disease 2019 pandemic which is estimated to substantially increase ALD-related morbidity and mortality.[2] The spectrum of ALD encompasses an array of conditions including alcohol-associated steatosis, steatohepatitis (ASH), fibrosis, cirrhosis, and hepatocellular carcinoma. Patients with prolonged alcohol use can present with histologic criteria of ASH at different stages of the disease.[3] ASH is characterized by significant steatosis, hepatocyte ballooning often with Mallory-Denk bodies, inflammatory cell infiltration, and chicken-wire like fibrosis. About 8% to 20% of patients with ASH progress to cirrhosis. Patients with underlying severe fibrosis or cirrhosis and excessive alcohol intake can present a form of acute-on-chronic liver failure (ACLF) called "alcohol-associated hepatitis (AH)." Most patients are diagnosed at later stages when disease becomes symptomatic. The histologic and clinical diagnosis of ACLF/AH patients comprises of

---

Department of Medicine, University of Massachusetts Chan Medical School, 364 Plantation Street, Worcester, MA 01605, USA
* Corresponding author.
E-mail address: pranoti.mandrekar@umassmed.edu

Clin Liver Dis 28 (2024) 647–661
https://doi.org/10.1016/j.cld.2024.06.005   liver.theclinics.com

prominent cholestasis that leads to an onset of jaundice, decompensated liver disease, malaise, and coagulopathy.[4] The susceptibility of development of ALD differs among heavy drinkers and several factors including female sex, obesity, environmental, genetic, and epigenetic have been considered. Current treatment options for ALD are limited to corticosteroid therapy and no Food and Drug Administration (FDA) approved drug is available. While some patients may respond to corticosteroids or cessation of alcohol drinking, others may benefit from liver transplantation. The pathogenesis of ALD is not completely understood. Studies over the past decades utilized pre-clinical animal models that failed to capture the pathologic features of ALD, and pointed to a therapeutic role for tumor necrosis factor α (TNFα). However, clinical studies targeting TNFα failed due to increased infections in AH patients.[5] Recent ongoing translational studies indicate new potential cellular and molecular therapeutic targets for AH.[6] Understanding the pathogenesis of ALD is crucial to ensure success in identifying pathogenic targets for future clinical development.

PATHOPHYSIOLOGY OF ALCOHOL-ASSOCIATED LIVER DISEASE

The pathogenesis of ALD is multifactorial and complex and depends on the stage of the disease. Alcohol is absorbed by the gut and primarily metabolized by hepatocytes. Alcohol is metabolized to acetaldehyde via alcohol dehydrogenase and cytochrome P450 2E1 (CYP2E1), which forms protein and DNA adducts. Increased CYP2E1 activity results in oxidative stress due to generation of reactive oxygen species (ROS) and also shifts the cellular redox potential by increasing nicotinamide adenine dinucleotide phosphate hydrogen (NADPH) to influence de novo lipid synthesis in hepatocytes.[7] In addition, alcohol metabolism leads to glutathione depletion, mitochondrial damage, lipid peroxidation, and innate immune responses. Besides its direct effects on hepatocytes, liver resident macrophages play a crucial role in ALD. Alcohol alters the gut microbiome and increases gut permeability resulting in translocation of bacterial products for instance lipopolysaccharide (LPS) into the portal circulation, activation of macrophages, and production of inflammatory cytokines. Subsequently, these cytokines recruit and/or activate other non-parenchymal cells such as neutrophils, natural killer T (NKT) cells, T cells, natural killer (NK) cells, and mucosal-associated invariant T (MAIT) cells contributing to progression of liver injury. Chronic alcohol exposure also modulates epigenetic mechanisms including alterations in microRNA and chromatin modifications.

MECHANISMS ASSOCIATED WITH FATTY LIVER INJURY

The earliest response to chronic alcohol drinking is steatosis characterized by the deposition of fat in hepatocytes due to de novo lipogenesis, reduced β-oxidation of fatty acids, impaired export of lipoproteins, and enhanced uptake of free fatty acids from the plasma (**Fig. 1**). De novo lipogenesis is regulated by glycolysis and conversion of pyruvate to citrate which is eventually used to synthesize fatty acids. The crucial transcription factors that regulate de novo lipogenesis in the liver include sterol regulatory element-binding protein 1c (SREBP-1c), early growth response-1 (Egr-1), and carbohydrate response element binding protein (ChREBP) are all activated by chronic alcohol in the liver. [8] Activation of SREBP-1c induces lipogenic genes such as fatty acid synthase (FAS), acyl coA carboxylase (ACC-1 and ACC-2), ATP citrate lyase, and stearoyl coA desaturase 1 (SCD1) to facilitate fatty acid synthesis. Subsequently, the synthesis of triglycerides (glycerolipid) from fatty acids is facilitated by key acetyltransferases such as diacylglycerol acyltransferase (DGAT) and glycerol-phosphate acyltransferase (GPAT) and phosphatide phosphatases such as lipin-1.

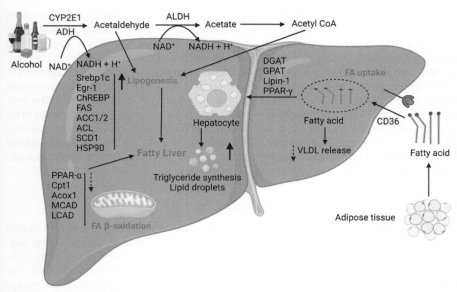

Fig. 1. Mechanisms of alcohol-associated fatty liver. Alcohol is primarily metabolized by alcohol dehydrogenase (ADH) and cytochrome P450 2E1 (CYP2E1) to produce acetaldehyde which is further metabolized by aldehyde dehydrogenase (ALDH) to produce acetate and acetyl-CoA. During the metabolism of alcohol, nicotinamide adenine dinucleotide (NAD)$^+$ gets converted to nicotinamide adenine dinucleotide hydrogen (reduced) NADH and H$^+$. Chronic alcohol consumption leads to accumulation of hepatic triglycerides and development of fatty liver by different pathways including increased lipogenesis, decreased fatty acid (FA) β-oxidation, and increased FA uptake. Alcohol consumption and acetaldehyde formation contribute to increased lipogenesis via upregulation of several lipogenic genes such as Srebp1c, Egr-1, ChREBP, FAS, ACC1/2, ACL, SCD1 as well as heat shock proteins (HSP90). Alcohol consumption leads to decreased FA-β-oxidation by downregulating expression of peroxisome proliferator-activated receptor α (PPAR-α), carnitine palmitoyltransferase 1 (CPT1), acyl-CoA-oxidase-1 (Acox-1), medium-chain acyl-CoA dehydrogenase (MCAD), long-chain acyl-CoA dehydrogenase (LCAD). Alcohol consumption leads to increased hepatic FA uptake from adipose tissue by upregulation of fatty acid uptake receptor cluster of differentiation 36 (CD36). FAs accumulated in hepatocytes get esterified by diacylglycerol acyltransferase (DGAT), glycerol-phosphate acyltranserases (GPAT), Lipin-1, PPAR-γ to synthesize triglycerides and formation of lipid droplets in the hepatocyte which is exaggerated by decreased release of very low-density lipoprotein (VLDL) triglycerides. (Created with BioRender.com.).

Alcohol upregulates lipin-1, facilitates cytosolic accumulation of the lipin-1 protein, enhances phosphatidic acid phosphohydrolase activity, and promotes lipogenesis via inhibition of adenosine monophosphate (AMP)-activated protein kinase (AMPK).[8] Further, alcohol-mediated inhibition of sirtuin-1 also facilitates increased SREBP-1c and elevated lipogenesis. Alcohol-mediated cellular stress also alters chaperones such as heat shock protein 90 (HSP90) to facilitate lipogenesis via SREBP-1c in ALD.[9]

Despite an increase in the supply of fatty acids for β-oxidation, alcohol negatively regulates β-oxidation genes via inhibition of peroxisome proliferator-activated receptor alpha (PPARα) signaling.[8,10] Alcohol reduces DNA binding activity of PPARα without affecting its expression and decreases target genes CPT-1, Acox, MCAD, LCAD. Alcohol also reduces expression of retinoid X receptor α (RXRα) which dimerizes with PPARα and is required for its activity. Alcohol metabolism increases NADPH and inhibits mitochondrial β-oxidation, causing mitochondrial depolarization impairing their ability to generate energy resulting in outer membrane leakage and inefficient fatty acid import. In addition, alcohol impairs adiponectin secretion from adipose tissue likely via TNFα and contributes to inhibition of β-oxidation.[8] Catabolism of lipid droplets termed as "lipophagy" is also impaired by chronic alcohol via decreasing transcription factor EB (TFEB), resulting in accumulation of triglycerides.[11] The liver exports triglycerides and cholesterol via export of very low-density lipoprotein (VLDL) particles. Alcohol impairs VLDL secretion by altering activity of an essential protein required for assembly of the VLDL particles.[12] Finally, alcohol facilitates uptake of circulating free fatty acids by upregulating transport receptor fatty acid translocase (FAT/CD36)[13] and promotes steatosis.

HEPATOCYTE DEATH AND REGENERATION

Various mechanisms of cell death have been identified including alcohol-mediated oxidative stress, endoplasmic reticulum stress, damage-associated molecular patterns (DAMPs)/pathogen-associated molecular patterns (PAMPs) as well as pro-inflammatory cytokines such as TNFα and dysregulation of autophagy in ALD. The intricate balance between adaptive pro-survival responses and cell death pathways determines hepatocyte cell fate. Several types of cell death mechanisms have been attributed to hepatocyte cell death including apoptosis, necroptosis, pyroptosis, and ferroptosis. The role of TNFα-mediated extrinsic apoptosis is shown in ALD.[14] Subsequent studies showed that interferon regulatory factor 3 (IRF3) mediates hepatocyte apoptosis in early ALD.[15] In addition to apoptotic cell death, necroptosis via receptor-interacting serine/threonine kinase 1 (RIP1)-RIP3 axis is facilitated by chronic alcohol, and RIP3 contributes to ALD in a RIP1-dependent manner.[16] There is growing evidence suggesting the role of pyroptosis cell death in ALD. The contribution of gasdermin D-caspase-11 in hepatocellular pyroptotic death is reported.[17] Alcohol-induced iron-dependent ferroptotic cell death is mediated by excessive lipid ROS accumulation and peroxidation, depletion of glutathione, and inactivation of glutathione peroxidase-4.[18] Based on the role of cell death mechanisms in ALD, several attempts to test interventions to target cell death have failed. For instance, trials with pan-caspase inhibitors were terminated due to lack of safe doses used and clinical trials testing selonosertib, an inhibitor of apoptosis signal-regulating kinase 1 (ASK1), did not show any beneficial outcomes in AH patients (NCT02854631).[19]

The regenerative capacity of the liver is crucial and promotes pro-survival and restorative functions. Alcohol exposure compromises the regenerative capacity of hepatocytes. Wingless/Integrated (WNT) signaling is regulated in ALD wherein upregulation of WNT5a and frizzled class receptor 5 (FZD5) occurs in moderate AH, and WNT5a is downregulated in severe AH, suggesting that liver regeneration occurs in moderate AH and dysregulation of regeneration is observed in severe AH.[20] Alcohol deregulates the Hippo/Yes-associated protein (YAP) pathway, by overactivation of YAP and down-regulation of epithelial splicing regulatory protein 2 and differential splicing of hepatocyte nuclear factor 4 alpha (HNF4α), resulting in defective periportal hepatocyte gene expression and liver progenitor activation and ductular reaction.[21–23] In addition, recent studies reported that genetic polymorphism of HNF4α in AH resulted in downregulation of target gene expression, important in hepatocyte differentiation.[21] In another study, Argemi and colleagues further identified the importance of HNF4α in the diagnosis and disease severity of AH.[24] However, the mechanistic and therapeutic effect of HNF4α in alcohol-associated hepatitis is still not well understood. In a recent study, Aguilar-Bravo et al identified increased CXCR4 and HNF4αP2 isoform, associated with hepatocyte dedifferentiation in alcohol-related liver disease (ALD) patients,[25] without any evidence of direct effect of CXCR4 on HNF4α. Additional studies targeting HNF4α-dependent gene expression could be beneficial to patients.

TRIGGERS OF INFLAMMATION IN ALCOHOL-ASSOCIATED LIVER DISEASE

Chronic alcohol alters innate and adaptive immune responses resulting in production of cytokines, chemokines, and pro-inflammatory mediators contributing to downstream activation of stellate cells culminating in fibrosis and cirrhosis (**Fig. 2**).

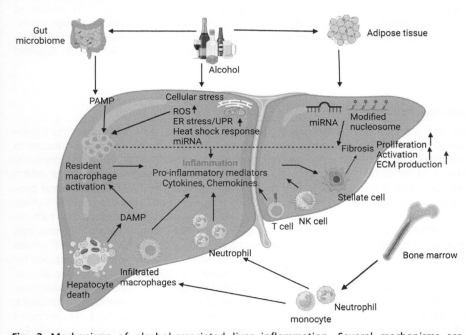

Fig. 2. Mechanisms of alcohol-associated liver inflammation. Several mechanisms are involved in alcohol-associated liver inflammation. Chronic alcohol consumption leads to leaky gut and release of gut-derived pathogen-associated molecular patterns (PAMPs) which bind to cell surface receptors on liver innate immune cells such as resident macrophages and trigger activation. Alcohol consumption results in hepatocyte death and release of damage-associated molecular patterns (DAMPs) that activate resident macrophages. Alcohol metabolism generates cellular stress including oxidative stress through reactive oxygen species, mitochondrial DNA, endoplasmic reticulum (ER) stress/unfolded protein response (UPR), and heat shock response/heat shock protein 90 (HSP90) which also trigger macrophage activation and release of cytokines and chemokines. Chronic alcohol-mediated chemokines promote migration of bone marrow-derived monocytes, macrophages, and neutrophils into the liver. Resident activated macrophages, T cells, NK cells as well as infiltrating neutrophils contribute to hepatic inflammation. Alcohol consumption also leads to the release of extra-hepatic factors from adipose tissue such as miRNA and modified nucleosome proteins and contribute to inflammation. Hepatic inflammation further activates stellate cells that proliferate and produce extracellular matrix (ECM) leading to fibrosis. (Created with BioRender.com.).

Extrahepatic Factors

The liver is connected to the gastrointestinal (GI) system via the portal vein, biliary system, and circulating soluble mediators. Commensal gut microbes preserve liver homeostasis, as well as generate metabolites leading to liver injury under pathologic conditions. Alcohol consumption compromises intestinal tight junctional proteins, increases permeability, and microbes and microbial components translocate via systemic circulation to the liver and trigger immune cell activation.[26] PAMPs derived from intestinal microbiota are recognized by different Toll-like receptors (TLRs) and nucleotide binding oligomerization domain (NOD)-like receptors (NLRs) expressed by immune cells and liver parenchymal cells resulting in release of various proinflammatory cytokines and chemokines.[27] In addition, many microbial metabolites such as short-chain fatty acids are detectable in the portal and systemic circulation in response to ethanol and can trigger ethanol-induced liver injury.[28] In advanced cirrhosis patients, low circulating levels of butyrate correlated with enhanced proinflammatory markers and serum endotoxin.[29] The gut microbial metabolite trimethylamine is also increased in AH patients and contributes to chronic ethanol-induced liver injury in murine models.[30]

Intrahepatic Factors

Alcohol is metabolized within the hepatocytes via alcohol dehydrogenase and microsomal ethanol-oxidizing system which utilizes CYP2E1 enzyme to oxidize ethanol to acetaldehyde, generating reactive oxygen species (ROS), and triggering oxidative stress to facilitate inflammation.[31,32] Oxidative stress damages hepatocytes which release DAMPs (eg, high mobility group box 1 protein [HMGB1]) and several proinflammatory cytokines and chemokines triggering neutrophil infiltration and activation. Consumption of alcohol also leads to endoplasmic reticulum (ER) stress, and in turn, alters unfolded protein response signaling to drive ALD pathogenesis.[33] In previous studies, Petrasek and colleagues observed that alcohol consumption led to ER stress via induction of IRF-3, a key component of the innate immune response mediated by the ER adaptor, stimulator of interferon genes (STING) resulting in hepatocyte apoptosis. However, the pathogenic role of IRF-3 in ALD was independent of inflammation or Type-I interferons.[15] Of note, is the role of cellular stress-mediated heat shock protein 90 (HSP90) in liver diseases. HSP90 functions as an important chaperone of LPS signaling and is required for production of pro-inflammatory cytokines. Earlier studies from our laboratory reported that chronic alcohol exposure differentially regulated HSP70 and HSP90 via heat shock factor 1 (HSF-1) activation. Inhibition of HSP90 regulated TNFα expression via HSF-1[34,35] in macrophages. In addition, pharmacologic inhibition of HSP90 by 17-dimethylaminoethylamino-17-demethoxygeldanamycin (17-DMAG) alleviated LPS-induced liver injury by down-regulation of pro-inflammatory cytokine, TNFα, and interleukin (IL)-6 likely via HSF-1 activation in the liver.[34] In both acute and chronic models of alcoholic liver injury (in human and experimental mice), HSP90 is elevated. Pharmacologic inhibition of HSP90 by 17-DMAG alleviated both acute and chronic alcohol-induced liver injury by ameliorating oxidative stress and downregulation of pro-inflammatory cytokine production.[9] In a more recent study, we reported the role of an ER stress-mediated chaperone of the HSP90 family, also called glycoprotein 96 (GP96)/heat shock protein 90B1 (HSP90B1)/glucose regulated protein 94 (GRP94) in ALD pathogenesis. We observed that GP96/GRP94 and GRP78/BiP are highly expressed in human alcohol-associated hepatitis livers as well as in mouse ALD livers with induction of GP96 prominent in alcohol-exposed macrophages. GP96 promoted alcohol-induced liver damage through activation of liver macrophage inflammatory responses, alteration in lipid homeostasis, and ER stress.[36]

DAMPs are crucial molecules responsible for inflammatory responses. The substantial presence of DAMPs promotes inflammation in ALD. In ALD, some of the DAMPs contributing to pro-inflammatory microenvironment include mitochondrial DNA, uric acid, ATP, and lipocalin 2 (LCN2).[37] Saha and colleagues recently found that patients with alcohol-associated hepatitis had higher level of HMGB1 and osteopontin compared to the healthy controls.[38] IL-33 released as an alarmin (or DAMP) after cell injury and/or necrosis is elevated in serum of ALD patients and acts through its receptor, IL-1 receptor like 1 /suppression of tumorigenicity 2 (ST2). During severe ALD, extracellular IL-33 release amplifies tissue inflammation by triggering the canonical IL-33/ST2L signaling in hepatic macrophages.[39] LCN2, also termed "neutrophil gelatinase-associated lipocalin (NGAL)," is highly expressed on hepatocytes upon stress and acts as a danger signal to promote ALD through ethanol-induced neutrophilic inflammation.[40]

In addition to PAMPs and DAMPs, epigenetic mechanisms such as microRNA and chromatin-modifying enzymes contribute to inflammation in ALD. Recently, Habash and colleagues summarized that upregulated microRNAs include miR-21 (hepatocellular carcinoma activation), miR-27a (macrophage 2 polarization), miR-34a (steatosis, inflammation), miR-182 (inflammation/chemokine release), miR-200a (hepatocyte apoptosis), miR-214 (hepatocyte oxidative stress), miR-217 (steatosis, inflammation), miR-291 (inflammation) in ALD. On the other hand, downregulated miRNA include miR-26a (hepatoprotective), miR-29 (antifibrotic), miR-122 (lipid metabolism, hypoxia inducible factor 1α regulation), miR-125b (ECM production/fibrosis), miR-126 (antifibrotic), miR-181b-3p (anti-inflammatory), miR-199 (anti-inflammatory), miR-223 (anti-inflammatory), and miR-378 (antifibrotic).[41] The role of DNA methylation is suggested in ALD. In a recent study, Shen and colleagues reported that aberrant DNA-methylation is associated with AH pathogenesis. They observed that the immunoreactive intensity of 5 mC was significantly higher in AH patients than normal controls.[42] In a recent study, Kusumanchi and colleagues reported that FK506-Binding Protein 51 plays an important role in alcohol-induced liver injury through the hippo pathway and chemokine (C-X-C Motif) ligand 1 signaling.[43] In the liver, alcohol induces epigenetic modifications through histone acetylation, methylation as well as phosphorylation. In a recent study, Argemi and colleagues reported that livers from alcoholic hepatitis patients show chromatin remodeling owing to defective hepatocyte nuclear factor-4a–dependent gene expression.[21]

IMMUNE CELLS AND CYTOKINES IN ALCOHOL-ASSOCIATED LIVER DISEASE
Innate Immune Cells

Portal LPS-mediated activation of macrophage is a hallmark of injury/inflammation, steatosis, and fibrogenesis in ALD. Generally, both resident Kupffer cells (KCs) and infiltrating macrophages exhibit strong plasticity regulating signals within their immune microenvironment in the liver. KCs play a pivotal role in the inflammatory response during ALD.[44] TLR4 expressed on immune cells and parenchymal cells recognizes LPS, activates downstream signaling cascades, and induces the activation of proinflammatory cytokines.[27] Further, a recent study reported that chronic alcohol consumption leads to the generation of mitochondrial double-stranded RNA (mtdsRNA) which activates TLR3 in KCs and thereby triggering the production of IL-1 by neighboring KCs promoting liver inflammation in ALD.[45] On the other hand, infiltrating macrophages are classified into 2 subgroups based on Ly6C expression. Ly6C^{hi} cells show a proinflammatory, tissue-damaging phenotype whereas Ly6C^{low} cells show an anti-inflammatory and tissue-protective phenotype. Wang and colleagues observed that the ratio of Ly6C^{hi}/Ly6C^{low} macrophages is higher in chronic-binge alcohol mice substantially aggravating liver injury.[46]

Recruitment of neutrophils in ALD is a critical process which is mediated by priming or activation, chemotaxis, adhesion, and transmigration.[47] There are reports that binge alcohol drinking significantly increased hepatic and circulating neutrophils in chronic ethanol-fed mice[48] and in human alcohol drinkers.[49] In a recent study, Cho and colleagues observed that alcohol can induce neutrophil extracellular trap (NET) formation in neutrophils. Moreover, they discovered 2 heterogenous population of neutrophils (low-density neutrophil and high-density neutrophil) in AH.[50] Furthermore, Ma and colleagues observed that neutrophil infiltration and hepatic neutrophil cytosolic factor 1 (NCF1) or p47phox expression is significantly increased in severe alcohol-associated hepatitis (SAH) patients indicating that NCF1-dependent ROS production triggers steatosis and hepatic inflammation through inhibition of AMPK and miR-223, respectively.[51]

Lymphoid and Innate Lymphoid Cells

Chronic alcohol alters T cells and contributes to adaptive immune dysfunction. Lin and colleagues reported that the intensity of the Th1 cell response is correlated with the severity of ALD.[52] Further, Almeida and colleagues observed that CD4$^+$ CD25^{hi} Tregs are markedly downregulated in the peripheral blood of patients with alcoholic hepatitis (AH) versus both healthy adults and chronic alcoholic patients without liver disease.[53] In a recent study, McTernan et al showed that alcohol-mediated shifts in T cell subsets are associated with changes in immune cell bioenergetics and promote naïve T cell differentiation to pro-inflammatory Th1 CD4$^+$ T cell.[54] Besides T cells, innate lymphoid cells (ILCs) which share similarities with T helper cells and cytotoxic T cells contribute to progression of ALD. In a recent study, Cheng and colleagues showed the interplay between liver ILC1 and NK cells in the development of alcoholic steatohepatitis.[55] However, evidence on the pathogenic or protective role of ILC2 and ILC3 in ALD warrants further investigation.

Previous studies reported decreased frequency of cytotoxic T lymphocytes and NK cells and degranulation capacity in the peripheral blood of alcoholic hepatitis patients compared to healthy controls.[56] Further, chronic alcohol consumption decreases the development and maturation of cytotoxic conventional NK cell (cNK) due to deficiency of IL-15, whereas IL-15/IL-15Rα treatment recovered ethanol-induced developmental defect in NK cells.[57] NKT cells can also trigger alcohol-associated liver injury via neutrophil infiltration and IL-1β.[58,59]

Circulating MAIT cells contribute to pathogenesis of ALD. Studies suggest that "leaky" gut in ALD triggers MAIT cell dysfunction and susceptibility to infection in these patients. Gu and colleagues observed that chronic-on-binge alcohol feeding in mice results in change in MAIT cell numbers and their phenotype in a tissue-specific manner, partially attributable to alcohol-associated dysbiosis.[60]

INTER-ORGAN CROSSTALK IN ALCOHOL-ASSOCIATED LIVER DISEASE

The crosstalk between the liver and various organs including gut, adipose tissue, and brain in ALD is being recognized (**Fig. 3**). The precise communication between these organs facilitates pathogenesis of ALD via mediators such as PAMPs and DAMPs, cytokines, and extracellular vehicles (EVs).

Inter-organ and inter-cellular communication via extracellular vesicles such as exosomes and microvesicles that contain microRNA, messenger RNA, long non-coding

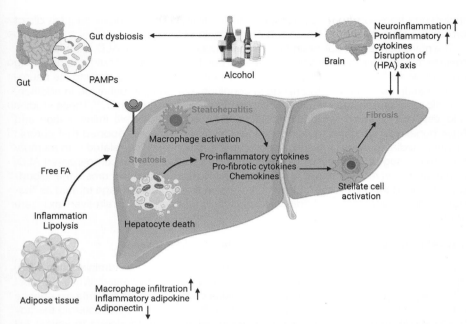

Fig. 3. Inter-organ crosstalk in alcohol-associated liver disease. Chronic alcohol consumption leads to steatosis, steatohepatitis, and fibrosis via several mechanisms. Crosstalk with multiple organs including adipose-liver, gut-liver, and brain-liver contributes to pathogenesis of alcohol-associated liver disease. Alcohol consumption induces lipolysis in adipose tissue as well as promotes inflammation in adipose tissue by releasing inflammatory adipokines, decreasing production of adiponectin, and macrophage infiltration. Inflamed adipose tissue releases free fatty acids into the portal circulation which enters the liver via fatty acid uptake receptors and contributes to steatosis. Excessive alcohol intake leads to gut dysbiosis and release of gut-derived PAMPs which bind to cell surface receptors on liver immune cells and trigger activation leading to inflammation. Alcohol consumption also promotes neuroinflammation through the release of pro-inflammatory cytokines and disruption of HPA axis. Excessive alcohol intake causes damage to hepatocytes, immune cell activation, and release of pro-inflammatory and pro-fibrotic cytokines and chemokines ultimately leading to fibrosis. (Created with BioRender.com.).

RNA, mitochondrial DNA, and mtdsRNA in ALD is increasingly evident.[61] Studies have shown that EVs containing CD40-L,[62] mtdsRNA[63] and proteins such as HSP90[64] during chronic alcohol feeding in mouse models can induce immune cell activation. The significance of EVs as biomarkers and/or therapeutic target requires further investigation. The crosstalk between gut and liver in pathophysiology of ALD is well established.[26] Modulating intestinal microbes using gut-microbe modulating agents and fecal microbial transplantation in AH patients are currently being investigated as therapeutic approaches complementary to current therapies.[26] Details of the role of the microbiome in ALD are discussed by Schnabl and colleagues in this series. Chronic alcohol directly impacts the adipose tissue and alters metabolic, endocrine, and immune functions. Alcohol is metabolized in adipocytes resulting in oxidative stress and adipocyte death eventually leading to increased inflammatory responses.[65] Studies show that increased TNFα and IL-10 in adipose tissue of AH patients correlate with severity of liver injury.[66] In addition, chronic alcohol-mediated adipose tissue lipolysis facilitates reverse triglyceride transport from adipose tissue to the liver.[66] These studies suggest direct crosstalk between adipose tissue and liver injury in ALD.

The novel concept of gut-brain-liver axis has been suggested in ALD. Circulating cytokines released by immune cells in the blood due to recognition of gut bacteria during chronic alcohol abuse can traverse to the central nervous system and induce neuro-inflammation associated with change in cognition and drinking behavior. In addition, chronic alcohol-mediated dysbiosis also leads to behavior disorder.[67] These studies suggest that targeting the gut microbiota may reduce systemic inflammation and have beneficial outcomes in alcohol dependence. Further, we reported that chronic alcohol-mediated liver injury and hippocampal IL-6 positively correlated with memory impairment suggesting an intrinsic brain-liver partnership.[68] In decompensated ALD, hepatocyte-derived ammonia and other neurotoxic substances cross the blood-brain barrier causing reverse neurologic impairment and brain damage termed as "hepatic encephalopathy."[69] Additional studies understanding brain-liver axis are warranted.

THERAPEUTIC TARGETS IN ALCOHOL-ASSOCIATED LIVER DISEASE

Despite several decades of research, there are no Food and Drug Administration (FDA) approved drugs for patients with AH and options are currently limited. While the most effective therapy for AH is abstinence or drinking cessation, most patients experience relapse and resume drinking.[70] The current standard of care is corticosteroid therapy which shows transient beneficial outcomes in patients with moderate to severe AH with increased risk of infections. AH patients are malnourished and nutritional supplementation especially in combination with corticosteroids improved survival and reduced bacterial infections.[71] Other pharmacologic therapies that were ineffective in AH patients are anti-TNF agents, growth factors, and antioxidants.[72] Patient prognosis in ALD is determined by whether the patient continues alcohol consumption and hence recent approaches use pharmacotherapy for alcohol use disorder in ALD.[73] Over the last few years, National Institutes of Alcohol Abuse and Alcoholism has supported several clinical trials based on mechanisms of ALD. These drugs are anti-inflammatory agents, drugs targeting gut-liver axis, antioxidants, and hepatocyte regeneration drugs. Several clinical trials are on-going with some promising outcomes so far. In a phase II clinical trial, IL-1R antagonist anakinra in combination with pentoxifylline and zinc provide similar benefits as corticosteroid therapy.[74] Granulocyte colony-stimulating factor (G-CSF) has been shown to mobilize CD34+ hematopoietic stem cells and increase hepatocyte growth factor; however, whether G-CSF improves liver function is unclear.[75] Since limited survival was noted in clinical trials using G-CSF, additional investigation is required. On the other hand, hepatoprotective recombinant IL-22 protein showed improved outcomes in AH in phase IIb clinical trials.[76] Details of current on-going trials and therapies are described by T. Morgan in Emerging Pharmacologic treatments in AH in this series.

SUMMARY

Understanding of the complex pathogenesis of alcohol-associated fatty liver injury and inflammation leading to fibrosis is growing rapidly. Cellular and molecular mechanisms identified so far include alcohol metabolism-associated oxidative stress due to reactive oxygen species, cellular stress and ER stress, gut-derived microbial factors, and cellular epigenetic events. Early alcohol-associated fatty liver injury occurs due to increased lipogenesis and fatty acid uptake and reduced fatty acid oxidation and release of VLDL particles. Activation of immune cells due to PAMPs and DAMPs contributes to inflammatory responses in the liver resulting in release of cytokines and chemokines that recruit circulating immune cells and promote disease progression. The role of inter-organ crosstalk in ALD is increasingly recognized. While several clinical trials are currently testing therapeutic agents targeting various pathways, additional investigation to understand combinatorial therapies to target pathogenic molecules and pathways simultaneously could be critical to effective treatments.

CLINICS CARE POINTS

- The spectrum and pathogenesis of alcohol associated liver disease is complex, multifactorial, and still not clearly understood.
- There are no FDA approved drugs available for the treatment of ALD and the current treatment options are restricted to corticosteroid therapy.
- In depth understanding of the pathogenesis of ALD is the need of the hour to identify novel therapeutic targets and drug development.
- Cellular and molecular signalling pathways associated with lipogenesis/FA uptake/FA oxidation, inflammation, cellular stress (oxidative, ER), epigenetic events, inter-organ crosstalk are being explored as therapeutic targets.
- Clinical trials of different investigational drugs are ongoing to understand the safety and efficacy of the drugs in AH patients.

DISCLOSURES

The authors have nothing to disclose. This work was supported by R01 grants (to P.M.) R01 AA17986-01A1 and R01 AA25289-01 from the National Institute on Alcohol Abuse and Alcoholism, United States (NIAAA), National Institute of Health (NIH), Bethesda, MD, USA

REFERENCES

1. Devarbhavi H, Asrani SK, Arab JP, et al. Global burden of liver disease: 2023 update. J Hepatol 2023;79(2):516–37.
2. Julien J, Ayer T, Tapper EB, et al. Effect of increased alcohol consumption during COVID-19 pandemic on alcohol-associated liver disease: a modeling study. Hepatology 2022;75(6):1480–90.
3. Gao B, Bataller R. Alcoholic liver disease: pathogenesis and new therapeutic targets. Gastroenterology 2011;141(5):1572–85.
4. Bataller R, Arab JP, Shah VH. Alcohol-associated hepatitis. N Engl J Med 2022; 387(26):2436–48.
5. Boetticher NC, Peine CJ, Kwo P, et al. A randomized, double-blinded, placebo-controlled multicenter trial of etanercept in the treatment of alcoholic hepatitis. Gastroenterology 2008;135(6):1953–60.
6. Mandrekar P, Bataller R, Tsukamoto H, et al. Alcoholic hepatitis: translational approaches to develop targeted therapies. Hepatology 2016;64(4):1343–55.
7. Donohue TM Jr. Alcohol-induced steatosis in liver cells. World J Gastroenterol 2007;13(37):4974–8.
8. You M, Arteel GE. Effect of ethanol on lipid metabolism. J Hepatol 2019;70(2): 237–48.

9. Ambade A, Catalano D, Lim A, et al. Inhibition of heat shock protein 90 alleviates steatosis and macrophage activation in murine alcoholic liver injury. J Hepatol 2014;61(4):903–11.

10. Purohit V, Gao B, Song BJ. Molecular mechanisms of alcoholic fatty liver. Alcohol Clin Exp Res 2009;33(2):191–205.

11. Thomes PG, Trambly CS, Fox HS, et al. Acute and chronic ethanol administration differentially modulate hepatic autophagy and transcription factor EB. Alcohol Clin Exp Res 2015;39(12):2354–63.

12. Sugimoto T, Yamashita S, Ishigami M, et al. Decreased microsomal triglyceride transfer protein activity contributes to initiation of alcoholic liver steatosis in rats. J Hepatol 2002;36(2):157–62.

13. Clugston RD, Yuen JJ, Hu Y, et al. CD36-deficient mice are resistant to alcohol- and high-carbohydrate-induced hepatic steatosis. J Lipid Res 2014;55(2): 239–46.

14. Pastorino JG, Hoek JB. Ethanol potentiates tumor necrosis factor-alpha cytotoxicity in hepatoma cells and primary rat hepatocytes by promoting induction of the mitochondrial permeability transition. Hepatology 2000;31(5):1141–52.

15. Petrasek J, Iracheta-Vellve A, Csak T, et al. STING-IRF3 pathway links endoplasmic reticulum stress with hepatocyte apoptosis in early alcoholic liver disease. Proc Natl Acad Sci U S A 2013;110(41):16544–9.

16. Roychowdhury S, McMullen MR, Pisano SG, et al. Absence of receptor interacting protein kinase 3 prevents ethanol-induced liver injury. Hepatology 2013;57(5): 1773–83.

17. Khanova E, Wu R, Wang W, et al. Pyroptosis by caspase11/4-gasdermin-D pathway in alcoholic hepatitis in mice and patients. Hepatology 2018;67(5): 1737–53.

18. Liu CY, Wang M, Yu HM, et al. Ferroptosis is involved in alcohol-induced cell death in vivo and in vitro. Biosci Biotechnol Biochem 2020;84(8):1621–8.

19. Tornai D, Szabo G. Emerging medical therapies for severe alcoholic hepatitis. Clin Mol Hepatol 2020;26(4):686–96.

20. Kim A, Wu X, Allende DS, et al. Gene deconvolution reveals aberrant liver regeneration and immune cell infiltration in alcohol-associated hepatitis. Hepatology 2021;74(2):987–1002.

21. Argemi J, Latasa MU, Atkinson SR, et al. Defective HNF4alpha-dependent gene expression as a driver of hepatocellular failure in alcoholic hepatitis. Nat Commun 2019;10(1):3126.

22. Bou Saleh M, Louvet A, Ntandja-Wandji LC, et al. Loss of hepatocyte identity following aberrant YAP activation: a key mechanism in alcoholic hepatitis. J Hepatol 2021;75(4):912–23.

23. Hyun J, Sun Z, Ahmadi AR, et al. Epithelial splicing regulatory protein 2-mediated alternative splicing reprograms hepatocytes in severe alcoholic hepatitis. J Clin Invest 2020;130(4):2129–45.

24. Argemi J, Kedia K, Gritsenko MA, et al. Integrated transcriptomic and proteomic analysis identifies plasma biomarkers of hepatocellular failure in alcohol-associated hepatitis. Am J Pathol 2022;192(12):1658–69.

25. Aguilar-Bravo B, Ariño S, Blaya D, et al. Hepatocyte dedifferentiation profiling in alcohol-related liver disease identifies CXCR4 as a driver of cell reprogramming. J Hepatol 2023;79(3):728–40.

26. Hartmann P, Seebauer CT, Schnabl B. Alcoholic liver disease: the gut microbiome and liver cross talk. Alcohol Clin Exp Res 2015;39(5):763–75.

27. Wang HJ, Gao B, Zakhari S, et al. Inflammation in alcoholic liver disease. Annu Rev Nutr 2012;32:343–68.
28. Couch RD, Dailey A, Zaidi F, et al. Alcohol induced alterations to the human fecal VOC metabolome. PLoS One 2015;10(3):e0119362.
29. Juanola O, Ferrusquía-Acosta J, García-Villalba R, et al. Circulating levels of butyrate are inversely related to portal hypertension, endotoxemia, and systemic inflammation in patients with cirrhosis. Faseb J 2019;33(10):11595–605.
30. Helsley RN, Miyata T, Kadam A, et al. Gut microbial trimethylamine is elevated in alcohol-associated hepatitis and contributes to ethanol-induced liver injury in mice. Elife 2022;11. https://doi.org/10.7554/eLife.76554.
31. Meroni M, Longo M, Rametta R, et al. Genetic and epigenetic modifiers of alcoholic liver disease. Int J Mol Sci 2018;19(12):3857.
32. Jiang Y, Zhang T, Kusumanchi P, et al. Alcohol metabolizing enzymes, microsomal ethanol oxidizing system, cytochrome P450 2E1, catalase, and aldehyde dehydrogenase in alcohol-associated liver disease. Biomedicines 2020;8(3):50.
33. Muralidharan S, Mandrekar P. Cellular stress response and innate immune signaling: integrating pathways in host defense and inflammation. J Leukoc Biol 2013;94(6):1167–84.
34. Ambade A, Catalano D, Lim A, et al. Inhibition of heat shock protein (molecular weight 90 kDa) attenuates proinflammatory cytokines and prevents lipopolysaccharide-induced liver injury in mice. Hepatology 2012;55(5):1585–95.
35. Mandrekar P, Catalano D, Jeliazkova V, et al. Alcohol exposure regulates heat shock transcription factor binding and heat shock proteins 70 and 90 in monocytes and macrophages: implication for TNF-alpha regulation. J Leukoc Biol 2008;84(5):1335–45.
36. Ratna A, Lim A, Li Z, et al. Myeloid endoplasmic reticulum resident chaperone GP96 facilitates inflammation and steatosis in alcohol-associated liver disease. Hepatol Commun 2021;5(7):1165–82.
37. Petrasek J, Iracheta-Vellve A, Saha B, et al. Metabolic danger signals, uric acid and ATP, mediate inflammatory cross-talk between hepatocytes and immune cells in alcoholic liver disease. J Leukoc Biol 2015;98(2):249–56.
38. Saha B, Tornai D, Kodys K, et al. Biomarkers of macrophage activation and immune danger signals predict clinical outcomes in alcoholic hepatitis. Hepatology 2019;70(4):1134–49.
39. Wang M, Shen G, Xu L, et al. IL-1 receptor like 1 protects against alcoholic liver injury by limiting NF-κB activation in hepatic macrophages. J Hepatol 2018;68(1):109–17.
40. Wieser V, Tymoszuk P, Adolph TE, et al. Lipocalin 2 drives neutrophilic inflammation in alcoholic liver disease. J Hepatol 2016;64(4):872–80.
41. Habash NW, Sehrawat TS, Shah VH, et al. Epigenetics of alcohol-related liver diseases. JHEP Rep 2022;4(5):100466.
42. Shen H, French BA, Tillman BC, et al. Increased DNA methylation in the livers of patients with alcoholic hepatitis. Exp Mol Pathol 2015;99(2):326–9.
43. Kusumanchi P, Liang T, Zhang T, et al. Stress-responsive gene FK506-binding protein 51 mediates alcohol-induced liver injury through the hippo pathway and chemokine (C-X-C Motif) ligand 1 signaling. Hepatology 2021;74(3):1234–50.
44. Mandrekar P, Szabo G. Signalling pathways in alcohol-induced liver inflammation. J Hepatol 2009;50(6):1258–66.
45. Lee JH, Shim YR, Seo W, et al. Mitochondrial double-stranded RNA in exosome promotes interleukin-17 production through toll-like receptor 3 in alcohol-associated liver injury. Hepatology 2020;72(2):609–25.

46. Wang M, You Q, Lor K, et al. Chronic alcohol ingestion modulates hepatic macrophage populations and functions in mice. J Leukoc Biol 2014;96(4):657–65.

47. Khan RS, Lalor PF, Thursz M, et al. The role of neutrophils in alcohol-related hepatitis. J Hepatol 2023;79(4):1037–48.

48. Bertola A, Park O, Gao B. Chronic plus binge ethanol feeding synergistically induces neutrophil infiltration and liver injury in mice: a critical role for E-selectin. Hepatology 2013;58(5):1814–23.

49. Li M, He Y, Zhou Z, et al. MicroRNA-223 ameliorates alcoholic liver injury by inhibiting the IL-6-p47(phox)-oxidative stress pathway in neutrophils. Gut 2017;66(4): 705–15.

50. Cho Y, Bukong TN, Tornai D, et al. Neutrophil extracellular traps contribute to liver damage and increase defective low-density neutrophils in alcohol-associated hepatitis. J Hepatol 2023;78(1):28–44.

51. Ma J, Guillot A, Yang Z, et al. Distinct histopathological phenotypes of severe alcoholic hepatitis suggest different mechanisms driving liver injury and failure. J Clin Invest 2022;132(14). https://doi.org/10.1172/jci157780.

52. Lin F, Taylor NJ, Su H, et al. Alcohol dehydrogenase-specific T-cell responses are associated with alcohol consumption in patients with alcohol-related cirrhosis. Hepatology 2013;58(1):314–24.

53. Almeida J, Polvorosa MA, Gonzalez-Quintela A, et al. Decreased peripheral blood CD4+/CD25+ regulatory T cells in patients with alcoholic hepatitis. Alcohol Clin Exp Res 2013;37(8):1361–9.

54. McTernan PM, Levitt DE, Welsh DA, et al. Alcohol impairs immunometabolism and promotes naïve T cell differentiation to pro-inflammatory Th1 CD4(+) T cells. Front Immunol 2022;13:839390.

55. Cheng C, Zhang Q, Li Y, et al. Interplay between liver type 1 innate lymphoid cells and NK cells drives the development of alcoholic steatohepatitis. Cellular and Molecular Gastroenterology and Hepatology 2023;15(1):261–74.

56. Støy S, Dige A, Sandahl TD, et al. Cytotoxic T lymphocytes and natural killer cells display impaired cytotoxic functions and reduced activation in patients with alcoholic hepatitis. Am J Physiol Gastrointest Liver Physiol 2015;308(4):G269–76.

57. Zhang H, Meadows GG. Exogenous IL-15 in combination with IL-15Rα rescues natural killer cells from apoptosis induced by chronic alcohol consumption. Alcohol Clin Exp Res 2009;33(3):419–27.

58. Mathews S, Feng D, Maricic I, et al. Invariant natural killer T cells contribute to chronic-plus-binge ethanol-mediated liver injury by promoting hepatic neutrophil infiltration. Cell Mol Immunol 2016;13(2):206–16.

59. Cui K, Yan G, Xu C, et al. Invariant NKT cells promote alcohol-induced steatohepatitis through interleukin-1β in mice. J Hepatol 2015;62(6):1311–8.

60. Gu M, Samuelson DR, Taylor CM, et al. Alcohol-associated intestinal dysbiosis alters mucosal-associated invariant T-cell phenotype and function. Alcohol Clin Exp Res 2021;45(5):934–47.

61. Hernández A, Arab JP, Reyes D, et al. Extracellular vesicles in NAFLD/ALD: from pathobiology to therapy. Cells 2020;9(4). https://doi.org/10.3390/cells9040817.

62. Verma VK, Li H, Wang R, et al. Alcohol stimulates macrophage activation through caspase-dependent hepatocyte derived release of CD40L containing extracellular vesicles. J Hepatol 2016;64(3):651–60.

63. Hirsova P, Ibrahim SH, Verma VK, et al. Extracellular vesicles in liver pathobiology: small particles with big impact. Hepatology 2016;64(6):2219–33.

64. Saha B, Momen-Heravi F, Furi I, et al. Extracellular vesicles from mice with alcoholic liver disease carry a distinct protein cargo and induce macrophage activation through heat shock protein 90. Hepatology 2018;67(5):1986–2000.
65. Parker R, Kim SJ, Gao B. Alcohol, adipose tissue and liver disease: mechanistic links and clinical considerations. Nat Rev Gastroenterol Hepatol 2018;15(1):50–9.
66. Naveau S, Cassard-Doulcier AM, Njiké-Nakseu M, et al. Harmful effect of adipose tissue on liver lesions in patients with alcoholic liver disease. J Hepatol 2010; 52(6):895–902.
67. Leclercq S, de Timary P, Delzenne NM, et al. The link between inflammation, bugs, the intestine and the brain in alcohol dependence. Transl Psychiatry 2017;7(2):e1048.
68. King JA, Nephew BC, Choudhury A, et al. Chronic alcohol-induced liver injury correlates with memory deficits: role for neuroinflammation. Alcohol 2020;83: 75–81.
69. Matsubara Y, Kiyohara H, Teratani T, et al. Organ and brain crosstalk: the liver-brain axis in gastrointestinal, liver, and pancreatic diseases. Neuropharmacology 2022;205:108915.
70. Altamirano J, López-Pelayo H, Michelena J, et al. Alcohol abstinence in patients surviving an episode of alcoholic hepatitis: prediction and impact on long-term survival. Hepatology 2017;66(6):1842–53.
71. Nguyen-Khac E, Thevenot T, Piquet MA, et al. Glucocorticoids plus N-acetylcysteine in severe alcoholic hepatitis. N Engl J Med 2011;365(19):1781–9.
72. Singal AK, Kamath PS, Gores GJ, et al. Alcoholic hepatitis: current challenges and future directions. Clin Gastroenterol Hepatol 2014;12(4):555–64, quiz e31-2.
73. Vannier AGL, Shay JES, Fomin V, et al. Incidence and progression of alcohol-associated liver disease after medical therapy for alcohol use disorder. JAMA Netw Open 2022;5(5):e2213014.
74. Szabo G, Mitchell M, McClain CJ, et al. IL-1 receptor antagonist plus pentoxifylline and zinc for severe alcohol-associated hepatitis. Hepatology 2022;76(4): 1058–68.
75. Spahr L, Lambert JF, Rubbia-Brandt L, et al. Granulocyte-colony stimulating factor induces proliferation of hepatic progenitors in alcoholic steatohepatitis: a randomized trial. Hepatology 2008;48(1):221–9.
76. Arab JP, Sehrawat TS, Simonetto DA, et al. An open-label, dose-escalation study to assess the safety and efficacy of IL-22 agonist F-652 in patients with alcohol-associated hepatitis. Hepatology 2020;72(2):441–53.

Gut Bacteria in Alcohol-Associated Liver Disease

Yongqiang Yang, PhD[a], Bernd Schnabl, MD[a,b],*

KEYWORDS

- Microbiota • Microbiome • FMT • Dysbiosis

KEY POINTS

- Alcohol-associated liver disease is linked to gut dysbiosis, characterized by an increase in harmful bacteria and a decrease in commensal species.
- Pathobionts and virulence factors contribute to the progression of alcohol-associated liver disease.
- Emerging treatments such as prebiotics, probiotics, postbiotics, synbiotics, phages, and fecal microbiota transplantation show promise in ameliorating chronic liver diseases.

INTRODUCTION

Alcohol-associated liver disease (ALD) is a substantial global public health concern, affecting an estimated 123 million individuals and contributing to approximately 25% of cirrhosis-related deaths.[1,2] This includes a spectrum of alcohol-related liver injuries such as alcohol-associated hepatitis, simple steatosis, steatohepatitis, hepatic fibrosis, cirrhosis, and liver cancer. Predictions suggest an additional 1 million deaths between 2019 and 2040 in the United States, with over a third of deaths occurring in individuals under the age of 55.[3] Alcohol consumption disrupts tight junction proteins in the gut, leading to increased intestinal permeability.[4,5] Consequently, this facilitates the translocation of microbial products such as lipopolysaccharide (LPS) and bacterial DNA into the portal circulation, eventually causing damage to the liver. In addition, viable bacteria are able to translocate across the gut barrier. Based on preclinical and clinical studies, the gut microbiota plays a pivotal role in the onset and progression of the ALD.[6] Although fungi and viruses also play an important role in liver disease, their contribution to ALD has been recently summarized by the authors and other groups.[6–9] In this review, the authors introduce dysbiosis in ALD and summarize the latest findings in terms of functional consequences of both pathobionts and commensals, and bacterial-based therapeutic targets.

[a] Department of Medicine, University of California San Diego, La Jolla, CA 92093, USA;
[b] Department of Medicine, VA San Diego Healthcare System, San Diego, CA 92161, USA
* Corresponding author. University of California San Diego, 9500 Gilman Drive, MC0063, La Jolla, CA 92093.
E-mail address: beschnabl@ucsd.edu

Clin Liver Dis 28 (2024) 663–679
https://doi.org/10.1016/j.cld.2024.06.008
1089-3261/24/Published by Elsevier Inc.

liver.theclinics.com

Alcohol-Associated Liver Disease

ALD is one of the most common liver diseases worldwide, and encompasses a disease spectrum of steatosis, steatohepatitis, fibrosis, and cirrhosis in a patient with harmful alcohol consumption.[2] Alcohol-associated hepatitis represents a severe cholestatic, acute-on-chronic form of ALD and is associated with the fastest disease progression.[10] Alcohol-associated hepatitis can be accompanied by bacterial infections, development of acute-on-chronic liver failure and multiorgan failure, culminating in high 90-day mortality rates of 20% to 50%.[11] Cirrhosis of the liver is the end stage of chronic liver disease and develops in approximately 10% to 20% of ALD patients. In 2017, an estimated 123 million individuals worldwide, and more than 2 million in the United States, were diagnosed with alcohol-associated cirrhosis. The in-hospital mortality rate among cirrhosis-related hospitalizations in the United States was 7.3% in 2016, and it increased to 13.4% among hospitalizations specifically due to alcohol-associated cirrhosis.[12] Notably, around 60% of hospitalizations related to complications of cirrhosis or acute-on-chronic liver failure were linked to alcohol-associated cirrhosis and alcohol-associated hepatitis.[13] There appears to be a growing global incidence of alcohol-associated hepatitis, particularly among young adults and women, incurring a heavy economic burden.[14]

The liver and intestine maintain communication through the portal vein, biliary system, and systemic circulation. Consequently, the liver stands as the first organ in our body exposed to metabolites and microbial components originating from the gut. Excessive alcohol consumption disrupts tight junctions in intestinal epithelial cells, leading to increased gut permeability, and translocation of microbes and microbial components to the liver (**Fig. 1**).[4,15] The dysfunction of the intestinal barrier plays a pivotal role in the pathogenesis and progression of alcohol-associated liver diseases by perpetuating hepatic inflammation, fibrosis, and portal hypertension. ALD is associated with alterations in the gut microbial composition. The modified composition of the gut microbiota also contributes to the progression of liver disease.

Gut Homeostasis and Dysbiosis

The gastrointestinal tract, an intricate ecosystem of microorganisms, contains more than a trillion of microbes. These microorganisms actively engage in digestion, metabolize various substances, and influence host immunity. The microbiota, along with its products, profoundly modulates physiology and pathophysiology of both the gut and the liver.[16]

The gut bacterial microbiome in individuals with liver disease shows compositional changes (dysbiosis), which is marked by an increase in harmful bacteria and a decrease in beneficial ones. This dysregulation intensifies with the severity of the disease and correlates with adverse liver and patient-related outcomes. Dysbiosis has been observed in both animal models and patients with ALD, influencing disease progression through various mechanisms.[17] Overall, at the phylum level, Bacteroidetes and Firmicutes of patients with alcohol use disorder are decreased, whereas Proteobacteria, Fusobacteria, and Actinobacteria are increased. At the family level, Ruminococcaceae decreases, while both Lachnospiraceae and Enterobacteriaceae increase.[4,18] Patients with alcohol-associated liver disease exhibit a dysbiotic gut microbiota characterized by reduced bacterial diversity, increased proportions of pathobionts such as enterococci, streptococci, and enterobacteria, and decreases in beneficial bacteria like *Akkermansia muciniphila* and *Faecalibacterium prausnitzii*.[19] A study comparing gut microbiota across diverse populations, including 122 patients with alcohol use disorder, 75 with ALD, 54 with non-alcoholic liver diseases, and 260

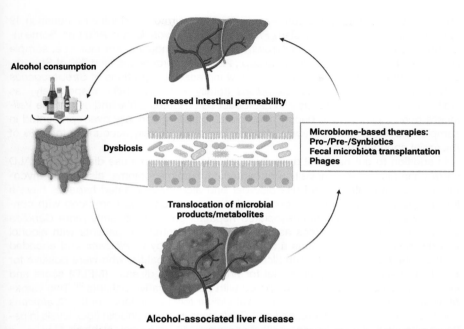

Alcohol-associated liver disease

Fig. 1. The role of the gut-liver axis in alcohol-associated liver disease and microbiome-based treatment. Excessive alcohol consumption can increase intestinal permeability, enabling the translocation of gut microbiota and their metabolites across the intestinal barrier to the liver via the portal vein, thereby promoting the progression of alcohol-associated liver disease. Microbiome-based treatments aim to restore the integrity of the intestinal barrier or target pathobionts to prevent the progression of alcohol-associated liver disease.

healthy controls, found consistent changes. There was a significantly lower abundance of multiple butyrate-producing families, including Ruminococcaceae, Lachnospiraceae, and Oscillospiraceae in patients with alcohol use disorder as compared with healthy controls, with further reductions in ALD as compared with patients with alcohol use disorder. Additionally, an increase in endotoxin-producing Proteobacteria was noted in patients with alcohol use disorder, with the ALD group showing the largest increase.[20] At the family level, a significant increase in bacteria from the Proteobacteria phylum, specifically Enterobacteriaceae and Burkholderiaceae, was observed. Another study reported a reduced abundance of beneficial bacteria such as Ruminococcaceae, *Faecalibacterium*, and *Prevotella*, associated with an increase in gram-negative bacteria, such as Proteobacteria, Enterobacteriaceae, and *Escherichia*. Most of the beneficial bacteria produce short-chain fatty acids, known to maintain and improve gut health.[21]

Several studies confirm that the gut microbial community in patients with alcohol-associated liver cirrhosis shows dysbiosis, characterized by an increased presence of Proteobacteria, particularly Gammaproteobacteria, and Bacilli. These shifts are paralleled by a reduction in commensal taxa such as Clostridia, Bacteroidetes, Ruminococcaceae, *Lactobacillus*, and *Bifidobacterium*. A significant decrease in levels of Lachnospiraceae, *Roseburia*, *Faecalibacterium*, and *Blautia* contributes to intestinal bacterial overgrowth. This, combined with the acetaldehyde-induced increase in intestinal permeability, results in elevated blood concentrations of endotoxins and activation of inflammatory cascades, likely contributing to liver damage.[22-24] At the species level, patients with alcohol-associated liver cirrhosis exhibit a reduction in 49 species from 13 genera, particularly *Prevotella, Paraprevotella*, and *Alistipes*. Some individuals also experience the outgrowth of certain pathogens. For instance, sample ALC_13 includes 68% of *Escherichia* spp., 22% of *Enterococcus*, and 7% of *Streptococcus*. Samples ALC_9 and ALC_20 show increased proportions of *Streptococcus salivarius* and *Streptococcus vestibularis* (totally 27% and 18%, respectively), as well as *Lactobacillus salivarius* and *Lactobacillus crispatus* (20% and 36%). The *Veillonella* genus, prevalent in buccal microbiota, is also abnormally overrepresented in sample ALC_9 (*Veillonella atypica, parvula*, and *dispar*, totally accounting for 17% of microbial abundance).[18]

In addition to gut bacterial dysbiosis, patients with alcohol use disorder and ALD show changes in the composition of the fecal fungal microbiome, also called mycobiome. Patients with alcohol use disorder and alcohol-associated hepatitis have a lower fungal diversity with a proportional increase in *Candida* compared with controls.[25] Patients with alcohol-associated hepatitis grew significantly more *Candida albicans* colonies in the feces as compared with controls or patients with alcohol use disorder.[26] Candidalysin is a heptatoxin secreted by *C. albicans* and encoded by the gene *ECE1*. Patients with alcohol-associated hepatitis, who were positive for *ECE1* in feces, had a higher model for end-stage liver disease (MELD) score and increased 90-day mortality as compared with *ECE1*-negative patients.[26] Two weeks of alcohol abstinence were associated with lower fecal abundance of the *C. albicans* and *C. zeylanoides,* and decreased anti-*C. albicans* immunoglobulin (IgG) levels in patients with alcohol use disorder, indicating reversibility of fungal dysbiosis.[27]

Gut Microbes Affect Liver Function

Gut dysbiosis has profound implications for the host. Notably, the composition of the intestinal microbiota is correlated with the fibrosis stage in patients with ALD.[28] The interconnection between the intestine and the liver is bidirectional: microorganisms and their products reach the liver through the lymph flow and portal blood flow. Conversely, bile produced in the liver is secreted into the intestine. The intestinal barrier serves as the initial defense mechanism against the penetration of pathogenic microorganisms and their products into circulation.[15] Bacteria and fungal products entering the bloodstream contribute to the onset and progression of ALD by activating signaling through pattern recognition receptors, initiating liver steatosis, cell death, and inflammation.[6,29] Under dysbiotic conditions, certain gut bacteria, such as *Enterococcus* species, expand and can adapt to evade mucosal immunity, translocating to mucocutaneous lymph nodes and the liver,[30] where bacterial clearance by periportally positioned Kupffer cells is impaired in the context of ALD and cirrhosis.[31,32]

In ALD, the presence of small intestinal bacterial overgrowth has been established, accompanied by a decrease in the number of bacteria from *Lactobacillus* species.[33] *Lactobacillus* species produce bactericidal substances that play a crucial role in maintaining the homeostasis of the intestinal microbiota, preventing the proliferation of pathogenic bacteria such as *Salmonella* and *Shigella* species. The metabolic byproducts of *Lactobacillus*, including short-chain fatty acids (SCFAs) such as butyrate, acetate, and propionate, contribute to the integrity of the intestinal barrier. Additionally, SCFAs serve as a source of energy for intestinal epithelial cells and play an immunologic role.[34,35]

Translocation of bacterial LPS to the peripheral circulation has been observed in both ethanol-induced and diet-induced steatotic liver diseases. However, the translocation of bacteria itself appears to be restricted to ethanol-induced liver disease.[36]

Notably, bacterial sphingolipids from the gut symbiont *Bacteroides thetaiotaomicron* have been found to transfer to the liver, reducing lipid accumulation by increasing beta-oxidation in mice.[37] Similarly, the health relevance of *F. prausnitzii, Christensenella minuta, Anaerobutyricum soehngenii*, and *Oxalobacter formigenes* was initially noted due to their low abundance in specific diseases, prompting further *in vivo* and mechanistic studies.[38]

Enterobacteriaceae plays a crucial role in the progression of liver diseases. In patients with hepatic encephalopathy, their presence has been linked to systemic inflammation and cognitive decline. Additionally, Enterobacteriaceae are implicated in the majority of cases of spontaneous bacterial peritonitis, a common infection in individuals with cirrhosis. Burkholderiaceae further exacerbates ethanol-associated inflammation, showing a significant correlation with interferon (IFN)-gamma-inducible protein 10 (IP-10 or CXCL10), which intensifies the inflammatory response in murine models of ALD.[20,39] Fusobacteria, the phylum exhibiting the largest increase in individuals with ALD compared with healthy controls, also contributes to inflammation. Furthermore, there is a higher abundance of Proteobacteria, a phylum encompassing many known human pathogens such as *Klebsiella, Enterobacter, Citrobacter, Salmonella, Escherichia coli, Shigella, Proteus*, and *Serratia* within the Enterobacteriaceae family.[5]

Pathobionts and Virulence Factors

Pathobionts are microorganisms that are typically commensal (harmless) in the microbiota but can become pathogenic (cause or promote disease) to the host under certain conditions or in specific contexts.[40] Understanding characteristics of pathobionts and the presence of virulence factors is crucial for comprehending their impact on the host. Moreover, evidence of bacterial translocation from the gut-colonized niche has been observed in patients with alcohol-associated hepatitis.[28] Virulence factors of translocated microbes can cause specific complications, and exotoxins, actively secreted microbial toxins targeting other bacteria or host cells, play a significant role. Cytolysin, a 2-subunit exotoxin secreted by *Enterococcus faecalis*,[41] has been associated with the severity of ethanol-induced liver disease in mouse models.[42] Ethanol feeding leads to the expansion of specific strains of *Enterococcus*, particularly in conditions where gastric acid is lacking.[42] Patients with alcohol-associated hepatitis carry significantly higher amounts of *E. faecalis* compared with individuals with or without alcohol use disorder.[43] The presence of gut-colonized cytolysin-positive *E. faecalis* predicts mortality of patients with alcohol-associated hepatitis.[43] Of note, this seems to be confined to alcohol-associated hepatitis, as cytolysin-positivity is not associated with increased disease severity or mortality in nonalcoholic fatty liver disease, acutely decompensated cirrhosis, or acute-on-chronic liver failure.[44,45] Cytolysin promotes ethanol-induced liver disease in preclinical models and causes direct hepatocyte death, likely through pore formation in the cell membrane. Detecting specific intestinal pathobionts has therapeutic implications, as targeted modulation of the intestinal microbiome and its products can improve alcohol-associated liver disease.[43,46]

Candidalysin is a fungal exotoxin secreted by the pathobiont *C. albicans*. It is associated with disease severity in patients with alcohol-associated hepatitis.[26] Candidalysin is directly toxic to cultured hepatocytes and causes disease exacerbation in a mouse model of ethanol-induced liver disease.[26] In addition, intestinal *C. albicans* causes priming of T helper 17 (Th17) cells. *C. albicans*-specific Th17 cells are increased in the circulation and present in the liver of patients with alcohol-associated liver disease.[47] Chronic ethanol administration in mice causes migration of *C. albicans*-reactive

Th17 cells from the intestine to the liver in mice, where they contribute to liver disease by secreting interleukin-17 (IL-17).[47]

Flagellin, a primary component of the bacterial flagellum, plays a crucial role in bacterial motility. In an animal study, flagellin-induced liver injury was observed in mice.[48] The swift immune responses to flagellin observed in various cell types, including hepatocytes, epithelial cells, monocytes, and dendritic cells, coupled with increased Proteobacteria found in studies related to ALD, could contribute to the progression of the disease in patients with ALD.[49]

Microbial-Based Therapies

Recognizing the pivotal role of gut microbiota homeostasis in the pathogenesis of ALD, therapeutic interventions targeting the microbiome show promise.[50] Use of prebiotics, probiotics, postbiotics, synbiotics, phages, and fecal microbiota transplantation (FMT) might lead to improvements in chronic liver diseases, including ALD and liver cirrhosis.[7,51] Clinical trials of microbiome-based therapies in alcohol-associated liver disease are summarized in **Table 1**.

Prebiotics, which are indigestible food ingredients, aid in intestinal peristalsis and stimulate the growth of specific bacteria. Studies have demonstrated that prebiotics can reduce ethanol-induced liver damage in mouse models by reducing bacterial overgrowth.[33] A randomized controlled clinical trial is using Profermin (a food for special medical purposes) to modulate the dysbiotic gut microbiota in patients with ALD (NCT03863730). Postbiotics, or microbe-derived metabolites, also show promise in the treatment of ALD.[52,53] In ALD and cirrhosis, impaired fermentation of carbohydrates into butyrate by Lachnospiraceae and Ruminococcaceae leads to lower butyrate concentrations in the blood, correlating with inflammation and disease progression.[54–56] Supplementation of butyrate via a synbiotics (F. prausnitzii and potato starch), tributyrin, or by gavage ameliorates intestinal barrier dysfunction and liver injury in preclinical models.[57–59] Live biotherapeutics, including genetically engineered bacteria, offer additional avenues for modulating the gut barrier. Limosilactobacillus reuteri engineered to produce interleukin-22 (IL-22), protective against experimental ethanol-induced liver disease in a toll-like receptor 7 (TLR7)-dependent manner,[60] induced the expression of regenerating islet-derived protein 3 gamma (Reg3g) (with antibacterial activity) in the intestine, reducing bacterial translocation to the liver, and preventing ethanol-induced liver disease in mice.[61] E. coli Nissle 1917, specifically engineered to produce aryl-hydrocarbon receptor agonists, reduced translocation of bacteria to the liver in mice following chronic plus binge ethanol.[62] However, preclinical findings on engineered bacteria require confirmation through interventional studies in humans.

Probiotics constitute a group of non-pathogenic microorganisms whose primary role is to modulate and maintain homeostasis of the intestinal microbiota. They demonstrate the ability to reduce inflammation, particularly in cases of ethanol-induced liver inflammation, and prevent gut barrier dysfunction. Various probiotic bacteria, such as Lactobacillus, Bifidobacteria, E. coli, Saccharomyces, Lactococcus, and A. muciniphila, are employed to mitigate or halt the progression of alcohol-associated liver diseases.[63,64] An example illustrating this is the use of a probiotic combination known as #VSL3, which includes Bifidobacterium breve, B. infantis, B. longum, L. acidophilus, L. paracasei, L. bulgaricus, L. plantarum, and Streptococcus thermophiles.[53,65] This compound probiotic effectively reversed acute ethanol-associated gut dysbiosis and maintained the integrity of the intestinal barrier by upregulating the production of mucus and the expression of tight junction proteins, consequently reducing LPS levels in the liver.[66]

Table 1
Clinical trials of microbiome-based therapies in alcohol-associated liver disease

Trial	Disease	Study Design	Treatment	Procedure	Country
Han et al,[73] 2015 (NCT01501162)	Alcohol-associated hepatitis	Multicenter, prospective, double-blind, randomized, and controlled	*Lactobacillus subtilis/ Streptococcus faecium*	Probiotics (n = 60) or placebo (n = 57) for 7 d	South Korea
Vatsalya et al,[74] 2023 (NCT01922895)	Alcohol use disorder and moderate alcohol-associated hepatitis	Randomized controlled	*Lactobacillus rhamnosus* GG (LGG)	All patients were randomized to receive either LGG (n = 24) or placebo (n = 22) orally once/day for 6 mo	USA
Li et al,[75] 2021	Alcohol-associated liver injury	Randomized, double-blind, and placebo-controlled	*Lactobacillus casei*	Supplementation of probiotics of high dose (n = 54) and low dose (n = 58) or placebo (n = 46) for 60 d	China
NCT05007470	Alcohol use disorder and alcohol-associated liver disease	Pilot randomized controlled	VSL#3	A randomized placebo (VSL#3 vs placebo) control trial will be performed in patients with AUD and ALD for 6 mo	USA
NCT03863730	Alcohol-associated liver disease	Randomized controlled	Profermin Plus	Patients will be randomized 1:1 to receive Profermin Plus versus Fresubin for 24 wk	Denmark
Sharma et al,[81] 2022 (NCT03827772)	Severe alcohol-associated hepatitis	Open-label, non-randomized	Fecal microbiota transplantation (FMT)	A single FMT (n = 13) session was administered as a freshly prepared stool suspension through a nasojejunal tube	India

(continued on next page)

Table 1
(*continued*)

Trial	Disease	Study Design	Treatment	Procedure	Country
Philips et al,[82] 2017	Severe alcohol-associated hepatitis	Pilot controlled	FMT	FMT (n = 8) through a nasoduodenal tube daily for 7 d	India
Pande et al,[83] 2023 (NCT03091010)	Severe alcohol-associated hepatitis	Randomized open-label	FMT	Patients were randomized to prednisolone (n = 60) for 28 d or healthy donor FMT (n = 60) through nasoduodenal tube daily for 7 d	India
NCT05006430	Severe alcohol-associated hepatitis	Randomized, parallel assignment, double-blind, and placebo-controlled	FMT	Patients will be randomly assigned in 1:1 where 25 patients will receive orally administered lyophilized PRIM-DJ2727 and standard of care and the other 25 patients will receive placebo and standard of care for 4 wk	USA
NCT05285592	Severe alcohol-associated hepatitis	Randomized, controlled, and open-label	FMT	Seven doses (30 gm 1 dose) of FMT will be given via a nasojejunal tube	India
Bajaj et al,[86] 2021 (NCT03416751)	Alcohol-associated cirrhosis with alcohol use disorder	Double-blind, randomized controlled	FMT	1:1 into receiving placebo or FMT enema from a donor enriched in *Lachnospiraceae* and *Ruminococcaceae*	USA
Bajaj et al,[94] 2017 (NCT02636647)	Cirrhosis and recurrent hepatic encephalopathy	Open-label, randomized controlled	FMT	FMT preceded by 5 d of broad-spectrum antibiotics vs standard of care	USA

Most studies investigated single strains as probiotics in ethanol-induced liver disease in preclinical models. A study isolated *Roseburia intestinalis* SNUG30017 from a healthy subject and investigated its roles in ethanol-induced liver disease. Administration of this singular strain resulted in a significant reduction in hepatic injury in ethanol-fed mice. Furthermore, it attenuated hepatic expression of inflammatory cytokines, such as the tumor necrosis factor (TNF) and the interleukin-1 beta (IL-1b), and modulated lipid transport. Additionally, *R. intestinalis* SNUG30017 restored intestinal barrier function in an ethanol feeding model by increasing the levels of occludin and mucin 2.[67] Furthermore, oral administration of *Phocaeicola dorei* and *Lactobacillus helveticus* reduced liver inflammation and intestinal barrier damage induced by ethanol administration in mice.[68]

A. muciniphila is a gram-negative anaerobic bacterium that colonizes the human gastrointestinal tract. Its ability to induce mucin production is crucial for maintaining intestinal integrity.[69] Multiple studies have established the connection between *A. muciniphila* and ALD.[19,70] In individuals with alcohol-associated hepatitis, there was a reduction in the abundance of fecal *A. muciniphila* compared with healthy controls, and this reduction correlated with the severity of hepatic disease. Oral supplementation of *A. muciniphila* successfully restored ethanol-induced depletion of intestinal *A. muciniphila* in mice.[19] *A. muciniphila* enhances gut barrier function by restoring the mucus layer thickness and the intestinal expression of the antimicrobial peptide Reg3g,[71] and alleviated ethanol-induced liver injury in mice.[72] Furthermore, *A. muciniphila* inhibited the proliferation of harmful bacteria, such as *E. coli* and *Helicobacter hepaticus*, induced by alcohol consumption, while promoting the growth of butyrate-producing and commensal bacteria, including *Paramuribaculum intestinale* and *Bacteroides ovatus*.[72]

Two clinical trials have used lactobacilli in patients with alcohol-associated hepatitis. In a multicenter, prospective, double-blind randomized, controlled clinical trial in South Korea (NCT01501162), hospitalized patients with alcohol-associated hepatitis and heavy drinking histories received probiotics (n = 60) or placebo (n = 57) for 7 days. Patients in the treatment group were administered *Lactobacillus subtilis/Streptococcus faecium* cultured probiotics, while those in the placebo group were given a placebo. Both groups were given standard alcohol detoxification therapies, including fluid therapy, a regular diet, thiamine, and milk thistle/silymarin capsules (450 mg/day) prior to admission to the hospital. Compared with the placebo group, the probiotic group showed significant improvement in serum albumin and TNF levels, while most of the other liver function tests improved in both groups.[73] In a clinical trial in the United States (NCT01922895), *Lactobacillus rhamnosus* GG (LGG) supplemental therapy (n = 24) was compared with a control placebo (n = 22) in patients with alcohol use disorder and moderate alcohol-associated hepatitis (MELD < 20). Following 180 days of therapy, there was a significant reduction in heavy drinking in patients treated with LGG. There was also a significant improvement in aspartate transaminase (AST):alanine transaminase (ALT) ratio and MELD score after 4 weeks.[74] In another randomized, double-blind, placebo-controlled trial conducted in China, 158 patients with alcohol-associated liver injury were randomized into 3 groups: a low-dose group receiving *Lactobacillus casei* strain Shirota (n = 58), a high-dose group of *L. casei* strain Shirota (n = 54), and a control group (n = 46) receiving a placebo without *L. casei* strain Shirota. Compared with the control group, the high-dose group showed a decrease in serum levels of triglyceride by 26.56% and low-density lipoprotein cholesterol by 23.83%. The group receiving high dose of *L. casei* strain Shirota showed improved liver function tests (AST, ALT, gamma-glutamyltransferase [GGT] and total bilirubin) as compared to baseline, while the low dose group showed decreased AST.[75]

Phages can specifically target bacteria and can be important therapies for alcohol-associated liver disease. There are 4 preclinical trials using phage therapy in liver diseases. For alcohol-associated liver disease, we found that patients with alcohol-associated hepatitis had significantly higher amounts of cytolysin-positive E. faecalis in the gut compared with individuals with or without alcohol use disorder.[43] Phages targeting cytolysin-positive E faecalis attenuate ethanol-induced liver disease in mice.[43] Two preclinical studies focused on phage therapy against alcohol-producing K pneumoniae in metabolic dysfunction-associated steatotic liver disease (MASLD). A total of 60% of MASLD patients carry high alcohol-producing K. pneumoniae in feces. Gavage of mice with high alcohol-producing K. pneumoniae or fecal microbiota containing high alcohol-producing K. pneumoniae from a patient induced steatohepatitis. Using phages targeting high alcohol-producing K. pneumoniae prior to FMT showed amelioration of liver disease.[76] Furthermore, the authors used phages targeting high alcohol-producing K. pneumoniae in mice by oral administration, which alleviated steatohepatitis caused by high alcohol-producing K. pneumoniae.[77] Another study used a lytic phage cocktail that targets K. pneumoniae associated with pathogenesis of experimental primary sclerosing cholangitis by oral administration in mice. Phages suppressed K. pneumoniae and attenuated liver inflammation and disease severity in hepatobiliary injury-prone mice.[78]

FMT is a promising future treatment option in patients with alcohol-associated hepatitis. FMT involves transplanting stool from a healthy individual to a patient suffering from a specific disease. Small retrospective cohort studies[79,80] and a prospective open-label study[81] have demonstrated improved survival in patients with severe alcohol-associated hepatitis who underwent FMT compared with standard of care. Another study in India monitored the 1-year survival of patients with alcohol-associated hepatitis who underwent FMT, revealing that 87.5% (7/8) of those who had FMT survived 1 year, compared with 33.3% (6/18) of control patients.[82] FMT treatment has been shown to be beneficial for patients with severe alcohol-associated hepatitis in a prospective randomized open-label clinical trial conducted over a period of 2 years among patients with chronic alcohol consumption for more than 5 years, who have continued to drink for the last 30 days and have been diagnosed with severe alcohol-associated hepatitis. Steroid-eligible patients with severe alcohol-associated hepatitis were randomized to prednisolone (n = 60) for 28 days or healthy donor FMT (n = 60) through nasoduodenal tube daily for 7 days. The primary outcome of the study, 90-day survival, was achieved by 56.6% patients in the prednisolone and 75% in the FMT group (P = .044). Survival was not significantly different at 180 and 365 days.[83] Ongoing larger randomized controlled trials (NCT05006430 and NCT05285592) are eagerly anticipated to provide further insights. Two placebo-controlled phase II/III trials are currently assessing the efficacy of encapsulated FMT in preventing redecompensation and death in cirrhosis (CHiFT; NCT04932577) and preventing infections in cirrhosis (PROMISE; ISRCTN17863382). Patients with liver cirrhosis (n = 20) received a single FMT enema with or without antibiotics. The results showed that FMT is a safe and well-tolerated procedure, enhancing the diversity of intestinal microbiota, the abundance of beneficial bacteria, and the intestinal barrier.[84] For patients with cirrhosis, careful consideration is essential to determine whether there is an increased risk of bacterial infections after FMT. A systematic review of the global incidence of FMT-related complications found that serious adverse events, including infections and deaths, occurred in 1.4% of cases, all in patients with structural mucosal barrier damage.[85] A recent randomized clinical trial of patients with alcohol use disorder and cirrhosis revealed increased microbial diversity with increased Ruminococcaceae and other SCFA-producing taxa post-FMT, but not with placebo. The investigators reported that FMT is safe and associated with short-term reduction in alcohol craving and consumption, and reduction in alcohol use-related events over 6 months.[86] In a retrospective study on FMT in 23 patients with alcohol-associated hepatitis-related acute-on-chronic liver failure (ACLF) who were ineligible for steroid therapy, an overall survival rate of 66% at 548 days of follow-up and a mean overall survival of 389 days were reported. The survival rates at lower and higher ACLF grades at the end of 548 days of follow-up were 72.7% and 58.3%, respectively.[87]

Furthermore, beyond regulating liver disease, gut microbiota plays a role in psychiatric disorders by interacting with the peripheral and central nervous systems and could potentially serve as a therapeutic target.[88] Details about the microbiota-gut-brain axis and gut-liver-brain axis have been extensively discussed in other reviews.[88–91] A few clinical trials have shown that probiotics and FMT can act as dual targets on both gut-liver and gut-brain axes. For instance, a randomized controlled trial administering LGG to patients with cirrhosis and minimal hepatic encephalopathy demonstrated improvement in microbial function and community, though no significant difference in cognitive performance was observed versus placebo.[92] Another double-blind clinical trial in India revealed that the intake of VSL#3 significantly reduced the risk of hospitalization for hepatic encephalopathy and complications of cirrhosis.[93] Additionally, a pilot randomized placebo-controlled trial (VSL#3 vs placebo) is set to be conducted in the United States, involving patients with alcohol use disorder and alcohol-associated liver disease for a duration of 6 months to examine the brain-gut-microbiome axis and sex-differences in severity (NCT05007470). Another open-label, randomized controlled trial of FMT in the United States showed that FMT preceded by 5 days of broad-spectrum antibiotics reduced hospitalizations, improved cognition and gut dysbiosis as compared with standard of care in patients with cirrhosis and recurrent hepatic encephalopathy.[94] It is essential to thoroughly investigate the factors such as treatment duration, dosage, and safety in future clinical trials.

SUMMARY

The onset and progression of ALD are closely linked to changes in gut microbiota. Various existing and experimental microbiome-based strategies aim to restore intestinal homeostasis in liver diseases. These approaches encompass the use of antimicrobials, prebiotics, probiotics, synbiotics, bacteriophage therapy, and FMT. Future directions in this field might involve strain-level profiling, functional genomics through deep metagenomics sequencing and culture-based whole-genome sequencing to better understand host-microbiome interactions during ALD and identify targets for microbiome-centered therapies.

CLINICS CARE POINTS

- The composition of the intestinal microbiota correlates with the fibrosis stage in patients with ALD.
- Fecal exotoxins from bacteria predict mortality in patients with alcohol-associated hepatitis.
- Probiotics show promising results in reducing heavy drinking and improving MELD score in patients with alcohol use disorder and moderate alcohol-associated hepatitis.
- FMT is a promising treatment option in patients with alcohol-associated hepatitis, but further clinical trials are required for confirmation.

ACKNOWLEDGMENTS

This work was supported by a NIH grants R01 AA024726, R01 AA020703, U01 AA026939, by Award Number BX004594 from the Biomedical Laboratory Research & Development Service of the VA Office of Research and Development (to B. Schnabl) and services provided by NIH centers P30 DK120515 and P50 AA011999.

DISCLOSURE

Conflicts of interest: B. Schnabl has been consulting for Ambys Medicines, Ferring Research Institute, Gelesis, HOST Therabiomics, Intercept Pharmaceuticals, Mabwell Therapeutics, Patara Pharmaceuticals, Surrozen and Takeda. B. Schnabl's institution UC San Diego has received research support from Axial Biotherapeutics, United States, BiomX, ChromoLogic, CymaBay Therapeutics, United States, Intercept Pharmaceuticals, United States, NGM Biopharmaceuticals, United States, Prodigy Biotech and Synlogic Operating Company. B. Schnabl is founder of Nterica Bio. UC San Diego has filed several patents with B. Schnabl as inventor related to this work.

Author contributions: Y. Yang wrote the review and B. Schnabl edited the article.

REFERENCES

1. Collaborators GBDC. The global, regional, and national burden of cirrhosis by cause in 195 countries and territories, 1990-2017: a systematic analysis for the Global Burden of Disease Study 2017. Lancet Gastroenterol Hepatol 2020;5(3): 245–66.
2. Singal AK, Mathurin P. Diagnosis and treatment of alcohol-associated liver disease: a review. JAMA 2021;326(2):165–76.
3. Julien J, Ayer T, Bethea ED, et al. Projected prevalence and mortality associated with alcohol-related liver disease in the USA, 2019-40: a modelling study. Lancet Public Health 2020;5(6):e316–23.
4. Leclercq S, Matamoros S, Cani PD, et al. Intestinal permeability, gut-bacterial dysbiosis, and behavioral markers of alcohol-dependence severity. Proc Natl Acad Sci U S A 2014;111(42):E4485–93.
5. Jew MH, Hsu CL. Alcohol, the gut microbiome, and liver disease. J Gastroenterol Hepatol 2023;38(8):1205–10.
6. Hsu CL, Schnabl B. The gut-liver axis and gut microbiota in health and liver disease. Nat Rev Microbiol 2023;21:719–33.
7. Fujiki J, Schnabl B. Phage therapy: targeting intestinal bacterial microbiota for the treatment of liver diseases. JHEP Rep 2023;5(12):100909.
8. Szostak N, Figlerowicz M, Philips A. The emerging role of the gut mycobiome in liver diseases. Gut Microb 2023;15(1):2211922.
9. Hartmann P, Schnabl B. Fungal infections and the fungal microbiome in hepatobiliary disorders. J Hepatol 2023;78(4):836–51.
10. Mathurin P, Beuzin F, Louvet A, et al. Fibrosis progression occurs in a subgroup of heavy drinkers with typical histological features. Aliment Pharmacol Ther 2007; 25(9):1047–54.
11. Bataller R, Arab JP, Shah VH. Alcohol-associated hepatitis. N Engl J Med 2022; 387(26):2436–48.
12. Hirode G, Saab S, Wong RJ. Trends in the burden of chronic liver disease among hospitalized US adults. JAMA Netw Open 2020;3(4):e201997.

13. Singal AK, Ahmed Z, Axley P, et al. Hospitalizations for acute on chronic liver failure at Academic compared to non-academic centers have higher mortality. Digest Dis Sci 2021;66(4):1306–14.

14. Singal AK, Arsalan A, Dunn W, et al. Alcohol-associated liver disease in the United States is associated with severe forms of disease among young, females and Hispanics. Aliment Pharmacol Ther 2021;54(4):451–61.

15. Lang S, Schnabl B. Microbiota and fatty liver disease-the known, the unknown, and the future. Cell Host Microbe 2020;28(2):233–44.

16. Pabst O, Hornef MW, Schaap FG, et al. Gut-liver axis: barriers and functional circuits. Nat Rev Gastroenterol Hepatol 2023;20(7):447–61.

17. Diaz LA, Arab JP, Louvet A, et al. The intersection between alcohol-related liver disease and nonalcoholic fatty liver disease. Nat Rev Gastroenterol Hepatol 2023;20(12):764–83.

18. Dubinkina VB, Tyakht AV, Odintsova VY, et al. Links of gut microbiota composition with alcohol dependence syndrome and alcoholic liver disease. Microbiome 2017;5(1):141.

19. Grander C, Adolph TE, Wieser V, et al. Recovery of ethanol-induced *Akkermansia muciniphila* depletion ameliorates alcoholic liver disease. Gut 2018;67(5):891–901.

20. Litwinowicz K, Gamian A. Microbiome alterations in alcohol use disorder and alcoholic liver disease. Int J Mol Sci 2023;24(3):2461.

21. Wu X, Fan X, Miyata T, et al. Recent advances in understanding of pathogenesis of alcohol-associated liver disease. Annu Rev Pathol 2023;18:411–38.

22. Chen YF, Yang FL, Lu HF, et al. Characterization of fecal microbial communities in patients with liver cirrhosis. Hepatology 2011;54(2):562–72.

23. Qin N, Yang FL, Li A, et al. Alterations of the human gut microbiome in liver cirrhosis. Nature 2014;513(7516):59–64.

24. Bajaj JS, Heuman DM, Hylemon PB, et al. Altered profile of human gut microbiome is associated with cirrhosis and its complications. J Hepatol 2014;60(5):940–7.

25. Lang S, Duan Y, Liu J, et al. Intestinal fungal dysbiosis and systemic immune response to fungi in patients with alcoholic hepatitis. Hepatology 2020;71(2):522–38.

26. Chu H, Duan Y, Lang S, et al. The *Candida albicans* exotoxin candidalysin promotes alcohol-associated liver disease. J Hepatol 2020;72(3):391–400.

27. Hartmann P, Lang S, Zeng S, et al. Dynamic changes of the fungal microbiome in alcohol use disorder. Front Physiol 2021;12:699253.

28. Fairfield B, Schnabl B. Gut dysbiosis as a driver in alcohol-induced liver injury. JHEP Rep 2021;3(2):100220.

29. Yang AM, Inamine T, Hochrath K, et al. Intestinal fungi contribute to development of alcoholic liver disease. J Clin Invest 2017;127(7):2829–41.

30. Duan Y, Chu H, Brandl K, et al. CRIg on liver macrophages clears pathobionts and protects against alcoholic liver disease. Nat Commun 2021;12(1):7172.

31. Yang Y, Nguyen M, Khetrapal V, et al. Within-host evolution of a gut pathobiont facilitates liver translocation. Nature 2022;607(7919):563–70.

32. Gola A, Dorrington MG, Speranza E, et al. Commensal-driven immune zonation of the liver promotes host defence. Nature 2021;589(7840):131–6.

33. Yan AW, Fouts DE, Brandl J, et al. Enteric dysbiosis associated with a mouse model of alcoholic liver disease. Hepatology 2011;53(1):96–105.

34. Sanna S, van Zuydam NR, Mahajan A, et al. Causal relationships among the gut microbiome, short-chain fatty acids and metabolic diseases. Nat Genet 2019; 51(4):600–5.

35. Chen P, Torralba M, Tan J, et al. Supplementation of saturated long-chain fatty acids maintains intestinal eubiosis and reduces ethanol-induced liver injury in mice. Gastroenterology 2015;148(1):203–214 e16.

36. Hsu CL, Wang Y, Duan Y, et al. Differences in bacterial translocation and liver injury in ethanol versus diet-induced liver disease. Dig Dis Sci 2023;68(7): 3059–69.

37. Le HH, Lee MT, Besler KR, et al. Host hepatic metabolism is modulated by gut microbiota-derived sphingolipids. Cell Host Microbe 2022;30(6):798–808.

38. Cani PD, Depommier C, Derrien M, et al. *Akkermansia muciniphila*: paradigm for next-generation beneficial microorganisms. Nat Rev Gastroenterol Hepatol 2022; 19(10):625–37.

39. Liang S, Zhong Z, Kim SY, et al. Murine macrophage autophagy protects against alcohol-induced liver injury by degrading interferon regulatory factor 1 (IRF1) and removing damaged mitochondria. J Biol Chem 2019;294(33):12359–69.

40. Jochum L, Stecher B. Label or concept - what is a pathobiont? Trends Microbiol 2020;28(10):789–92.

41. Haas W, Shepard BD, Gilmore MS. Two-component regulator of *Enterococcus faecalis* cytolysin responds to quorum-sensing autoinduction. Nature 2002; 415(6867):84–7.

42. Llorente C, Jepsen P, Inamine T, et al. Gastric acid suppression promotes alcoholic liver disease by inducing overgrowth of intestinal *Enterococcus*. Nat Commun 2017;8(1):837.

43. Duan Y, Llorente C, Lang S, et al. Bacteriophage targeting of gut bacterium attenuates alcoholic liver disease. Nature 2019;575(7783):505–11.

44. Hartmann P, Lang S, Schierwagen R, et al. Fecal cytolysin does not predict disease severity in acutely decompensated cirrhosis and acute-on-chronic liver failure. Hepatobiliary Pancreat Dis Int 2023;22(5):474–81.

45. Lang S, Demir M, Duan Y, et al. Cytolysin-positive *Enterococcus faecalis* is not increased in patients with non-alcoholic steatohepatitis. Liver Int 2020;40(4): 860–5.

46. Cabre N, Hartmann P, Llorente C, et al. IgY antibodies against cytolysin reduce ethanol-induced liver disease in mice. Hepatology 2023;78(1):295–306.

47. Zeng S, Rosati E, Saggau C, et al. *Candida albicans*-specific Th17 cell-mediated response contributes to alcohol-associated liver disease. Cell Host Microbe 2023;31(3):389–404, e7.

48. Xiao Y, Liu F, Yang J, et al. Over-activation of TLR5 signaling by high-dose flagellin induces liver injury in mice. Cell Mol Immunol 2015;12(6):729–42.

49. Leclercq S, de Timary P, Stärkel P. Targeting the gut microbiota to treat alcoholic liver diseases : evidence and promises. Acta Gastro-Enterol Belg 2020;83(4): 616–21.

50. Ratiner K, Ciocan D, Abdeen SK, Elinav E. Utilization of the microbiome in personalized medicine. Nat Rev Microbiol 2024;22(5):291–308.

51. Park JW, Kim SE, Lee NY, et al. Role of microbiota-derived metabolites in alcoholic and non-alcoholic fatty liver diseases. Int J Mol Sci 2021;23(1):426.

52. Mimee M, Citorik RJ, Lu TK. Microbiome therapeutics - advances and challenges. Adv Drug Deliver Rev 2016;105:44–54.

53. Forsyth CB, Farhadi A, Jakate SM, et al. *Lactobacillus* GG treatment ameliorates alcohol-induced intestinal oxidative stress, gut leakiness, and liver injury in a rat model of alcoholic steatohepatitis. Alcohol 2009;43(2):163–72.

54. Smirnova E, Puri P, Muthiah MD, et al. Fecal microbiome distinguishes alcohol consumption from alcoholic hepatitis but does not discriminate disease severity. Hepatology 2020;72(1):271–86.

55. Jin ML, Kalainy S, Baskota N, et al. Faecal microbiota from patients with cirrhosis has a low capacity to ferment non-digestible carbohydrates into short-chain fatty acids. Liver Int 2019;39(8):1437–47.

56. Juanola O, Ferrusquia-Acosta J, Garcia-Villalba R, et al. Circulating levels of butyrate are inversely related to portal hypertension, endotoxemia, and systemic inflammation in patients with cirrhosis. FASEB J 2019;33(10):11595–605.

57. Sheng L, Jena PK, Hu Y, et al. Hepatic inflammation caused by dysregulated bile acid synthesis is reversible by butyrate supplementation. J Pathol 2017;243(4): 431–41.

58. Cresci GA, Glueck B, McMullen MR, et al. Prophylactic tributyrin treatment mitigates chronic-binge ethanol-induced intestinal barrier and liver injury. J Gastroenterol Hepatol 2017;32(9):1587–97.

59. Roychowdhury S, Glueck B, Han Y, et al. A designer synbiotic attenuates chronic-binge ethanol-induced gut-liver injury in mice. Nutrients 2019;11(1):97.

60. Wang QL, Kim SY, Matsushita H, et al. Oral administration of PEGylated TLR7 ligand ameliorates alcohol-associated liver disease via the induction of IL-22. Proc Natl Acad Sci U S A 2021;118(1). e2020868118.

61. Hendrikx T, Duan Y, Wang YH, et al. Bacteria engineered to produce IL-22 in intestine induce expression of REG3G to reduce ethanol-induced liver disease in mice. Gut 2019;68(8):1504–15.

62. Kouno T, Zeng S, Wang Y, et al. Engineered bacteria producing aryl-hydrocarbon receptor agonists protect against ethanol-induced liver disease in mice. Alcohol Clin Exp Res 2023;47(5):856–67.

63. Mishra G, Singh P, Molla M, et al. Harnessing the potential of probiotics in the treatment of alcoholic liver disorders. Front Pharmacol 2023;14:1212742.

64. Gu Z, Liu Y, Hu S, et al. Probiotics for alleviating alcoholic liver injury. Gastroenterol Res Pract 2019;2019:9097276.

65. Chang B, Sang L, Wang Y, et al. The protective effect of VSL#3 on intestinal permeability in a rat model of alcoholic intestinal injury. BMC Gastroenterol 2013;13:151.

66. Liu H, Kang X, Yang X, et al. Compound probiotic ameliorates acute alcoholic liver disease in mice by modulating gut microbiota and maintaining intestinal barrier. Probiotics Antimicrob Proteins 2023;15(1):185–201.

67. Seo B, Jeon K, Moon S, et al. Roseburia spp. abundance associates with alcohol consumption in humans and its administration ameliorates alcoholic fatty liver in mice. Cell Host Microbe 2020;27(1):25–40 e6.

68. Eom JA, Jeong JJ, Han SH, et al. Gut-microbiota prompt activation of natural killer cell on alcoholic liver disease. Gut Microb 2023;15(2):2281014.

69. Zhao Q, Yu J, Hao Y, et al. *Akkermansia muciniphila* plays critical roles in host health. Crit Rev Microbiol 2023;49(1):82–100.

70. Grander C, Grabherr F, Spadoni I, et al. The role of gut vascular barrier in experimental alcoholic liver disease and *A. muciniphila* supplementation. Gut Microb 2020;12(1):1851986.

71. Everard A, Belzer C, Geurts L, et al. Cross-talk between *Akkermansia muciniphila* and intestinal epithelium controls diet-induced obesity. Proc Natl Acad Sci U S A 2013;110(22):9066–71.
72. Fang C, Cheng J, Jia W, et al. *Akkermansia muciniphila* ameliorates alcoholic liver disease in experimental mice by regulating serum metabolism and improving gut dysbiosis. Metabolites 2023;13(10):1057.
73. Han SH, Suk KT, Kim DJ, et al. Effects of probiotics (cultured *Lactobacillus subtilis/Streptococcus faecium*) in the treatment of alcoholic hepatitis: randomized-controlled multicenter study. Eur J Gastroenterol Hepatol 2015;27(11):1300–6.
74. Vatsalya V, Feng W, Kong M, et al. The beneficial effects of *Lactobacillus* GG therapy on liver and drinking assessments in patients with moderate alcohol-associated hepatitis. Am J Gastroenterol 2023;118(8):1457–60.
75. Li X, Liu Y, Guo X, et al. Effect of *Lactobacillus casei* on lipid metabolism and intestinal microflora in patients with alcoholic liver injury. Eur J Clin Nutr 2021;75(8):1227–36.
76. Yuan J, Chen C, Cui J, et al. Fatty liver disease caused by high-alcohol-producing *Klebsiella pneumoniae*. Cell Metab 2019;30(4):675–88.
77. Gan L, Feng Y, Du B, et al. Bacteriophage targeting microbiota alleviates non-alcoholic fatty liver disease induced by high alcohol-producing *Klebsiella pneumoniae*. Nat Commun 2023;14(1):3215.
78. Ichikawa M, Nakamoto N, Kredo-Russo S, et al. Bacteriophage therapy against pathological *Klebsiella pneumoniae* ameliorates the course of primary sclerosing cholangitis. Nat Commun 2023;14(1):3261.
79. Philips CA, Ahamed R, Rajesh S, et al. Long-term outcomes of stool transplant in alcohol-associated hepatitis-analysis of clinical outcomes, relapse, gut microbiota and comparisons with standard care. J Clin Exp Hepatol 2022;12(4):1124–32.
80. Philips CA, Phadke N, Ganesan K, et al. Corticosteroids, nutrition, pentoxifylline, or fecal microbiota transplantation for severe alcoholic hepatitis. Indian J Gastroenterol 2018;37(3):215–25.
81. Sharma A, Roy A, Premkumar M, et al. Fecal microbiota transplantation in alcohol-associated acute-on-chronic liver failure: an open-label clinical trial. Hepatol Int 2022;16(2):433–46.
82. Philips CA, Pande A, Shasthry SM, et al. Healthy donor fecal microbiota transplantation in steroid-ineligible severe alcoholic hepatitis: a pilot study. Clin Gastroenterol Hepatol 2017;15(4):600–2.
83. Pande A, Sharma S, Khillan V, et al. Fecal microbiota transplantation compared with prednisolone in severe alcoholic hepatitis patients: a randomized trial. Hepatol Int 2023;17(1):249–61.
84. Bajaj JS, Salzman NH, Acharya C, et al. Fecal microbial transplant capsules are safe in hepatic encephalopathy: a phase 1, randomized, placebo-controlled trial. Hepatology 2019;70(5):1690–703.
85. Marcella C, Cui B, Kelly CR, et al. Systematic review: the global incidence of faecal microbiota transplantation-related adverse events from 2000 to 2020. Aliment Pharmacol Ther 2021;53(1):33–42.
86. Bajaj JS, Gavis EA, Fagan A, et al. A randomized clinical trial of fecal microbiota transplant for alcohol use disorder. Hepatology 2021;73(5):1688–700.
87. Philips CA, Augustine P, Padsalgi G, et al. Only in the darkness can you see the stars: severe alcoholic hepatitis and higher grades of acute-on-chronic liver failure. J Hepatol 2019;70(3):550–1.

88. Morkl S, Butler MI, Holl A, et al. Probiotics and the microbiota-gut-brain Axis: focus on psychiatry. Curr Nutr Rep 2020;9(3):171–82.
89. Westfall S, Lomis N, Kahouli I, et al. Microbiome, probiotics and neurodegenerative diseases: deciphering the gut brain axis. Cell Mol Life Sci 2017;74(20): 3769–87.
90. Smith ML, Wade JB, Wolstenholme J, et al. Gut microbiome-brain-cirrhosis axis. Hepatology 2023. https://doi.org/10.1097/HEP.0000000000000344.
91. Ding JH, Jin Z, Yang XX, et al. Role of gut microbiota via the gut-liver-brain axis in digestive diseases. World J Gastroenterol 2020;26(40):6141–62.
92. Bajaj JS, Heuman DM, Hylemon PB, et al. Randomised clinical trial: *Lactobacillus* GG modulates gut microbiome, metabolome and endotoxemia in patients with cirrhosis. Aliment Pharmacol Ther 2014;39(10):1113–25.
93. Dhiman RK, Rana B, Agrawal S, et al. Probiotic VSL#3 reduces liver disease severity and hospitalization in patients with cirrhosis: a randomized, controlled trial. Gastroenterology 2014;147(6):1327–37, e3.
94. Bajaj JS, Kassam Z, Fagan A, et al. Fecal microbiota transplant from a rational stool donor improves hepatic encephalopathy: a randomized clinical trial. Hepatology 2017;66(6):1727–38.

Beyond the Liver
Neurologic Manifestations of Alcohol Use

Jiannan Huang, MD[a], Ibrahim Munaf Ahmed, MD[a],
Tian Wang, MD[b,c], Chencheng Xie, MD[a,d],*

KEYWORDS

- Alcohol withdrawal • Alcohol intoxication • Wernicke encephalopathy
- Korsakoff syndrome • Alcohol-related dementia • Cerebellar degeneration
- Peripheral neuropathy • Hepatic encephalopathy

KEY POINTS

- The acute alcohol-related complications are related to the imbalance of inhibitory and excitatory neurotransmitters.
- Alcohol direct toxicity could be exacerbated by thiamine deficiency, which induces neuronal loss and shrinkage and leads to chronic neurologic disorders.
- Distinguishing alcohol-related neurologic complications from hepatic encephalopathy remains clinically challenging, and thorough history-taking and physical examination are crucial.

INTRODUCTION

Alcohol, one of the oldest and most commonly abused substances, poses a substantial health burden.[1] In 2016, it was the leading risk factor for both disability-adjusted life-years and death among the age group between 15 and 49 years, and ranked the seventh risk factor for the entire population globally.[2]

Alcohol primarily impacts the liver due to its central role in alcohol metabolism, making it highly susceptible to alcohol-induced injury. However, alcohol's extensive distribution throughout the body also contributes to extrahepatic toxicity and various diseases. Neurologic effects associated with alcohol use are among the many

a Department of Internal Medicine, University of South Dakota Sanford School of Medicine, 1400 West 22nd Street, Sioux Falls, SD 57105, USA; b Department of Neurology, Georgetown University, Washington, DC, USA; c Georgetown University Medical Center, Comprehensive Epilepsy Center, MedStar Georgetown University Hospital, MedStar Southern Maryland Hospital Center, 10401 Hospital Drive, Suite 102, Clinton, MD 20735, USA; d Division of Hepatology, Avera McKennan Hospital & University Health Center, 1315 South Cliff Avenue, Suite 1200 Plaza 3, Sioux Falls, SD 57105, USA
* Corresponding author. Division of Hepatology, Avera McKennan Hospital & University Health Center, 1315 South Cliff Avenue, Suite 1200 Plaza 3, Sioux Falls, SD 57105.
E-mail address: Chencheng.xie@usd.edu

Clin Liver Dis 28 (2024) 681–697
https://doi.org/10.1016/j.cld.2024.06.004
liver.theclinics.com
1089-3261/24/© 2024 Elsevier Inc. All rights reserved, including those for text and data mining, AI training, and similar technologies.

extrahepatic complications with neuropsychiatric manifestations ranging from mild cognitive impairment to significant disorientation and ranging from acute impact, including intoxication/withdrawal, to long-term neurologic impairments. These manifestations, frequently encountered in clinical practice, can closely resemble hepatic encephalopathy (HE), thus complicating both diagnosis and management. Alcohol-related neurologic complications also impact the decision-making of liver transplantation for patients with end-stage liver disease. Therefore, addressing alcohol's extrahepatic neurologic manifestations is imperative in the comprehensive management of alcohol-associated liver disease.

PATHOPHYSIOLOGY

Alcohol rapidly enters the circulation with a large volume of distribution in the body.[3] It readily crosses the blood–brain barrier because of its lipophilicity and widely interacts with neurotransmitter receptors. An imbalance between the inhibitory gamma-aminobutyric acid (GABA) receptors and excitatory glutamate receptors, particularly the excitatory N-methyl-D-aspartate (NMDA) type, is implicated in various neurologic manifestations.[4] Acute and chronic alcohol use can precipitate neurologic reactions by disrupting the neurotransmitter balance. Notably, acute consumption quickly prompts GABA receptor agonism, resulting in its anxiolytic, sedative, and disinhibitory effects across multiple brain regions.[4–6] Central nervous system (CNS) adaptation involves reducing GABA receptor sensitivity coupled with the upregulation of NMDA receptor activity.[7] In chronic and regular alcohol consumers, the heightened GABA activity is counterbalanced by an increased glutamate activity.[4] However, when alcohol is cleared or when its level lowers in the system after acute cessation or a decrease in drinking behaviors, the neurotransmitter equilibrium can be disrupted again and lead toward the direction of heightened autonomic excitability and psychomotor agitation (**Fig. 1**).[4]

Chronic exposure to ethanol has been known to cause significant loss and shrinkage of cortical neurons due to direct neurotoxicity.[8] Thiamine deficiency, commonly induced by chronic alcohol use through poor diet and impaired gastrointestinal absorption, can further exacerbate these effects. Moreover, the activity of thiamine-metabolizing enzymes in the CNS is also compromised by chronic alcohol exposure.[9] Thiamine deficiency leads to a decrease in α-ketoglutarate-dehydrogenase activity in astrocytes, which in turn reduces glucose utilization and increases vulnerability to oxidative stress.[10] This deficiency can also overstimulate microglia, thereby facilitating neuronal injury. Additionally, thiamine shortage impairs the synthesis of acetylcholine, rendering cholinergic neurons more susceptible and accelerating cognitive decline, potentially hastening the progression to dementia.[10] In cases where an alcoholic patient correcting hypoglycemia without pretreatment with thiamine, the risk of lactic acidosis and cellular damage increases due to an inefficient tricarboxylic acid (TCA) cycle, potentially exacerbating Wernicke encephalopathy (WE; **Fig. 2**).[11]

Other micronutrient deficiencies may also play a role in causing neurologic complications. Vitamin B12 maintains the function of a few critical enzymes, such as homocysteine methyltransferase and methylmalonyl-CoA mutase, in the neuronal myelin synthesis process. Thus, vitamin B12 deficiency could disrupt the maintenance of myelin integrity and cause demyelination.[12] Zinc deficiency, for example, impacts synaptic function and neurotransmitter metabolism.[13] Magnesium is another commonly deficient electrolyte in patients with alcohol use disorder (AUD), and magnesium could block the calcium channel in the NMDA receptor to suppress glutamate-related

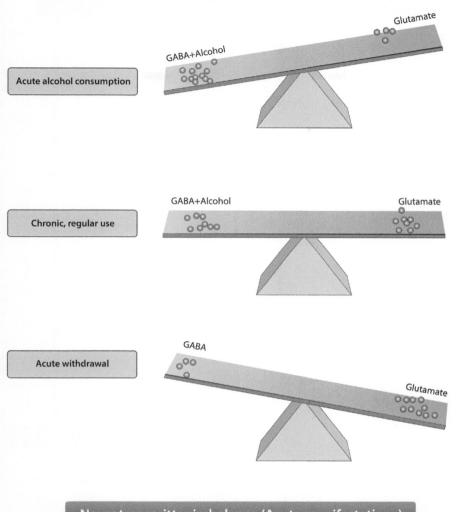

Fig. 1. Neurotransmitter imbalance in alcohol-related acute neurologic complications. Acute alcohol consumption leads to GABA receptor agonism, overpowering the excitatory glutamate activities. In chronic and regular alcohol consumers, the adaption of the CNS could counterbalance the GABA by upregulating glutamate activity and achieving a new balance. In acute withdrawal, the sudden shift of this balance toward the other side leads to heightened neurologic excitability. GABA, gamma-aminobutyric acid. (Figure modified from the work of Dr.Valenzuela CF[4]; with permission.)

excitatory signaling, thus protecting neurons from excitotoxicity-related oxidative stress or cell death.[14]

The pathophysiology mentioned earlier of alcohol-induced neurologic conditions is distinct from HE, which results from liver insufficiency and portal-systemic shunting. The distinction is crucial as it necessitates different treatment strategies.

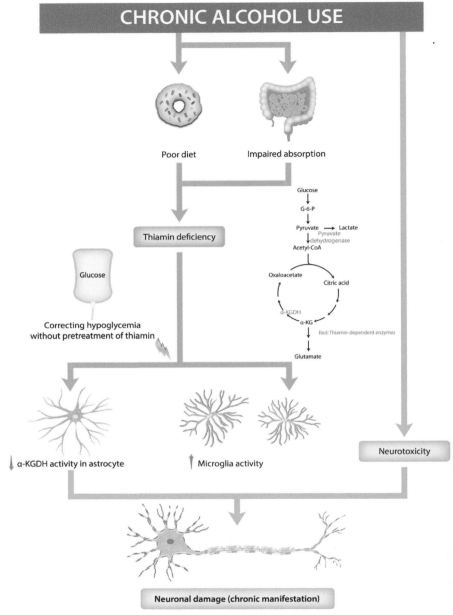

Fig. 2. Pathophysiology of chronic alcohol-related neurologic disorders. In chronic alcohol consumers, neuronal damage is mediated by both direct alcohol neurotoxicity and thiamin deficiency. Thiamin is essential for several key enzymes (*red*) in the TCA cycle, also known as the Krebs cycle. The inefficiency in the Krebs cycle caused by thiamin deficiency can be further exacerbated by correcting hypoglycemia without pretreatment of thiamin and can cause decreased alpha-ketoglutarate dehydrogenase activity and enhanced microglia activity. The direct toxicity to neurons and dysregulation of the neural supporting cells lead to neuronal damage, therefore causing chronic alcohol-related neurologic manifestations. G-6-P, glucose 6-phosphate; α-KG, alpha ketoglutarate; α-KGDH, alpha ketoglutarate dehydrogenase.

CLINICAL MANIFESTATIONS
Part I: Acute Complications

Excessive alcohol intake gives rise to various acute neurologic complications. Acute alcohol intoxication (AAI) and alcohol withdrawal syndrome (AWS) are caused by direct alcohol effects on the CNS and are commonly encountered in the emergency department. However, altered mental status (AMS) can also be caused by alcohol via various indirect mechanisms. For instance, alcohol is responsible for 28% of falls and 64% of violent events that result in traumatic brain injury.[15] Additionally, acute thiamine metabolism alteration on chronic deficiency can lead to WE, also referred to as Gayet-Wernicke encephalopathy in some European countries, which is characterized by a triad of confusion, ataxia, and oculomotor disturbances.[16] Moreover, alcohol use is often related to demyelination (such as central pontine myelinolysis, or Marchiafava–Bignami syndrome involving the corpus callosum) and metabolic alterations such as hypothermia, hypoglycemia, ketoacidosis or lactic acidosis, and electrolytes disturbances, all of which can lead to acute metabolic encephalopathy.[17] Alcohol effects can also exacerbate underlying systemic diseases, leading to AMS through cardiovascular complications such as hypotension, tachycardia, myocardial injury, and arrhythmias, often referred to as "holiday heart syndrome."[18] Furthermore, it can involve other organ systems, including the respiratory, gastrointestinal, and hepatobiliary systems, due to various mechanisms such as infectious, inflammatory (eg, pneumonia, aspiration, gastritis, and pancreatitis), thrombosis (like portal vein thrombosis), and hemorrhagic (such as Mallory–Weiss syndrome). This section will focus on reviewing AAI, AWS, and WE.

Acute alcohol intoxication

AAI is a clinical diagnosis of exclusion. As the name suggests, it manifests as transitory symptoms that arise from excessive alcohol intake. Common clinical manifestations involving psychological and neurologic aspects include impairment in cerebral functions, including judgment, memory, emotions, behaviors, and mental status. Common cerebellar signs include slurred speech, incoordination, ataxia, and nystagmus.[19]

A comprehensive diagnosis of AAI should include recognizing typical signs and symptoms, ruling out other serious mimics (eg, head trauma and metabolic imbalances), and assessing the severity. Similar neurologic manifestations can often be observed in other mimickers and should be differentiated. Because alcohol intoxication may co-occur with the use of other substances, thorough screening for substance misuse is essential. Metabolic derangements in ketones, blood glucose, and electrolytes are common in alcohol users due to their altered metabolism, especially when other comorbidities exist. Trauma is frequently presented under the influence of alcohol, leading to head injuries such as concussion or intracranial bleeding. When encephalopathy precludes detailed history-taking, a broad differential diagnosis must be considered to exclude CNS infection, stroke, seizures, and major cardiopulmonary events.

The severity of AAI can be categorized by blood alcohol concentration (BAC) levels, with symptoms ranging from mild to life-threatening. Manifestations overlapping is common across different stages. Mild AAI, with BAC between 50 and 100 mg/dL, typically involves social disinhibition, relaxation, euphoria, and increased talkativeness. Notably, mild AAI can be caused by as little as 2 to 3 standard alcoholic drinks (14 g of ethanol). Although it may not require medical intervention, it increases the risk of injury from falls and trauma. Moderate AAI develops with BAC between 100 mg/dL and 200 mg/dL and presents with more pronounced neurologic deficits, such as ataxia, hyperreflexia, incoordination, nystagmus, slurred speech, and so forth. Severe

AAI, indicated by BAC levels exceeding 200 mg/dL, may lead to significant autonomic disturbances (hypothermia and hypotension), respiratory depression, stupor, and cardiac arrest, which often necessitates health care. Episodic amnesia, often anterograde, is a useful marker indicative of a large amount and rapid rate of drinking. Complete (or "en bloc") amnesia represents global neurologic impairment, but fragmentary amnesia can occur with moderate AAI. Life-threatening intoxication occurs at BAC levels above 300 mg/dL and varies depending on individual tolerance.[20]

The treatment of moderate or severe AAI is centered on supportive care in a hospital setting. This may include the use of pharmacologic agents as well as nonpharmacologic measures such as physical restraints and one-on-one care to prevent self-harm or harm to others. Airway protection is important, entailing aspiration prevention and mechanical ventilation in an appropriate clinical context. Hypotension is a common cardiovascular complication in AAI due to volume depletion, vasodilation (autonomic deficiency), potential underlying cardiac condition, or cirrhosis. Fluid resuscitation, cardiac monitoring, and electrolyte correction are pivotal, especially in acute settings. Other supportive care essentially focuses on normalizing physiologic status and symptomatic treatment, which commonly involve treating hypothermia, hypoglycemia, acid–base state, nausea, vomiting, and so forth. One special consideration is vitamin replacement, given the potential chronic malnutrition in patients with AUD. High-dose thiamine is generally encouraged and is critical before glucose infusion to avoid precipitating WE. Alcohol-specific medications are rarely used. Among them, metadoxine, a pyrrolidone carboxylate of pyridoxine that accelerates ethanol metabolism and clearance and restores ATPs, has been approved in Europe.[21] Other drugs, such as dihydromyricetin[22] and biomimetic nanocomplexes,[23] are currently under investigation, but no clinical trial has been conducted in acute intoxication treatment.

Alcohol withdrawal syndrome
Although AWS and AAI present clinically in distinct ways, they can manifest as a continuum within the disease process due to the dynamic pathophysiology involving neurotransmitter imbalances. AWS typically presents with two or more symptoms, including autonomic hyperactivity, hand tremor, insomnia, gastroenterology upset, and the presence of transient visual, tactile, or auditory hallucinations or illusions, agitation, anxiety, and severe form could present as generalized tonic-clonic seizures. For a diagnosis to be considered, these symptoms must cause significant distress or impair the individual's social or occupational ability and rule out other causes that might mimic the presentation.[19] Notably, symptoms often develop while BAC remains high, even in the intoxication range in individuals with developed alcohol tolerance. About 59.3% of patients with AUD develop withdrawal manifestations upon reducing or ceasing alcohol consumption.[24] A history of AWS[25] and higher BAC levels[26] are predictive of developing withdrawal symptoms. Scoring systems such as the Prediction of Alcohol Withdrawal Severity Scale[27] and the admission Alcohol Use Disorders Identification Test-Piccinelli Consumption[28] can be used for their high sensitivity and specificity in predicting AWS. The presence of thrombocytopenia and hypokalemia on admission is the most predictive indicator of developing severe AWS,[25] which is defined by withdrawal delirium and/or seizures. Delirium tremens (DT) is characterized by rapid-onset fluctuating disturbances of attention and cognition in the setting of alcohol withdrawal.[29] Visual and/or auditory hallucinations are common in DT, but isolated withdrawal hallucinosis can also occur without acute attention deficits (**Fig. 3**). Withdrawal seizures, colloquially known as "rum fits," typically occur in prolonged heavy alcohol drinkers.[30] Distinct from other seizure mechanisms such as structural or metabolic alteration-related, withdrawal seizures are induced by neurotransmitter

balance shifts, therefore, typically manifest as generalized tonic–clonic convulsions.[30] DT and withdrawal seizures are the most dangerous components of AWS and usually necessitate admission to an intensive care unit (ICU).[6] The symptoms and signs can manifest several hours to days after the last alcoholic drink. Mild and common symptoms include tremors, insomnia, diaphoresis, agitation, nausea, and vomiting, which can occur as early as 6 hours following alcohol cessation (see **Fig. 3**).

Diagnosing AWS can be challenging due to frequently incomplete or unreliable patient histories. The presence of sedative medications, metabolic imbalances, and trauma can further complicate the clinical picture. AWS is a clinical diagnosis of exclusion, and it is pivotal to distinguish it from other mimickers. A wide range of differential diagnoses should include considerations for cardiopulmonary, gastrointestinal, psychiatric, and neurologic disorders. Patients with severe AWS are often managed in the ICU. Manifestations of DTs may resemble conditions such as sepsis or paroxysmal sympathetic hyperactivity, which are prevalent in medical ICUs and neurointensive care units. Therefore, physicians should be vigilant about cognitive biases. Not all encephalopathic patients with an alcohol withdrawal history have AWS. Ensuring thorough history-taking with an emphasis on recent alcohol use is critical to discerning AWS from other life-threatening illnesses.

While the administration of alcohol can alleviate withdrawal symptoms and is often utilized by patients as self-treatment, it is not a feasible treatment in health care facilities due to the barrier of titrating dosage appropriately and the potential adverse effects. The mainstay of AWS management is supportive care in conjunction with benzodiazepines, which is the conventional pharmacologic therapy. Symptom-triggered dosing of benzodiazepines is generally preferred over scheduled dosing,[6] as it often results in a lower total dosage and shortened treatment duration.[31] The Clinical Institute Withdrawal Assessment for Alcohol–Revised is a widely implemented clinical tool to gauge the severity and guide the administration of benzodiazepines.[32] Alternatively, the Minnesota Detoxification Scale (MINDS) offers the benefit of not requiring subjective information from patients.[33] Because of this, MINDS-based protocols such as the Yale Alcohol Withdrawal Protocol (YAWP)[34] or the modified YAWP (midazolam-based instead of lorazepam-based) are preferred in ICU settings or when the patient could not participate in the frequent assessment.[6] The frequency of the assessment can be as often as less than an hour and can be decreased to hourly or every 4 to 6 hours when patients are stabilized with mild symptoms. No single benzodiazepine has been noted for its efficacy in reducing mortality. Chlordiazepoxide was considered to be the most effective agent in early studies with fewer subjects[35]; however, a newer meta-analysis demonstrated comparable efficacy and safety profiles among various benzodiazepines in both scheduled and symptom-triggered manner.[36] The selection of benzodiazepines should be dictated by the pharmacokinetics and side effects. Longer acting benzodiazepines, such as chlordiazepoxide, offer a smoother withdrawal process but can be limited by the lack of intravenous formulation. On the contrary, midazolam can be favored in the ICU due to its fast onset, very short half-life (2–6 hours), and staff's familiarity with its use. Lorazepam is favored in patients with liver diseases because it undergoes minimal hepatic first-pass metabolism and is generally well tolerated.[37,38]

In cases where benzodiazepine treatment is insufficient, other medications can be considered, including those that potentiate GABA receptor activity or downregulate glutamate activity, such as barbiturates, valproic acid, propofol, gabapentin, carbamazepine, baclofen, and ketamine. Among these alternatives, phenobarbital has received increasing support in the literature as a noninferior monotherapy for AWS.[39] The advantages include superior neurochemistry (glutamate activity inhibition as well as GABA activation), reliable efficacy and pharmacokinetics, a wide therapeutic index, and sustained efficacy allowing self-tapering.[40] Dexmedetomidine, a central α-2 receptor agonist, may serve as an adjuvant sedative with the benefit of sparing respiratory inhibition and allowing arousal during sedation. Combined with benzodiazepine-based therapy, it could more effectively decrease delirium compared with benzodiazepine-based therapy alone.[41]

Wernicke encephalopathy

WE is commonly discussed along with Korsakoff syndrome (KS) due to a shared etiology of thiamine deficiency, which is commonly linked to chronic alcohol use. However, they are very distinctive in acuity and reversibility. It is also worth noticing that WE may be unmasked or precipitated by medical treatment such as refeeding or improperly correcting hypoglycemia. If left untreated, irreversible neuronal injury and structural damage in WE would occur within 2 weeks.[42] Despite being well-recognized, WE remain underdiagnosed, with autopsy studies indicating diagnosis rates as low as 20% to 25%.[42] This low rate may be an exaggeration due to inadequate sign elicitation, documentation, and data collection in those retrospective studies. Nevertheless, the diagnosis can be missed and is likely challenged by numerous confounders in patients with acute alcoholic encephalopathy and a lack of effective laboratory tests. The classic triad of symptoms—acute confusion, nystagmus (ophthalmoplegia), and ataxia—is only present in 10% of patients with WE.[43] The most widely accepted operational criteria were proposed by Caine and colleagues, which include 4 conditions (dietary deficiency, oculomotor abnormalities, cerebellar dysfunction, and altered mental state/mild memory impairment) in regular assessment of suspected WE, with 2 out of 4 solidifying the diagnosis. Although not specific, this criteria increased the diagnosis sensitivity from 22% (based on the classic triad) to 85%.[44] There are no diagnostic laboratory tests for WE. MRI might demonstrate abnormalities such as decreased T1 with contrast enhancement and increased T2 and fluid-attenuated inversion recovery signals indicative of acute lesions, often symmetrically distributed in the thalamus, periaqueductal, hypothalamus, periaqueductal gray matter, third ventricle, and cerebral cortex. Periventricular regions containing defective blood–brain barrier is a hallmark of WE due to its high thiamine-related oxidative and glucose metabolism rate. Mammillary body hemorrhage and diffusion restriction change, while not an acute marker, is also a typical finding associated with WE. Characteristic WE findings on MRI can be seen in half of the cases and are relatively specific (93%) to the diagnosis.[45,46]

Given the safety and affordability of treatment, a low threshold for empirical treatment of WE is recommended. The cornerstone of treatment is thiamine supplementation. Data suggesting a superior regimen of a certain dose, route, frequency, or duration are lacking. There is no consensus on optimum thiamine dosing. A systemic review analyzed 6 studies dated before 2021 and did not find outcome differences in regimens containing thiamine 100 mg or greater administered in a route other than orally (intravenous or intramuscular); the heterogeneity of each study caused challenges to elude definitive consensus. However, researchers recommend high-dose parental thiamine greater than 100 mg to treat patients with confirmed alcohol-induced WE.[47] Folic acid supplementation is also recommended in the acute phase of alcohol-induced WE. Multiple research studies and guidelines have suggested aggressive protocols that start with intravenous 500 mg 3 times daily for 3 to 5 days, followed by intravenous 250 mg daily for at least 3 to 5 additional days, and/or followed by oral doses.[48] A typical response to thiamine therapy is quick improvement in ophthalmoplegia within days to weeks, delayed recovery in gait disturbances, and even

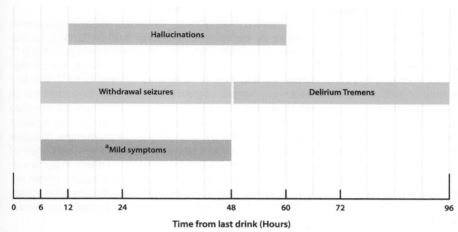

Fig. 3. A typical timeframe of alcohol withdrawal manifestations from the time of the last alcoholic drink or significant reduction in alcohol use. [a]Mild symptoms include tremors, diaphoresis, agitation, gastrointestinal symptoms, insomnia, and so forth. Hallucinations can occur within 12 to 60 hours after either a significant reduction or cessation of alcohol, while withdrawal seizures are typically observed within the range of 6 to 48 hours. DT have a later onset around the timeframe of 48 to 96 hours.

slower and potentially incomplete improvement in mental status.[10] Unfortunately, some patients experience lasting cognitive deficits, such as the amnesia characteristic of KS.

Part II: Chronic Complications

Korsakoff syndrome

KS, also known as Korsakoff psychosis—though the latter term has become less common—is typically the result of chronic nutritional depletion such as untreated thiamine deficiency and is a sequela of WE.[49] Approximately 80% of untreated patients with WE eventually develop KS.[43] KS is classified under the category of "alcohol-induced major neurocognitive disorder, amnestic confabulatory type" by DSM-5.[19] This definition can be misleading as KS is neither necessarily caused by alcohol use nor always present with confabulation.[50] The hallmark of KS is impairment in memory that is disproportionate to other cognitive functions, and patients might be alert and oriented.[50] Context memory deficit, both anterograde and retrograde, is often significantly impaired in KS.[51] Spatial and temporal context confusions lead to most instances of confabulations, which is considered a pathognomonic sign of KS.[50,51] Additionally, KS also comprises psychological manifestations that often include impaired executive dysfunction, flattened affect, apathy, and lack of illness insight.[50]

To date, no pharmacologic treatments have shown efficacy in treating KS. Clinical trials found no improvement in memory using clonidine[52] and inconsistent results with fluvoxamine treatment.[53,54] Consequently, treatment primarily emphasizes cognitive rehabilitation to enhance the patients' remaining cognitive abilities.[55] The most affected memory in KS is declarative memory ("knowing what"), which can lead to significant impairment in many patients' daily living activities. As procedural learning ("knowing how") is usually preserved in KS, thus there is growing evidence that memory rehabilitation may hold promises by improving their autonomy through learning procedures.[55]

Alcohol-related dementia

Alcohol use is one of the most common risk factors for dementia, especially at earlier ages.[56,57] Although the contemporary definition of this condition by DSM-5 further classified the subtypes (nonamnestic type vs confabulating-amnestic type),[19] alcohol-related dementia (ARD) is still an umbrella term that contains the consequences of both thiamine deficiency and long-term ethanol neurotoxicity.[58] The key feature of ARD is the persistence of multiple cognitive deficits after the cessation of prolonged alcohol use, excluding all other causes of dementia.[58,59] Physicians should be aware of the descriptive nature of the diagnosis of ARD and caution against hampering further investigation of the etiology and alternative diagnoses. Despite the observed correlation between heavy alcohol use and an increased incidence of dementia later in life, a direct causal link remains unconfirmed.[60,61] Detailed neurocognitive assessments often uncover subtler cognitive impairments, particularly within executive functions.[62] Evidence suggests that excessive alcohol consumption may induce white matter loss in the brain's frontal regions, as well as reduced metabolic activity observed in PET scans.[63,64]

Cerebellar degeneration

Alcohol-related cerebellar degeneration is considered to be one of the leading causes of acquired cerebellar ataxia and likely results from both the direct neurotoxic effects of alcohol and thiamine deficiency.[65] This condition can manifest acutely or chronically, with gait abnormalities often being the initial symptom. These gait issues can, sometimes, be incorrectly attributed to AAI. As the condition progresses, other cerebellar symptoms such as double vision (diplopia), speech difficulties (dysarthria), instability of the trunk, and incoordination of the limbs (limb ataxia) may emerge.[66] The diagnosis relies heavily on patients' detailed medical history and physical examination, with neuroimaging often revealing atrophy in the anterior superior vermis of the cerebellum.[67] More advanced stages of the disease may show greater loss of brain volume. The cornerstone of management includes abstaining from alcohol, addressing nutritional deficits, and engaging in physical therapy to improve motor function. Although recovery tends to be limited and further degeneration can occur with ongoing alcohol consumption, early intervention and sustained abstinence can help mitigate the progression of symptoms.[66]

Subacute combined degeneration

Subacute combined degeneration (SCD), although not directly caused by alcohol consumption, often occurs in the context of excessive alcohol use due to associated malnutrition, leading to vitamin B12 deficiency. SCD affects the CNS, specifically the dorsal (posterior) and lateral columns of the spinal cord; presenting with neurologic signs could be categorized as sensory dysfunction, including paresthesia in the early stage and loss of proprioception in the later stage, as well as motor dysfunction, include stiffness as early sign, and slowly progressive muscle weakness, and associated with hyperreflexia and spasticity, and progressed to paraplegia, quadriplegia, or incontinence. In addition, if the spinocerebellar tract is involved, it could present gait due to sensory ataxia.[12] SCD might present additional symptoms related to vitamin B12 deficiency, such as psychiatric disturbances, macrocytic anemia, glossitis, and laboratory check indicated low serum vitamin B12 level.[12]

Vitamin B12 supplementation has been proven effective for treating SCD. A systemic review of observational studies indicates that supplementation halts the progression of neurologic deficits, with complete resolution and improvement of signs and symptoms in approximately 14% and 86%, respectively, of patients with SCD.[68]

Peripheral neuropathy

Patients with AUD frequently exhibit neuropathic manifestations such as paresthesia, weakness, and ataxia. Although these signs and symptoms may appear similar, the underlying pathologies related to alcohol can differ in their anatomic location. It is crucial to distinguish between peripheral and central causes.

Alcohol-associated peripheral neuropathy can develop either acutely, as in the case of high radial nerve entrapment (HRNE), also known as "Saturday night palsy," where upper extremity weakness follows prolonged compression of the radial nerve above the radial groove, or insidiously, as a length-dependent and slowly progressive disorder. HRNE is typically managed conservatively, and the prognosis is usually good, with full recovery in 2 to 3 months.[69] Chronic peripheral neuropathy typically impairs sensory nerves in the lower extremities first, with motor or autonomic symptoms appearing as the condition progresses.[70] The pathogenesis includes direct neurotoxic effects of chronic alcohol exposure and deficiencies in essential micronutrients such as folate, thiamin, B6, and B12. Factors like hyperglycemia and, less frequently, heavy metal contamination in beverages may also contribute.[71] The severity of peripheral neuropathy correlates with the amount and duration of alcohol consumption. Clinically, patients may present with symmetric sensory deficits in distal lower extremities, often accompanied by neuropathic pain, diminished deep tendon reflexes, and weakness.[72]

A detailed history and physical examination are helpful when assessing neuropathy in patients with AUD. Initial evaluations typically include screening for diabetes, checking micronutrient levels, serum protein electrophoresis, and thyroid function tests. Electrophysiological testing in alcohol-related neuropathy usually demonstrates axonal neuropathy in sensory nerves. Histologic features of sural nerve biopsy usually show a small fiber predominant axonal loss.[73] Management strategies for alcohol-related peripheral neuropathy focus on supportive care, addressing nutritional deficiencies, promoting alcohol abstinence, and relieving neuropathic pain with medications like gabapentin, tricyclic antidepressants, or serotonin-norepinephrine reuptake inhibitors.[74]

DIFFERENTIATING ALCOHOL-RELATED NEUROLOGIC TOXICITY AND HEPATIC ENCEPHALOPATHY

Clinicians often encounter the challenge of differentiating between alcohol-related neurologic toxicity and HE, as both conditions share common symptoms like lethargy, extrapyramidal symptoms, seizures, and coma. It is important to recognize that HE is diagnosed by exclusion, necessitating the ruling out of other factors that could cause AMS. This task becomes particularly challenging when there is concurrent alcohol use, complicating the process of reaching a definitive diagnosis. Ultimately, the differential diagnosis is made clinically with high vigilance and familiarity with various conditions, thorough history-taking, and physical examination. A good hint for alcohol-related neurologic complications is the amount and duration of alcohol intake, as a high blood alcohol level coupled with a history of recent drinking suggests alcohol-induced disorders like AAI and AWS, and a significant amount of alcohol usage is often associated with these chronic alcohol-related neurologic disorders. On the other hand, HE is typically more probable in patients exhibiting signs of advanced liver disease, like decompensated cirrhosis or severe alcohol hepatitis, and thus could present with many physical stigmata related to liver dysfunction, such as jaundice, palmar erythema, spider telangiectasia, caput medusae, ascites, lower extremity edema, sarcopenia, fetor hepaticus, coagulopathy, and so forth. Frailty, sarcopenia, and malnutrition are commonly observed in patients with cirrhosis, stemming from the cirrhosis itself and related complications, including portal hypertension, HE, and ascites, through complex mechanisms. Nevertheless, chronic alcohol exposure is a risk factor for frailty, sarcopenia, and malnutrition.[75] Clinical context and history dictate the likelihood of each category between alcohol-related neurologic disorders and HE. Key findings in examinations could further help differentiate them. Bilateral asterixis, that is, negative myoclonus, is a frequent and early symptom of HE and is a relatively sensitive but nonspecific sign of HE, which can be presented in other metabolic or structural neurologic abnormalities, hypercapnia, hypoxia, and antiepileptics medication.[76] Thus, asterixis might be helpful in grading HE severity and monitoring response to treatment while differentiating diagnosis value is controversial. The symptoms of AWS delirium share similarities with worsening HE in terms of clinical presentation and physical examination. However, distinct characteristics of alcohol-withdrawal delirium, not seen in HE, include a pronounced and rhythmic tremor, loud shouting, and dysautonomia, such as cold sweats.[77] KS and WE might present with a mental acuity decline similar to HE. However, KS featured confabulation and profound anterograde amnesia, and WS is characterized as ophthalmoplegia, gaze-evoked nystagmus, and ataxia, which would be helpful to differentiate from HE.[77]

Ammonia has neurotoxicity and needs to be converted to urea through the urea cycle. However, in advanced liver disease, ammonia accumulates due to liver insufficiency and bypasses the liver into the systemic circulation by shunting, and an elevated ammonia level could result in neuronal dysfunction and decreased excitatory neurotransmission.[77] Sarcopenia is commonly associated with patients with cirrhosis, and in addition to the liver as an ammonia disposal organ, ammonia could be converted to glutamate in muscle. Thus, patients with sarcopenia have a relatively higher level of ammonia, and multiple studies indicated a relatively higher risk of HE among cirrhosis patients with sarcopenia status.[78] However, ammonia metabolism is intricate, involving various organs/tissues, such as blood cells and kidneys, on top of the mentioned liver and muscles. Accurate measurement of blood ammonia levels has logistical challenges and variability, depending on the blood's origin, sample handling, and analysis procedures.[79] Ammonia level might also aid in risk stratification for mortality.[80] However, it is neither a diagnostic marker nor guide therapy for HE in clinical practice.[81,82]

Significant pattern alternation in the electroencephalographic (EEG) presented in HE, and triphasic waves are associated with worsened outcomes in patients with HE.[77,83] However, findings on EEG are not specific, and the clinical rationale to utilize EEG in assessing patients with encephalopathy is to rule out nonconvulsive status epilepticus rather than as a differentiating tool for HE.[77] Noncontrast computed tomography (CT) can reveal generalized or localized cerebral edema and rule out other CNS pathologies. MRI has a similar role but is superior in detecting cerebral edema. WE might have characteristic changes on MRI that might be distinct from HE.[45,46] However, neither CT nor MRI has specific pathognomonic findings as diagnostic modalities for HE.[82]

While the multifaceted nature of these conditions and the presence of comorbidities can complicate the diagnostic process, it should not hold back starting prompt empiric treatment to cover broad possibilities. Patients' response to specific interventions may also provide retrospective confirmation of the diagnosis.

SUMMARY

The pathophysiology of alcohol's impact on the nervous system is complicated and multifaceted. The imbalance between inhibitory and excitatory neurotransmitters intrigues wide-spectrum neurologic disorders related to alcohol use. Chronic alcohol exposure leads to direct neurotoxic effects on the brain, including neuronal loss and shrinkage. Furthermore, alcohol-induced thiamine deficiency exacerbates these neurotoxic effects, leading to conditions like WE and KS. Differentiating alcohol-related neurologic toxicity from HE remains a clinical challenge due to overlapping symptoms. However, thorough history-taking, including alcohol use patterns and detailed physical examinations, is crucial in guiding the diagnosis. While certain modalities like EEG and MRI can aid in differentiating diagnosis to a certain extent, their value in clinical practice remains controversial.

CLINICS CARE POINTS

Early identification and thiamin administration:
- Be vigilant for signs of alcohol-related neurologic disorders in patients with an alcohol history. Administer thiamine prophylactically in patients with heavy alcohol use, especially before glucose administration, to prevent WE.

Awareness of chronic complications:
- Recognize the potential for chronic complications like KS, cerebellar degeneration, and peripheral neuropathy in long-term alcohol users.

Differentiating alcohol-related neurologic disorders:
- Distinguish among alcohol withdrawal, intoxication, WE, KS, and HE based on clinical history and physical examination.

DISCLOSURE

All authors have no commercial or financial conflicts of interest to disclose. There are no funding sources to disclose for this article.

REFERENCES

1. Khaderi SA. Introduction: alcohol and alcoholism. Clin Liver Dis 2019;23(1):1–10.
2. GBDA Collaborators. Alcohol use and burden for 195 countries and territories, 1990-2016: a systematic analysis for the Global Burden of Disease Study 2016. Lancet 2018;392(10152):1015–35.
3. Norberg A, Jones AW, Hahn RG, et al. Role of variability in explaining ethanol pharmacokinetics: research and forensic applications. Clin Pharmacokinet 2003;42(1):1–31.
4. Valenzuela CF. Alcohol and neurotransmitter interactions. Alcohol Health Res World 1997;21(2):144–8.
5. Harrison NL, Skelly MJ, Grosserode EK, et al. Effects of acute alcohol on excitability in the CNS. Neuropharmacology 2017;122:36–45.
6. Farrokh S, Roels C, Owusu KA, et al. Alcohol withdrawal syndrome in neurocritical care unit: assessment and treatment challenges. Neurocrit Care 2021;34(2):593–607.
7. Holloway HC, Hales RE, Watanabe HK. Recognition and treatment of acute alcohol withdrawal syndromes. Psychiatr Clin North Am 1984;7(4):729–43.
8. Brust JC. Ethanol and cognition: indirect effects, neurotoxicity and neuroprotection: a review. Int J Environ Res Public Health 2010;7(4):1540–57.
9. Langlais PJ. Alcohol-related thiamine deficiency: impact on cognitive and memory functioning. Alcohol Health Res World 1995;19(2):113–21.

10. Wijnia JW. A clinician's view of Wernicke-Korsakoff Syndrome. J Clin Med 2022; 11(22).
11. Singleton CK, Martin PR. Molecular mechanisms of thiamine utilization. Curr Mol Med 2001;1(2):197–207.
12. Qudsiya Z, De Jesus O. Subacute combined degeneration of the spinal cord. Treasure Island, FL: StatPearls; 2024.
13. Skalny AV, Skalnaya MG, Grabeklis AR, et al. Zinc deficiency as a mediator of toxic effects of alcohol abuse. Eur J Nutr 2018;57(7):2313–22.
14. Kirkland AE, Sarlo GL, Holton KF. The role of magnesium in neurological disorders. Nutrients 2018;10(6).
15. Maas AIR, Menon DK, Manley GT, et al. Traumatic brain injury: progress and challenges in prevention, clinical care, and research. Lancet Neurol 2022;21(11): 1004–60.
16. Slim S, Ayed K, Triki W, et al. Gayet-Wernicke's encephalopathy complicating prolonged parenteral nutrition in patient treated for colonic cancer - a case report. BMC Nutr 2022;8(1):83.
17. Wolfe M, Menon A, Oto M, et al. Alcohol and the central nervous system. Pract Neurol 2023;23(4):273–85.
18. Mirijello A, Sestito L, Lauria C, et al. Echocardiographic markers of early alcoholic cardiomyopathy: six-month longitudinal study in heavy drinking patients. Eur J Intern Med 2022;101:76–85.
19. American Psychiatric Association. Diagnostic and statistical manual of mental disorders: DSM-5. 5th edition. Washington, DC: American Psychiatric Association; 2013.
20. D'Angelo A, Petrella C, Greco A, et al. Acute alcohol intoxication: a clinical overview. Clin Ter 2022;173(3):280–91.
21. Haass-Koffler CL, Akhlaghi F, Swift RM, et al. Altering ethanol pharmacokinetics to treat alcohol use disorder: can you teach an old dog new tricks? J Psychopharmacol 2017;31(7):812–8.
22. Shen Y, Lindemeyer AK, Gonzalez C, et al. Dihydromyricetin as a novel anti-alcohol intoxication medication. J Neurosci 2012;32(1):390–401.
23. Liu Y, Du J, Yan M, et al. Biomimetic enzyme nanocomplexes and their use as antidotes and preventive measures for alcohol intoxication. Nat Nanotechnol 2013; 8(3):187–92.
24. Schuckit MA, Danko GP, Smith TL, et al. A 5-year prospective evaluation of DSM-IV alcohol dependence with and without a physiological component. Alcohol Clin Exp Res 2003;27(5):818–25.
25. Goodson CM, Clark BJ, Douglas IS. Predictors of severe alcohol withdrawal syndrome: a systematic review and meta-analysis. Alcohol Clin Exp Res 2014; 38(10):2664–77.
26. Kapur JH, Rajamanickam V, Fleming MF. Can the blood alcohol concentration be a predictor for increased hospital complications in trauma patients involved in motor vehicle crashes? Int J Environ Res Public Health 2010;7(3):1174–85.
27. Wood E, Albarqouni L, Tkachuk S, et al. Will this hospitalized patient develop severe alcohol withdrawal syndrome?: the rational clinical examination systematic review. JAMA 2018;320(8):825–33.
28. Pecoraro A, Ewen E, Horton T, et al. Using the AUDIT-PC to predict alcohol withdrawal in hospitalized patients. J Gen Intern Med 2014;29(1):34–40.
29. Schuckit MA. Recognition and management of withdrawal delirium (delirium tremens). N Engl J Med 2014;371(22):2109–13.

30. Rogawski MA. Update on the neurobiology of alcohol withdrawal seizures. Epilepsy Curr 2005;5(6):225–30.
31. Daeppen JB, Gache P, Landry U, et al. Symptom-triggered vs fixed-schedule doses of benzodiazepine for alcohol withdrawal: a randomized treatment trial. Arch Intern Med 2002;162(10):1117–21.
32. Sullivan JT, Sykora K, Schneiderman J, et al. Assessment of alcohol withdrawal: the revised clinical institute withdrawal assessment for alcohol scale (CIWA-Ar). Br J Addict 1989;84(11):1353–7.
33. DeCarolis DD, Rice KL, Ho L, et al. Symptom-driven lorazepam protocol for treatment of severe alcohol withdrawal delirium in the intensive care unit. Pharmacotherapy 2007;27(4):510–8.
34. Heavner JJ, Akgün KM, Heavner MS, et al. Implementation of an ICU-specific alcohol withdrawal syndrome management protocol reduces the need for mechanical ventilation. Pharmacotherapy 2018;38(7):701–13.
35. Holbrook AM, Crowther R, Lotter A, et al. Meta-analysis of benzodiazepine use in the treatment of acute alcohol withdrawal. CMAJ (Can Med Assoc J) 1999;160(5): 649–55.
36. Bahji A, Bach P, Danilewitz M, et al. Comparative efficacy and safety of pharmacotherapies for alcohol withdrawal: a systematic review and network meta-analysis. Addiction 2022;117(10):2591–601.
37. Trifu S, Țibîrnă A, Costea RV, et al. A multidisciplinary approach to the management of liver disease and alcohol disorders in psychiatric settings (Review). Exp Ther Med 2021;21(3):271.
38. LiverTox. National institute of health. Available at: http://LiverTox.nih.gov. [Accessed 26 December 2023].
39. Nisavic M, Nejad SH, Isenberg BM, et al. Use of phenobarbital in alcohol withdrawal management - a retrospective comparison study of phenobarbital and benzodiazepines for acute alcohol withdrawal management in general medical patients. Psychosomatics 2019;60(5):458–67.
40. Umar Z, Haseeb Ul Rasool M, Muhammad S, et al. Phenobarbital and alcohol withdrawal syndrome: a systematic review and meta-analysis. Cureus 2023; 15(1):e33695.
41. Woods AD, Giometti R, Weeks SM. The use of dexmedetomidine as an adjuvant to benzodiazepine-based therapy to decrease the severity of delirium in alcohol withdrawal in adult intensive care unit patients: a systematic review. JBI Database System Rev Implement Rep 2015;13(1):224–52.
42. Sechi G, Serra A. Wernicke's encephalopathy: new clinical settings and recent advances in diagnosis and management. Lancet Neurol 2007;6(5):442–55.
43. Sinha S, Kataria A, Kolla BP, et al. Wernicke encephalopathy-clinical pearls. Mayo Clin Proc 2019;94(6):1065–72.
44. Caine D, Halliday GM, Kril JJ, et al. Operational criteria for the classification of chronic alcoholics: identification of Wernicke's encephalopathy. J Neurol Neurosurg Psychiatry 1997;62(1):51–60.
45. Antunez E, Estruch R, Cardenal C, et al. Usefulness of CT and MR imaging in the diagnosis of acute Wernicke's encephalopathy. AJR Am J Roentgenol 1998; 171(4):1131–7.
46. Sullivan EV, Pfefferbaum A. Neuroimaging of the wernicke-Korsakoff syndrome. Alcohol Alcohol Mar-Apr 2009;44(2):155–65.
47. Smith H, McCoy M, Varughese K, et al. Thiamine dosing for the treatment of alcohol-induced wernicke's encephalopathy: a review of the literature. J Pharm Technol 2021;37(2):107–13.

48. Pruckner N, Baumgartner J, Hinterbuchinger B, et al. Thiamine substitution in alcohol use disorder: a narrative review of medical guidelines. Eur Addict Res 2019;25(3):103–10.

49. Kopelman MD, Thomson AD, Guerrini I, et al. The Korsakoff syndrome: clinical aspects, psychology and treatment. Alcohol Alcohol Mar-Apr 2009;44(2):148–54.

50. Arts NJ, Walvoort SJ, Kessels RP. Korsakoff's syndrome: a critical review. Neuropsychiatr Dis Treat 2017;13:2875–90.

51. Kessels RP, Kopelman MD. Context memory in Korsakoff's syndrome. Neuropsychol Rev 2012;22(2):117–31.

52. O'Carroll RE, Moffoot A, Ebmeier KP, et al. Korsakoff's syndrome, cognition and clonidine. Psychol Med 1993;23(2):341–7.

53. O'Carroll RE, Moffoot AP, Ebmeier KP, et al. Effects of fluvoxamine treatment on cognitive functioning in the alcoholic Korsakoff syndrome. Psychopharmacology (Berl) 1994;116(1):85–8.

54. Martin PR, Adinoff B, Lane E, et al. Fluvoxamine treatment of alcoholic amnestic disorder. Eur Neuropsychopharmacol 1995;5(1):27–33.

55. Oudman E, Nijboer TC, Postma A, et al. Procedural learning and memory rehabilitation in Korsakoff's Syndrome - a review of the literature. Neuropsychol Rev 2015;25(2):134–48.

56. Harvey RJ, Skelton-Robinson M, Rossor MN. The prevalence and causes of dementia in people under the age of 65 years. J Neurol Neurosurg Psychiatry 2003; 74(9):1206–9.

57. Picard C, Pasquier F, Martinaud O, et al. Early onset dementia: characteristics in a large cohort from academic memory clinics. Alzheimer Dis Assoc Disord 2011; 25(3):203–5.

58. Cheng C, Huang CL, Tsai CJ, et al. Alcohol-related dementia: a systemic review of epidemiological studies. Psychosomatics 2017;58(4):331–42.

59. Schmidt KS, Gallo JL, Ferri C, et al. The neuropsychological profile of alcohol-related dementia suggests cortical and subcortical pathology. Dement Geriatr Cogn Disord 2005;20(5):286–91.

60. Rehm J, Hasan OSM, Black SE, et al. Alcohol use and dementia: a systematic scoping review. Alzheimer's Res Ther 2019;11(1):1.

61. Sabia S, Fayosse A, Dumurgier J, et al. Alcohol consumption and risk of dementia: 23 year follow-up of Whitehall II cohort study. Bmj 2018;362:k2927.

62. Montgomery C, Fisk JE, Murphy PN, et al. The effects of heavy social drinking on executive function: a systematic review and meta-analytic study of existing literature and new empirical findings. Hum Psychopharmacol 2012;27(2):187–99.

63. Kril JJ, Halliday GM, Svoboda MD, et al. The cerebral cortex is damaged in chronic alcoholics. Neuroscience 1997;79(4):983–98.

64. Adams KM, Gilman S, Koeppe RA, et al. Neuropsychological deficits are correlated with frontal hypometabolism in positron emission tomography studies of older alcoholic patients. Alcohol Clin Exp Res 1993;17(2):205–10.

65. Shanmugarajah PD, Hoggard N, Currie S, et al. Alcohol-related cerebellar degeneration: not all down to toxicity? Cerebellum Ataxias 2016;3:17.

66. Laureno R. Nutritional cerebellar degeneration, with comments on its relationship to Wernicke disease and alcoholism. Handb Clin Neurol 2012;103:175–87.

67. Anderson CM, Rabi K, Lukas SE, et al. Cerebellar lingula size and experiential risk factors associated with high levels of alcohol and drug use in young adults. Cerebellum 2010;9(2):198–209.

68. Vasconcelos OM, Poehm EH, McCarter RJ, et al. Potential outcome factors in subacute combined degeneration: review of observational studies. J Gen Intern Med 2006;21(10):1063–8.
69. Węgiel A, Karauda P, Zielinska N, et al. Radial nerve compression: anatomical perspective and clinical consequences. Neurosurg Rev 2023;46(1):53.
70. Julian T, Glascow N, Syeed R, et al. Alcohol-related peripheral neuropathy: a systematic review and meta-analysis. J Neurol 2019;266(12):2907–19.
71. Chopra K, Tiwari V. Alcoholic neuropathy: possible mechanisms and future treatment possibilities. Br J Clin Pharmacol 2012;73(3):348–62.
72. Sosenko JM, Soto R, Aronson J, et al. The prevalence and extent of vibration sensitivity impairment in men with chronic ethanol abuse. J Stud Alcohol 1991; 52(4):374–6.
73. Bosch EP, Pelham RW, Rasool CG, et al. Animal models of alcoholic neuropathy: morphologic, electrophysiologic, and biochemical findings. Muscle Nerve 1979; 2(2):133–44.
74. Watson JC, Dyck PJ. Peripheral neuropathy: a practical approach to diagnosis and symptom management. Mayo Clin Proc 2015;90(7):940–51.
75. Lai JC, Tandon P, Bernal W, et al. Malnutrition, frailty, and sarcopenia in patients with cirrhosis: 2021 practice guidance by the American association for the study of liver diseases. Hepatology 2021;74(3):1611–44.
76. Ellul MA, Cross TJ, Larner AJ. Asterixis. Pract Neurol 2017;17(1):60–2.
77. Wijdicks EF. Hepatic encephalopathy. N Engl J Med 2016;375(17):1660–70.
78. Jindal A, Jagdish RK. Sarcopenia: ammonia metabolism and hepatic encephalopathy. Clin Mol Hepatol 2019;25(3):270–9.
79. Deutsch-Link S, Moon AM, Jiang Y, et al. Serum ammonia in cirrhosis: clinical impact of hyperammonemia, utility of testing, and national testing trends. Clin Ther 2022;44(3):e45–57.
80. Bhatia V, Singh R, Acharya SK. Predictive value of arterial ammonia for complications and outcome in acute liver failure. Gut 2006;55(1):98–104.
81. Haj M, Rockey DC. Ammonia levels do not guide clinical management of patients with hepatic encephalopathy caused by cirrhosis. Am J Gastroenterol 2020; 115(5):723–8.
82. American Association for the Study of Liver D, European Association for the Study of the L. Hepatic encephalopathy in chronic liver disease: 2014 practice guideline by the European association for the study of the liver and the American association for the study of liver diseases. J Hepatol 2014;61(3):642–59.
83. Ficker DM, Westmoreland BF, Sharbrough FW. Epileptiform abnormalities in hepatic encephalopathy. J Clin Neurophysiol 1997;14(3):230–4.

Diagnosis of Alcohol Use Disorder and Alcohol-Associated Liver Disease

Katie Witkiewitz, PhD[a],*, Anne C. Fernandez, PhD[b],
Ellen W. Green, MD, PhD[c], Jessica L. Mellinger, MD, MSc[b,d]

KEYWORDS

- Alcohol use disorder • Alcohol dependence • Harm reduction
- Alcohol-associated liver disease • Alcohol-associated hepatitis
- Liver transplantation

KEY POINTS

- Alcohol use disorder (AUD) is among the most common psychiatric disorders and excessive drinking is attributable to 5.1% of the global burden of disease and injury.
- Most individuals with AUD never receive treatment and the primary reasons for not seeking treatment include not wanting to stop drinking, lack of access to treatment, and concerns about stigma.
- Alcohol-associated liver disease (ALD) is also increasing, and there is growing research on the need for coordinated medical and psychosocial care for individuals with AUD and/or ALD. Early intervention can reduce alcohol use and prevent progression to alcohol-associated hepatitis.
- Liver transplantation is effective in treating ALD, including alcohol-associated hepatitis.

INTRODUCTION

Alcohol has been consumed by humans and non-human animals for as long as we have historical records, with earliest evidence of human alcohol consumption dating back to 7000 BC.[1] Paleogenetic analyses have identified that a mutation in the enzyme alcohol dehydrogenase class 4, which improved primates' ability to metabolize alcohol, first appeared over 10 million years ago.[2] In present day, alcohol is the most commonly used psychoactive substance worldwide. Data from 2017 indicate

[a] Center on Alcohol, Substance Use, and Addictions, University of New Mexico, 2650 Yale Boulevard Southeast, Albuquerque, NM 87106, USA; [b] Department of Psychiatry, University of Michigan, 1500 East Medical Center Drive, Ann Arbor, MI 48109, USA; [c] Division of Gastroenterology & Hepatology, University of North Carolina, 130 Mason Farm Road, Bioinformatics Building CB# 7080, Chapel Hill, NC 27599-7080, USA; [d] Department of Medicine, University of Michigan
* Corresponding author.
E-mail address: katiew@unm.edu

Clin Liver Dis 28 (2024) 699–713
https://doi.org/10.1016/j.cld.2024.06.009
1089-3261/24/© 2024 Elsevier Inc. All rights reserved, including those for text and data mining, AI training, and similar technologies.

liver.theclinics.com

47% of the world population are current drinkers of alcohol, and the adult per-capita consumption of alcohol is estimated at 6.5 L of per alcohol per adult.[3]

Given the high level of consumption worldwide, it follows that alcohol use disorder (AUD) is one of the most prevalent psychiatric disorders, globally. Recent estimates of global lifetime prevalence of AUD have been estimated at 8.6%[4] (range: 3.8% to 97.1% within individual countries). There are also tremendous human and social costs of AUD. More than 3 million people die annually worldwide due to causes related to alcohol, and alcohol is attributable to 5.1% of the global burden of disease and injury.[5]

One of the many factors that has contributed to the burden of harmful alcohol use and AUD worldwide is the lack of treatment access and very low rates of seeking treatment for alcohol-related problems. The majority of individuals who engage in harmful alcohol use and those with AUD will never seek treatment[6] with recent estimates of 17.3% of individuals with AUD worldwide receiving AUD treatment services and even lower rates in lower and middle income countries.[7] The primary reasons for not seeking treatment include not wanting to stop drinking, lack of access to treatment, and concerns about stigma.[6]

Given high rates of AUD and lack of treatment, it is not surprising that alcohol-associated liver disease (ALD) is also a prevalent and costly disease. Previously thought of as a disease of older, white males, recent changes have demonstrated a marked and disproportionate increase in ALD in younger people, females, and some minoritized racial and ethnic groups. While overall ALD prevalence is approximately 8.1% in the United States, the prevalence of more severe forms of ALD has risen disproportionately over time, with an increase in more advanced ALD from 2.2% to 6.6% from 2001 to 2016.[8] In the United States, cirrhosis-related mortality increased 65% from 1999 to 2016 and was driven almost entirely by ALD.[9] The most severe form of ALD, alcohol-associated hepatitis, which carries a 30% to 50% mortality rate at 6 months, has also increased in recent years, particularly during the coronavirus disease 2019 (COVID-19) pandemic which saw a 60% increase in waitlisting and transplants for alcohol-associated hepatitis.[10,11] Increased alcohol use, especially amongst females and young people, has fueled the rising ALD rates. Metabolic-associated steatotic liver disease, a liver disease similar to ALD histologically, occurs in the presence of the metabolic syndrome (obesity, hypertension, diabetes, dyslipidemia) and results in synergistic damage to the liver.[10] Liver disease from both alcohol use and metabolic syndrome has been termed MetALD,[12] and rising rates of metabolic syndrome and obesity in the United States are almost certainly contributing to the increase in MetALD.

DIAGNOSIS OF ALCOHOL USE DISORDER

The diagnosis of AUD has shifted substantially over the past 74 years. The first edition of the Diagnostic and Statistical Manual for Mental Disorders (DSM) published by the American Psychiatric Association in 1952[13] described "alcoholism" within a broader classification of Sociopathic Personality Disorder. The second edition of the DSM, published in 1968,[14] included text descriptions for problems caused by alcohol use that were divided into 3 categories: alcohol dependence, episodic excessive drinking, and habitual excessive drinking. In the 1970s Feighner[15] and Spitzer[16] published diagnostic criteria for the disease of "alcoholism" based on observational research studies to inform research and practice.[17] The third and fourth editions of the DSM would take a similar approach of creating diagnostic categories based on symptoms, with the designation of alcohol abuse and alcohol dependence as separate diagnostic categories.[18,19] In 2013, the fifth edition of the DSM was published[20] and AUD was considered a single diagnosis, based on endorsing 2 or more of 11 criteria (**Fig. 1**) measuring impaired control over alcohol use, social and occupational impairment from drinking, alcohol use that causes harm, and physiologic consequences of heavy drinking. DSM-5 also added a severity continuum based on the number of criteria endorsed such that individuals can now be classified as mild (2–3 criteria), moderate (4–5 criteria), or severe (6 or more criteria).

The International Classification of Diseases (ICD), published by the World Health Organization (WHO), has followed a similar trajectory as the DSM. The diagnosis of alcohol dependence in ICD-11[21] changed from prior versions of the ICD and also was a point of departure from the 11 criteria of DSM-5, as shown in **Fig. 1**, with only 3 diagnostic features and at least 2 required for a diagnosis: impaired control over alcohol use, alcohol interferes with life and often continues despite problems,

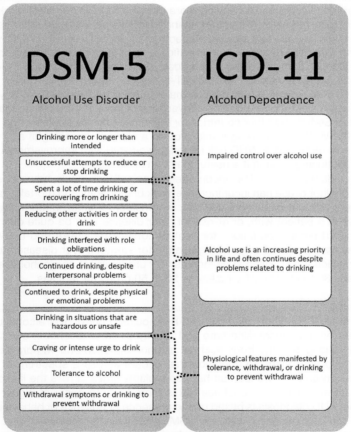

Fig. 1. Criteria for the diagnosis of alcohol use disorder in the Diagnostic and Statistical Manual for Mental Disorders-5 and alcohol dependence in the International Classification of Diseases-11, with both systems using a past 12-month time frame for presence of criteria. Dotted lines indicate conceptual overlap in criteria between the 2 systems.

and physiologic features indicative of neuroadaptations to alcohol.[22] ICD-11 has better concordance with earlier versions of the ICD and DSM-IV, and DSM-5 may be inclusive of a larger group of people with problems related to alcohol.[23]

Harmful Alcohol Use

Alcohol use occurs across a spectrum. As alcohol use increases in quantity and frequency so does the risk of developing or worsening medical conditions (eg, liver disease), mental health problems, and AUD. Heavy alcohol use is also more likely to lead to acute health risks such as accidents and injuries. These harms from alcohol use increase in a dose dependent fashion. For this reason, alcohol-related harm or risk is typically defined as the quantity and frequency of standard drinks consumed over a given time interval (eg, average standard drinks a day in the past month).

In the United States, the National Institute on Alcohol Abuse and Alcoholism (NIAAA) defines harmful alcohol use as having more than 4 (males)/3 (females) drinks on any day or more than 14 (males)/7 (females) standard drinks per week. Another useful definition that takes into account a broader spectrum of alcohol risk is the WHO risk drinking levels.[24] The WHO defines 4 sex-specific levels of drinking risk, based on average grams of alcohol consumed per day (g/day), that correspond to low (1–40 g/day males; 1–20 g/day females), medium (41–60 g/day males; 21–40 g/day females), high (61–100 g/day males; 41–60 g/day females), or very high risk (>100 g/day males; > 60 g/day for females). Corresponding conversions of these cut-offs to standard drinks in the United States and other countries for these cut-offs are available and shown in **Table 1**. The WHO risk drinking levels provide a clinically meaningful and validated endpoint, and reduction in WHO risk level is associated with improvements in health and liver functioning making it a useful metric in clinical care.[25–27]

Drinking reductions should be encouraged among all individuals, however even very low levels of alcohol use can incur increased risk of morbidity and mortality, and there is no current amount of alcohol use that is considered safe. Furthermore, harmful alcohol use in a patient with, or at-risk for, liver disease may be quite different than these standard recommendations for healthy adults. The NIAAA and the WHO risk drinking levels, somewhat align with guidance for steototic liver disease subclassification, for which ALD is defined as increasingly predominant as alcohol use reaches and exceeds 30 to 60 g/day for males, or 20 to 50 g/day for females.

Alcohol Use Disorder

AUD is a medical condition characterized by impaired control over alcohol use, consequences from use, increasing time and priority given to alcohol in one's life, and physiologic changes in the body such as alcohol tolerance and withdrawal. AUD is also a chronic and relapsing condition that occurs across a spectrum of severity. AUD remission and recurrence can happen multiple times across the lifespan. AUD can occur at any level of alcohol use but is more likely to occur at higher levels of alcohol use. AUD diagnosis is based on the presence or absence of behavioral symptoms and can be diagnosed using the DSM-5[20] or ICD-11,[21] shown in **Fig. 1**. Those who do not meet AUD diagnostic criteria for 3 months are considered in early remission, and those who do not meet criteria for 12 months are considered in sustained remission.

Assessment

Alcohol consumption and AUD should be evaluated at regular intervals. Regular assessment can lead to timely intervention and treatment given that changes in alcohol use and return to drinking are common even after a period of abstinence. In

Table 1
World health organization risk drinking levels converted to standard drink sizes

	Low Risk	Medium Risk	High Risk	Very High Risk
World Health Organization Drinking Risk Levels (for males)				
Drinks per day (in grams)	1–40 g	41–60 g	61–100 g	101+ g
Drinks per day (in Australia, Germany, France, 10 g)	1–4 drinks	4.1–6 drinks	6.1–10 drinks	10.1+ drinks
Drinks per day (in United Kingdom, Iceland standard drinks, 8 g)	1–5 drinks	5.1–7.5 drinks	7.6–12.5 drinks	12.6+ drinks
Drinks per day (in US standard drinks, 14 g)	1–2.9 drinks	3.0–4.3 drinks	4.4–7.1 drinks	7.2+ drinks
World Health Organization Drinking Risk Levels (for females)				
Drinks per day (in grams)	1–20 g	21–40 g	41–60 g	61+ g
Drinks per day (in Australia, Germany, France, 10 g)	1–2 drinks	2.1–4 drinks	4.1–6 drinks	6.1+ drinks
Drinks per day (in United Kingdom, Iceland standard drinks, 8 g)	1–2.5 drinks	2.6–5 drinks	5.1–7.5 drinks	7.6+ drinks
Drinks per day (in US standard drinks, 14 g)	1–1.4 drinks	1.5–2.8 drinks	2.9–4.3 drinks	4.4+ drinks

addition to standard clinical interviews, we recommend 3 types of assessment to capture key alcohol-related information: (1) self-report questionnaires and interviews that assess alcohol consumption, (2) AUD symptom assessments, and (3) alcohol-related biomarkers.

Alcohol consumption should be assessed using validated alcohol screening instruments. These instruments are often short and easy to embed into measurement-based care digitally or given in person at clinics. One such instrument is the AUDIT-C,[28] a 3-item assessment of alcohol quantity and frequency. Alternatively, the 10-item AUDIT[29] assesses alcohol use as well as domains related to AUD symptoms. The Timeline Follow-Back is a gold standard for measuring frequency and intensity of alcohol consumption using a calendar-based method.[30]

For patients who drink at any level of risk, a full diagnostic assessment of AUD should occur via clinical interview by a trained provider for diagnostic accuracy. Common comorbid conditions, such as depression, anxiety, and other substance use disorders, should also be assessed. This may require the involvement of a psychosocial team member, or referral to an addiction specialist. However, when this is not possible we recommend using a brief alcohol symptom checklist[31] or using the AUDIT to assess domains relevant to AUD symptoms which can inform clinical decision making.

Direct alcohol biomarkers are also recommended.[32] Phosphatidylethanol (PEth) is a highly specific and sensitive biomarker that can detect alcohol use or cessation over a 3 to 4 week period.[33] Interpretive guidelines for PEth levels provide ability to categorize consumption levels corresponding to no/light, moderate, or heavy alcohol consumption.[34] PEth has been shown to correspond with objective measures of alcohol consumption.[35] Other biomarkers, such as urine ethyl glucuronide or urine ethyl sulfate, are relatively common and inexpensive and can detect alcohol use in the past 3 to 5 days. With patient consent, family members or loved ones can also be useful sources of information when assessing alcohol use to corroborate self-report or when an individual is unable to self-report (eg, cognitively impaired or unconscious).

DIAGNOSIS OF ALCOHOL-ASSOCIATED LIVER DISEASE

The era of deepened understanding of ALD pathophysiology abutted the first liver transplantation in humans by Thomas Starzl in 1963.[36] Though early attempts yielded short survival durations and a brief international moratorium on the surgery, improvement in immunosuppression with cyclosporine extended survival in the late 1970s and liver transplantation was accepted by the American Association of the Study of Liver Diseases (AASLD) in November 1982. It was approved by the National Institutes of Health Consensus Development Conference the following June, including ALD as an appropriate liver transplantation indication if alcohol abstinence was achieved giving rise to the informal recommendation of 6 months of alcohol abstinence as a liver transplantation prerequisite.[37–39]

Liver transplantation for ALD, though hampered by stigma, was undertaken but considered exceptionally challenging in the 1980s with the perspective that increased risk of complications due to malnourishment and infection, and overall lower survival was noted.[40–42] Advocates of liver transplantation in ALD emerged, including Starzl, who published not only on the equal post-operative survival with cyclosporine immunosuppression in patients with ALD as compared to those with other causes of liver failure in 1988.[43] As heterogeneity developed among liver transplantation centers in approach to liver transplantation in ALD, physicians from the University of Michigan Alcohol Research Center proposed a pre-liver transplantation evaluation based on 4 domains (diagnosis, patient/family recognition of the disease, social stability, and prognostic factors) on the basis that pre-operative abstinence did not predict surgical or return to drinking outcomes.[44] This group went on to demonstrate excellent, equivalent survival of 45 patients with ALD requiring liver transplantation who underwent multidisciplinary evaluation, and only 2 patients were found to return to hazardous alcohol use.[45]

The growth of liver transplantation for ALD indications continued to revolve around the controversy of the pre-transplant sobriety period.[46] This was most notably restrictive of liver transplantation for patients suffering from severe alcohol-associated hepatitis. This barrier to transplant for alcohol-associated hepatitis was prominently challenged by the 2011 French-Belgian study which demonstrated 70% survival of the 26 carefully selected patients with alcohol-associated hepatitis as compared to the dismal 20% of the matched controls, and that return to alcohol was late and rare.[47] The ACCELERATE-AH consortium then re-demonstrated 94%, 1-year survival of 147 patients transplanted for severe alcohol-associated hepatitis.[48]

As the AASLD sought to decrease stigma by reforming its lexicon, "alcoholic" for "alcohol-associated,[49]" and encourage concomitant AUD treatment,[50,51] the COVID-19 pandemic ignited the rates of AUD and ALD in the United States and doubled the rates of liver transplantation for alcohol-associated hepatitis.[52,53] This prompted the proposal from the Dallas Consensus Conference of criteria to evaluate patients for liver transplantation in alcohol-associated hepatitis.[54] Understanding of AUD and return to use after liver transplantation in patients transplanted for ALD indications continues to evolve, with further nuanced means of monitoring[55,56] and understanding of patterns of post-liver transplantation return to alcohol use.[57] There continues to be lack of consensus in the liver transplantation field and in the AUD research field, generally, regarding how to define relapse, slip, versus return to heavy drinking.[58]

ALD comprises a spectrum of liver damage. The earliest form of liver damage from alcohol use is steatosis, or fatty liver. Steatosis from alcohol occurs in most patient (>90%) when chronically consuming 20 to 50 g per day for females or 60 to 80 g per day for males for at least 2 weeks.[49] With 4 to 6 weeks of total abstinence, steatosis can resolve. With continued heavy drinking, however, approximately 20% to 40% of these patients who develop steatosis will go on to develop inflammation (steatohepatitis) and scarring (fibrosis). Grades F3 and F4 are considered advanced chronic liver disease (ACLD) as such patients have increased risk of mortality over time.[59] Patients who have cirrhosis but who have not developed symptoms of portal hypertension (eg, ascites, variceal bleeding, jaundice, or hepatic encephalopathy) are termed compensated cirrhosis or compensated ACLD (cACLD) and those who have developed such symptoms are considered decompensated ACLD or decompensated cirrhosis. Decompensated cirrhosis portends significantly worse prognosis overall.[59] However, for those with ACLD secondary to alcohol use, complete alcohol cessation can lead to recompensation and fibrosis regression.[59] Finally, the most severe form of liver disease, alcohol-associated hepatitis, which is defined by clinical diagnosis and biopsy,[60] can occur at any timepoint in the spectrum of liver disease, though most frequently co-occurs with cirrhosis.[61] Alcohol-associated hepatitis is a severe hepatic and systemic inflammation that occurs in the presence of heavy alcohol use, but is likely influenced by other factors, such as genetic predispositions as well.

The diagnosis of ALD involves assessing levels of alcohol use and AUD, as noted above, and diagnosing the stage of ALD. Earlier stages of ALD, particularly steatosis, may be challenging to diagnose as these early stages are usually asymptomatic and may not be accompanied by liver enzyme changes. In some cases, physical examination will disclose an enlarged liver by palpation. Common liver enzyme elevations of aspartate aminotransferase (AST) and gamma-glutamyl transferase may indicate the presence of alcohol use. Other liver enzyme elevations (alanine aminotransferase [ALT], alkaline phosphatase, and/or bilirubin) may also be elevated with steatohepatitis and more advanced stages, though this is not uniform. Diagnosis of steatosis can be made with imaging such as ultrasound, computed tomography, or MRI. Liver biopsy is not required for steatosis diagnosis typically.

Staging of fibrosis can be performed using non-invasive tests (NITs) or liver biopsy. NITs are more popular due to their relative ease of performance and the avoidance of liver biopsy and its potential complications. Commonly performed laboratory tests, such as the FIB-4, performed reasonably well for ruling in advanced ALD with specificity of 89% to 91% for F3-F4 fibrosis and negative predictive value of 88%, but with poorer sensitivity (58%–71%).[62] The Enhanced Liver Fibrosis test, also performed well with comparable specificity and slightly improved sensitivity, but is not widely available in the United States. NITs based on elastography, an imaging-based examination that uses vibration to determine liver stiffness, have traditionally performed even better than laboratory-based NITs, but have the disadvantage of being more costly and less widely available. Transient elastography performs well to diagnosis advanced CLD (F3 or F4) with sensitivity and specificity over 90% and a negative predictive value of 96%.[62] Though no formal care pathways exist for guiding the diagnosis of ALD, initial evaluation for staging ALD should start with basic laboratories, including liver enzymes (AST, ALT, alkaline phosphatase, and bilirubin) as well as a complete blood count to obtain platelet counts to enable calculation of a FIB-4 score. A FIB-4 score greater than or equal to 3.25 should prompt further evaluation with transient elastography and a potential referral to gastroenterology or hepatology for further diagnostic evaluation for ACLD. Lower than normal platelet levels may denote the presence of portal hypertension so should be investigated further with imaging. Cirrhosis may be directly seen on imaging, but the absence of cirrhotic morphology of the liver does not rule out the presence of F3-F4 fibrosis. Patients with evidence of cirrhosis by NIT, physical examination, clinical symptoms (eg, ascites, jaundice), or imaging should be referred to hepatology for further evaluation.

SUMMARY

Alcohol is widely consumed in society and many individuals worldwide meet criteria for harmful use of alcohol and/or AUD. Alcohol can affect all human organ systems and any medical provider may find themselves as first to learn of a patient's struggle with alcohol use, necessitating universal preparation of medical professionals, either through education and intent to treat or up-to-date referral options at hand. ALD is also common and increasing with rising rates of drinking in some population groups, and with increases in metabolic diseases. There are many diagnostic tools for AUD and ALD, and clinicians are encouraged to use these tools to intervene early in the progression of AUD and/or ALD. Integrated medical and psychosocial care has been highly effective in supporting patients with AUD and ALD in achieving recovery and as such the standard of care has become specialized multidisciplinary clinics.[44,49,63] Patients with AUD and ALD can recovery through early, coordinated intervention, reductions in stigma, and through careful management with integrated medical and psychosocial care. AUD treatment is effective even for those with advanced ALD with reduced risk of decompensation and patient mortality.[64–66] Future research on integrated treatments and how to best support patients with AUD and ALD is needed.

CLINICS CARE POINTS

- *There is "no wrong door" by which patients access addiction care—all physicians can treat addiction, regardless of sub-specialization.* Despite acknowledgment of previous deficits in addiction care training by surveyed gastroenterologists,[67] it has been demonstrated further training is available and effective. Modalities have included interdisciplinary institutional didactics,[68] participation in immersive programs like ASAM's Fundamentals of Addiction Medicine course, addiction-specific conferences such as ASAM or AMERSA or state-chapter meetings, in-person or on society platforms like AASLD's Liver Learning,[69] or formal subspecialty training in Addiction Medicine or Addiction Psychiatry.[70] NIAAA also offers a core resource on alcohol with free continuing education credit.[71]

- *Words matters, utilize clinically accurate and medically appropriate language.* Stigma is a significant barrier for patients with AUD toward building rapport with medical teams and enabling access to care.[72] It is imperative physicians, staff, and researchers avoid terms of negative bias when speaking and documenting encounters involving patients with AUD as word choice influences perceptions and judgments resulting in disparate outcomes.

- *Screen universally, and by evidence-based means, early and often.* Screening for problematic alcohol use is recommended across the care continuum from emergency departments, to primary care clinics, to hospitals, to sub-specialist hepatology offices.[49] Ideally, a brief assessment such as the AUDIT-C is used to assess whether a person is drinking any alcohol, and whether the level of use necessitates advice about risk and/or further clinical intervention. Given even low levels of alcohol use increase risk of morality in those with ALD it is critical to assess all individuals regularly for alcohol use, even after periods of abstinence.[49]

- *Diagnose AUD with DSM-5 criteria, if adding a diagnosis, disclose to the patient and document criteria met.* The DSM-5 can be used to create a single diagnosis of AUD with mild, moderate, and severe sub-classifications. Transparency with diagnosis is important to allow for a shared understanding of illness and impacts, support rapport and alliance, as well as empower patients and promote agency.

- *Offer treatment early and often.* Only 1 in 3 patients with AUD is offered evidence-based AUD medications despite good efficacy and tolerability.[73] However, response to treatment is heterogeneous among patients and additionally given the chronic recurrent nature of AUD, may necessitate multiple treatment attempts to achieve sustained remission.[73] Together this means providers must be prepared to offer treatment for AUD when patient indicates interest and be prepared to revisit gently and often.

- *Document extent of patient education and AUD treatment offered during alcohol-related health care interactions, as these impact future treatment options.* With the adoption and recapitulation of the Dallas Consensus Conference around transplant in severe alcohol-associated hepatitis across United States institutions, it is important to manage all alcohol-related health care interactions in light of future impacts on transplant candidacy. Given criteria related to alcohol-associated hepatitis recommend consideration for liver transplantation be given only with "*first* presentation with decompensated alcohol-related liver disease" and criteria related to AUD caution against "repeated unsuccessful attempts at addiction rehabilitation" and "acceptance of ALD diagnosis with insight," it is imperative that counseling and treatment options, progress, or complications be explicitly addressed in medical record documentation.[54]

- *Make space for ambivalence.* Motivational interviewing offers a framework to support behavior change through and emphasis on empathy of the provider, approaching with curiosity by rolling with resistance, and partnering patients instead of lecturing in clinical case to promote "change-talk" by our patients which often leads to better outcomes.

- *Multidisciplinary care is the standard for AUD in ALD given the biopsychosocial complexity of these patients.* Integrated medical and psychosocial care has been highly effective in supporting patients with AUD and ALD in achieving recovery and as such the standard of care has become specialized multidisciplinary clinics.[44,49,63]

- *Concurrently address concomitant mood disorders.* Up to 60% of patients with AUD have a concurrent mental illness, most commonly depression, anxiety, and post-traumatic stress disorder.[74] Dual treatment of AUD with other psychiatric diagnoses is recommended.

- *Concurrently address nutrition deficiencies.* The neurotoxic effects of alcohol are compounded by replacement of nutrients and create additional challenges in care engagement for patients suffering from neurologic deficits from thiamine deficiency, anemia-related fatigue, and protein-malnutrition fragility. Given this, all patients at risk of malnutrition should receive thiamine and folate replacement and high protein dietary supplementation if alcohol-associated hepatitis or cirrhosis is suspected.[75]

- *Make space to discuss—and a plan to address—slips and return to use before they happen.* It is important to discuss and plan with patients around inadvertent alcohol use in order to minimize alcohol-related harms and regain recovery in as short a duration as possible. It is important to support a patient's understanding of their triggers resulting in craving or use, and increase healthy coping and care-seeking behaviors.

DISCLOSURE

K. Witkiewitz has received travel and speaker fees in the past 5 years from the Alcohol Clinical Trials Initiative (ACTIVE) Workgroup which has been supported previously, but not in the past 36 months, by Abbott/Abbvie, Amygdala Neurosciences, Arbor Pharmaceuticals, GSK, Janssen, Lilly, Mitsubishi, Pfizer, and Schering Plow, but in the past 36 months its activities were supported by Alkermes, Dicerna, Ethypharm, Indivior, Kinnov Therapeutics, Lundbeck, Otsuka, and Pear Therapeutics. J.L. Mellinger has consulted for GlaxoSmithKline. This research was supported by R01AA022328 (PI Wltkiewitz) from the National Institute on Alcohol Abuse and Alcoholism.

REFERENCES

1. Vidrih R, Hribar J. Mead: the oldest alcoholic beverage. In: Kristbergsson K, Oliveira J, editors. Traditional foods: General and consumer aspects. Integrating food science and engineering knowledge into the food chain. Springer US; 2016. p. 325–38. https://doi.org/10.1007/978-1-4899-7648-2_26.
2. Carrigan MA, Uryasev O, Frye CB, et al. Hominids adapted to metabolize ethanol long before human-directed fermentation. Proc Natl Acad Sci USA 2015;112(2):458–63. https://doi.org/10.1073/pnas.1404167111.
3. Manthey J, Shield KD, Rylett M, et al. Global alcohol exposure between 1990 and 2017 and forecasts until 2030: a modelling study. Lancet 2019;393(10190):2493–502. https://doi.org/10.1016/S0140-6736(18)32744-2.
4. Glantz MD, Bharat C, Degenhardt L, et al. The epidemiology of alcohol use disorders cross-nationally: findings from the World Mental Health Surveys. Addict Behav 2020;102:106128. https://doi.org/10.1016/J.ADDBEH.2019.106128.
5. World Health Organization. Global status report on alcohol and health 2018. Geneva, Switzerland: World Health Organization; 2018.
6. Lipari RN, Park-Lee E. Key substance use and mental health indicators in the United States: results from the 2019 national survey on drug use and health. Substance Abuse and Mental Health Services Administration 2020.
7. Mekonen T, Chan GCK, Connor J, et al. Treatment rates for alcohol use disorders: a systematic review and meta-analysis. Addiction 2021;116(10):2617–34. https://doi.org/10.1111/add.15357.

8. Dang K, Hirode G, Singal AK, et al. Alcoholic liver disease epidemiology in the United States: a retrospective analysis of 3 US databases. ACG 2020;115(1): 96. https://doi.org/10.14309/ajg.0000000000000380.

9. Tapper EB, Parikh ND. Mortality due to cirrhosis and liver cancer in the United States, 1999-2016: observational study. BMJ 2018;362:k2817. https://doi.org/10.1136/bmj.k2817.

10. Han S, Yang Z, Zhang T, et al. Epidemiology of alcohol-associated liver disease. Clin Liver Dis 2021;25(3):483–92. https://doi.org/10.1016/j.cld.2021.03.009.

11. Anderson MS, Valbuena VSM, Brown CS, et al. Association of COVID-19 with new waiting list registrations and liver transplantation for alcoholic hepatitis in the United States. JAMA Netw Open 2021;4(10):e2131132. https://doi.org/10.1001/jamanetworkopen.2021.31132.

12. Kanwal F, Neuschwander-Tetri BA, Loomba R, et al. Metabolic dysfunction-associated steatotic liver disease (MASLD): update and impact of new nomenclature on the AASLD clinical practice guidance on nonalcoholic fatty liver disease. Hepatology 2023. https://doi.org/10.1097/HEP.0000000000000670. Published online.

13. American Psychiatric Association. Mental disorders: diagnostic and statistical manual. Washington, DC: Mental Hospital Service; 1952.

14. American Psychiatric Association. Diagnostic and statistical manual of mental disorders. 2nd Edition. Washington, DC: American Psychiatric Association; 1968.

15. Feighner JP, Robins E, Guze SB, et al. Diagnostic criteria for use in psychiatric research. Arch Gen Psychiatry 1972;26(1):57–63. https://doi.org/10.1001/archpsyc.1972.01750190059011.

16. Spitzer RL, Endicott J, Robins E. Research diagnostic criteria: rationale and reliability. Arch Gen Psychiatry 1978;35(6):773–82. https://doi.org/10.1001/archpsyc.1978.01770300115013.

17. Hasin D. Classification of alcohol use disorders. Alcohol Res Health 2003; 27(1):5–17.

18. American Psychiatric Association. Diagnostic and statistical manual of mental disorders. 4th edition. Washington, DC: Author, DSM-IV; 1994.

19. American Psychiatric Association. Diagnostic and statistical manual of mental disorders. 3rd edition. Washington, DC: Author, DSM-III; 1980.

20. American Psychiatric Association. Diagnostic and statistical manual of mental disorders, 5th edition (DSM-5). Diagnostic and Statistical Manual of Mental Disorders 2013;280. https://doi.org/10.1176/appi.books.9780890425596.744053, 4th edition TR. Published online.

21. World Health Organization (WHO). International classification of diseases, eleventh revision (ICD-11). Geneva, Switzerland: World Health Organization; 2021.

22. Saunders JB, Degenhardt L, Reed GM, et al. Alcohol use disorders in ICD-11: past, present, and future. Alcohol Clin Exp Res 2019;43(8):1617–31. https://doi.org/10.1111/acer.14128.

23. Slade T, Mewton L, O'Dean S, et al. DSM-5 and ICD-11 alcohol use disorder criteria in young adult regular drinkers: lifetime prevalence and age of onset. Drug Alcohol Depend 2021;229(Pt B):109184. https://doi.org/10.1016/j.drugalcdep.2021.109184.

24. World Health Organization (WHO). International guide for monitoring alcohol consumption and related harm. Geneva, Switzerland: World Health Organization; 2000.

25. Witkiewitz K, Hallgren KA, Kranzler HR, et al. Clinical validation of reduced alcohol consumption after treatment for alcohol dependence using the World

Health Organization risk drinking levels. Alcohol Clin Exp Res 2017;41(1):179–86. https://doi.org/10.1111/ACER.13272.

26. Knox J, Wall M, Witkiewitz K, et al. Reduction in nonabstinent WHO drinking risk levels and change in risk for liver disease and positive AUDIT-C scores: prospective 3-year follow-up results in the U.S. general population. Alcohol Clin Exp Res 2018;42(11):2256–65. https://doi.org/10.1111/acer.13884.

27. Witkiewitz K, Kranzler HR, Hallgren KA, et al. Drinking risk level reductions associated with improvements in physical health and quality of life among individuals with alcohol use disorder. Alcohol Clin Exp Res 2018;42(12):2453–65. https://doi.org/10.1111/acer.13897.

28. Bush K, Kivlahan DR, McDonell MB, et al. For the ambulatory care quality improvement project (ACQUIP). The AUDIT alcohol consumption questions (AUDIT-C): an effective brief screening test for problem drinking. Arch Intern Med 1998;158(16):1789–95. https://doi.org/10.1001/archinte.158.16.1789.

29. Saunders JB, Aasland OG, Babor TF, et al. Development of the alcohol use disorders identification test (AUDIT): WHO collaborative project on early detection of persons with harmful alcohol consumption–II. Addiction 1993;88(6):791–804.

30. Sobell LC, Sobell MB. In: Litten RZ, Allen JP, editors. Timeline follow-back: a technique for assessing self-reported alcohol consumption. Human Press; 1992. Available at: http://search.proquest.com/psycinfo/docview/618232357/13607B0066F5980EE41/1?accountid=14902.

31. Hallgren KA, Matson TE, Oliver M, et al. Practical assessment of alcohol use disorder in routine primary care: performance of an alcohol symptom checklist. J Gen Intern Med 2022;37(8):1885–93. https://doi.org/10.1007/s11606-021-07038-3.

32. Cabezas J, Lucey MR, Bataller R. Biomarkers for monitoring alcohol use. Clin Liver Dis (Hoboken) 2016;8(3):59–63. https://doi.org/10.1002/cld.571.

33. Khanna S, Shah NL, Argo CK. Use of phosphatidylethanol testing in patients with liver disease. Am J Gastroenterol 2023. https://doi.org/10.14309/ajg.0000000000002537.

34. Ulwelling W, Smith K. The PEth blood test in the security environment: what it is; why it is important; and interpretative guidelines. J Forensic Sci 2018;63(6):1634–40. https://doi.org/10.1111/1556-4029.13874.

35. Hahn JA, Fatch R, Barnett NP, et al. Phosphatidylethanol vs transdermal alcohol monitoring for detecting alcohol consumption among adults. JAMA Netw Open 2023;6(9):e2333182. https://doi.org/10.1001/jamanetworkopen.2023.33182.

36. Archives & Special Collections of the University Library System. University of Pittsburgh. the official Dr. Thomas E. Starzl web site: Dr. Francis D. Moore. Available at: https://www.starzl.pitt.edu/people/moore.html. [Accessed 7 January 2024].

37. National Institutes of Health. National Institutes of health consensus development conference statement: liver transplantation–June 20-23, 1983. Hepatology 1984;4(1 Suppl):107S–10S.

38. Starzl TE. History of clinical transplantation. World J Surg 2000;24(7):759–82. https://doi.org/10.1007/s002680010124.

39. Mitchell MC, Maddrey WC. Changing times in liver transplantation for alcohol-associated liver disease. JAMA Intern Med 2019;179(3):348–50. https://doi.org/10.1001/jamainternmed.2018.6532.

40. Macdougall BR, Calne RY, McMaster P, et al. Survival and rehabilitation after orthotopic liver transplantation. Lancet 1980;1(8182):1326–8. https://doi.org/10.1016/s0140-6736(80)91785-7.

41. Scharschmidt BF. Human liver transplantation: analysis of data on 540 patients from four centers. Hepatology 1984;4(1 Suppl):95S–101S. https://doi.org/10.1002/hep.1840040723.
42. Maddrey WC, Friedman LS, Munoz SJ, et al. Transplantation of the liver, chapter 2: selection of the patient for liver transplantation and timing of surgery. Elsevier; 1988. Available at: https://catalog.lib.unc.edu/catalog/UNCb3910287.
43. Starzl TE, Van Thiel D, Tzakis AG, et al. Orthotopic liver transplantation for alcoholic cirrhosis. JAMA 1988;260(17):2542–4.
44. Beresford TP, Turcotte JG, Merion R, et al. A rational approach to liver transplantation for the alcoholic patient. Psychosomatics 1990;31(3):241–54. https://doi.org/10.1016/S0033-3182(90)72160-3.
45. Lucey MR, Merion RM, Henley KS, et al. Selection for and outcome of liver transplantation in alcoholic liver disease. Gastroenterology 1992;102(5):1736–41. https://doi.org/10.1016/0016-5085(92)91737-o.
46. Beresford TP. Psychiatric assessment of alcoholic candidates for liver transplantation,. In: Liver transplantation & the alcoholic patient : medical, surgical and psychosocial issues. Cambridge, UK: Cambridge University Press; 1994. p. 29–49.
47. Mathurin P, Moreno C, Samuel D, et al. Early liver transplantation for severe alcoholic hepatitis. N Engl J Med 2011;365(19):1790–800. https://doi.org/10.1056/NEJMoa1105703.
48. Lee BP, Mehta N, Platt L, et al. Outcomes of early liver transplantation for patients with severe alcoholic hepatitis. Gastroenterology 2018;155(2):422–30.e1. https://doi.org/10.1053/j.gastro.2018.04.009.
49. Crabb DW, Im GY, Szabo G, et al. Diagnosis and treatment of alcohol-associated liver diseases: 2019 practice guidance from the American association for the study of liver diseases. Hepatology 2020;71(1):306–33. https://doi.org/10.1002/hep.30866.
50. Addolorato G, Mirijello A, Barrio P, et al. Treatment of alcohol use disorders in patients with alcoholic liver disease. J Hepatol 2016;65(3):618–30. https://doi.org/10.1016/j.jhep.2016.04.029.
51. Addolorato G, Leggio L, Ferrulli A, et al. Effectiveness and safety of baclofen for maintenance of alcohol abstinence in alcohol-dependent patients with liver cirrhosis: randomised, double-blind controlled study. Lancet 2007;370(9603):1915–22. https://doi.org/10.1016/S0140-6736(07)61814-5.
52. Deutsch-Link S, Jiang Y, Peery AF, et al. Alcohol-associated liver disease mortality increased from 2017 to 2020 and accelerated during the COVID-19 pandemic. Clin Gastroenterol Hepatol 2022;20(9):2142–4.e2. https://doi.org/10.1016/j.cgh.2022.03.017.
53. Bittermann T, Mahmud N, Abt P. Trends in liver transplantation for acute alcohol-associated hepatitis during the COVID-19 pandemic in the US. JAMA Netw Open 2021;4(7):e2118713. https://doi.org/10.1001/jamanetworkopen.2021.18713.
54. Asrani SK, Trotter J, Lake J, et al. Meeting report: the Dallas consensus conference on liver transplantation for alcohol associated hepatitis. Liver Transpl 2020;26(1):127–40. https://doi.org/10.1002/lt.25681.
55. Mueller GC, Fleming MF, LeMahieu MA, et al. Synthesis of phosphatidylethanol–a potential marker for adult males at risk for alcoholism. Proc Natl Acad Sci U S A 1988;85(24):9778–82. https://doi.org/10.1073/pnas.85.24.9778.
56. Isaksson A, Walther L, Hansson T, et al. Phosphatidylethanol in blood (B-PEth): a marker for alcohol use and abuse. Drug Test Anal 2011;3(4):195–200. https://doi.org/10.1002/dta.278.

57. Lee BP, Im GY, Rice JP, et al. Patterns of alcohol use after early liver transplantation for alcoholic hepatitis. Clin Gastroenterol Hepatol 2022;20(2):409–18.e5. https://doi.org/10.1016/j.cgh.2020.11.024.

58. Sliedrecht W, Roozen H, de Waart R, et al. Variety in alcohol use disorder relapse definitions: should the term "relapse" Be abandoned? J Stud Alcohol Drugs 2022; 83(2):248–59. https://doi.org/10.15288/jsad.2022.83.248.

59. de Franchis R, Bosch J, Garcia-Tsao G, et al. Baveno VII - renewing consensus in portal hypertension. J Hepatol 2022;76(4):959–74. https://doi.org/10.1016/j.jhep.2021.12.022.

60. Crabb DW, Bataller R, Chalasani NP, et al. Standard definitions and common data elements for clinical Trials in patients with alcoholic hepatitis: recommendation from the NIAAA alcoholic hepatitis consortia. Gastroenterology 2016;150(4): 785–90. https://doi.org/10.1053/j.gastro.2016.02.042.

61. Ventura-Cots M, Argemi J, Jones PD, et al. Clinical, histological and molecular profiling of different stages of alcohol-related liver disease. Gut 2022;71(9): 1856–66. https://doi.org/10.1136/gutjnl-2021-324295.

62. Thiele M, Madsen BS, Hansen JF, et al. Accuracy of the enhanced liver fibrosis test vs FibroTest, elastography, and indirect markers in detection of advanced fibrosis in patients with alcoholic liver disease. Gastroenterology 2018;154(5): 1369–79. https://doi.org/10.1053/j.gastro.2018.01.005.

63. Mellinger JL, Winder GS, Fernandez AC, et al. Feasibility and early experience of a novel multidisciplinary alcohol-associated liver disease clinic. J Subst Abuse Treat 2021;130:108396. https://doi.org/10.1016/j.jsat.2021.108396.

64. Vannier AGL, Shay JES, Fomin V, et al. Incidence and progression of alcohol-associated liver disease after medical therapy for alcohol use disorder. JAMA Netw Open 2022;5(5):e2213014. https://doi.org/10.1001/jamanetworkopen.2022.13014.

65. Rogal S, Youk A, Zhang H, et al. Impact of alcohol use disorder treatment on clinical outcomes among patients with cirrhosis. Hepatology 2020;71(6):2080–92. https://doi.org/10.1002/hep.31042.

66. Rabiee A, Mahmud N, Falker C, et al. Medications for alcohol use disorder improve survival in patients with hazardous drinking and alcohol-associated cirrhosis. Hepatol Commun 2023;7(4):e0093. https://doi.org/10.1097/HC9.0000000000000093.

67. Im GY, Mellinger JL, Winters A, et al. Provider attitudes and practices for alcohol screening, treatment, and education in patients with liver disease: a survey from the American association for the study of liver diseases alcohol-associated liver disease special interest group. Clin Gastroenterol Hepatol 2021;19(11): 2407–16.e8. https://doi.org/10.1016/j.cgh.2020.10.026.

68. Johnson E, Ghosh M, Daniels VJ, et al. The development and evaluation of a provider-focused educational intervention about alcohol use disorder in patients with cirrhosis. Can Liver J 2023;6(3):295–304. https://doi.org/10.3138/canlivj-2022-0036.

69. Winters AC, Aby ES, Fix OK, et al. Joining the fight: enhancing alcohol treatment education in hepatology. Clinical Liver Disease 2021;18(5):225–9. https://doi.org/10.1002/cld.1127.

70. Haque LY, Fiellin DA. Bridging the gap: dual fellowship training in addiction medicine and digestive diseases. Dig Dis Sci 2022;67(7):2721–6. https://doi.org/10.1007/s10620-022-07478-9.

71. National Institute on Alcohol Abuse and Alcoholism. The healthcare professional's core resource on alcohol. Available at: https://www.niaaa.nih.gov/health-professionals-communities/core-resource-on-alcohol.
72. Ashford RD, Brown AM, McDaniel J, et al. Biased labels: an experimental study of language and stigma among individuals in recovery and health professionals. Subst Use Misuse 2019;54(8):1376–84. https://doi.org/10.1080/10826084.2019.1581221.
73. Witkiewitz K, Litten RZ, Leggio L. Advances in the science and treatment of alcohol use disorder. Sci Adv 2019;5(9):eaax4043. https://doi.org/10.1126/sciadv.aax4043.
74. SAMHSA. Substance use disorder treatment for people with Co-occurring disorders. Treatment improvement protocol (TIP) series, No. 42. 2020. Available at: https://store.samhsa.gov/sites/default/files/pep20-02-01-004.pdf.
75. Peterson BD, Stotts M. Beyond the banana bag: treating nutritional deficiencies of alcohol withdrawal syndrome. Practical gastro 2021. Available at: https://practicalgastro.com/2021/08/18/beyond-the-banana-bag-treating-nutritional-deficiencies-of-alcohol-withdrawal-syndrome/. [Accessed 7 January 2024].

Noninvasive Tests in Assessment of Patients with Alcohol-Associated Liver Disease

Lukas Otero Sanchez, MD, PhD[a,b,*],
Christophe Moreno, MD, PhD[a,b,*]

KEYWORDS

- Alcohol-associated liver disease • Screening strategy • Non-invasive tests
- Liver fibrosis • Steatosis

KEY POINTS

- Diagnosis of alcohol-associated liver disease (ALD) often occurs at an advanced stage, with over half exhibiting steatohepatitis or cirrhosis at liver biopsy. Moreover, at the time of liver cirrhosis diagnosis, more than 75% of patients present with liver-related complications.
- There is a crucial need to improve early detection of ALD, as notably the survival benefit of alcohol abstinence and medical interventions wanes in more advanced stages. Moreover, prompt screening for liver fibrosis in at-risk patients for ALD has shown a short-term and long-term beneficial impact on alcohol consumption levels.
- This review aims to summarize available noninvasive testing methods that are clinically available for assessing patients with ALD, including notably steatosis and fibrosis. Secondarily, all of this will be integrated within the framework of a practical clinical approach.

INTRODUCTION

Diagnosis of patients with alcohol-associated liver disease (ALD) often occurs at an advanced stage, with over half exhibiting steatohepatitis or cirrhosis at liver biopsy.[1] Moreover, at the time of liver cirrhosis diagnosis, more than 75% of patients present with liver-related complications.[2] Considering this, there is a crucial need to improve

---

Financial support: L. Otero Sanchez is a postdoctoral research fellow supported by Fonds Erasme for Medical Research, Belgium.

[a] Department of Gastroenterology, Hepatopancreatology and Digestive Oncology, Hôpital Universitaire de Bruxelles, C.U.B. Hôpital Erasme, Université Libre de Bruxelles, Brussels, Belgium; [b] Laboratory of Experimental Gastroenterology, Université Libre de Bruxelles, Brussels, Belgium
* Corresponding authors.
E-mail addresses: lukas.oterosanchez92@gmail.com (L.O.S.); christophe.moreno@hubruxelles. be (C.M.)

early detection of ALD, as notably the survival benefit of alcohol abstinence and medical interventions wanes in more advanced stages.[3]

Liver fibrosis stage remains the key determinant of patient's liver prognosis and shapes the management strategy. This underscores why both invasive and noninvasive tests (NITs) have been primarily dedicated to quantifying and staging the extent of liver fibrosis. Liver biopsy remains the gold standard method for staging fibrosis in populations with ALD and non-ALD; however, it has several drawbacks. These include its invasiveness, resulting in 30% to 50% of patients experience mild complications such as pain or transient vasovagal reactions. Additionally, there is a 0.1% to 0.7% risk of potential life-threatening complications, such as serious hemorrhage or pneumothorax.[4,5] Moreover, its accuracy for liver fibrosis assessment may be limited due to potential high interobserver and intraobserver variability, and a lack of representativeness in the sampling, leading to over-staging or under-staging. Finally, it is a timely and costly procedure with limited availability. For these reasons, liver biopsy is generally not recommended in routine clinical practices for all patients with suspected ALD.

Since the late 1990s, there has been a growing interest in identifying noninvasive markers associated with fibrosis and its progression, primarily assessed in populations with viral hepatitis C, but also in populations with ALD.[6,7] Since then, numerous clinical and biological markers have been developed to quantify other key histologic features, notably steatosis and steatohepatitis. Additionally, these markers have also been designed not only to predict liver histology components but also to predict disease progression and patient prognosis, thereby reshaping several aspects of international clinical practice guidelines. NITs are traditionally categorized into two main groups: (1) serologic markers, including "indirect" biomarkers reflecting hepatic injury or portal hypertension indirectly, and "direct" markers measuring components directly involved in the fibrogenesis process, and (2) liver stiffness (LS) measurement tools using ultrasound or magnetic resonance-based elastography techniques.[8]

This review aims to summarize available NIT methods that are clinically available for assessing patients with ALD, including notably steatosis and fibrosis. Additionally, all of this will be integrated within the framework of a practical clinical approach.

NONINVASIVE MARKERS OF HISTOLOGIC FEATURES IN ALCOHOL-ASSOCIATED LIVER DISEASE

The spectrum of ALD encompasses a wide range, extending from simple steatosis to steatohepatitis, fibrosis, and liver cirrhosis. The prototypical hallmark of ALD histology includes four key lesions: steatosis (predominantly macrovesicular), lobular inflammation, hepatocellular ballooning, and fibrosis.[9] Given that steatosis represents the earliest stage in the disease spectrum and is fully reversible after periods of abstinence, while liver fibrosis stands out as the pivotal histologic parameter for outcomes, research efforts have predominantly focused on developing noninvasive markers for their detection and quantification.

Noninvasive Assessment of Liver Steatosis in Patients with Alcohol-Associated Liver Disease

Liver steatosis is characterized by an excess of lipid droplets within the cytoplasm in more than 5% of hepatocytes. While almost all patients with heavy chronic alcohol consumption will develop steatosis, only a small fraction, representing 5% to 10%, will progress to liver cirrhosis within 5 years.[10] Additionally, individuals with alcohol-associated simple steatosis still show a 2.5-fold higher risk of mortality compared to control individuals.[11] This emphasizes the significance of evaluating and quantifying steatosis through NITs in populations with chronic alcohol consumption. This applies not only to risk stratification but also to enhance disease awareness among both patients and health care providers, potentially leading to increased delivery of brief interventions.

Ultrasound-based methods

B-mode ultrasonography remains the most widely used approach as an initial screen for steatosis due to its high diagnostic accuracy for the presence of moderate-to-severe steatosis ($\geq$ 30%). Classically used criteria to assess the presence of steatosis include[1] liver-to-kidney contrast,[2] parenchymal brightness,[3] deep beam attenuation,[4] bright vessel walls, and[5] gallbladder wall definition. Notably, the imaging criterion with the highest sensitivity for diagnosing moderate-to-severe steatosis (~ 98%) is liver-to-kidney contrast, while specificity remains comparable across the various criteria (93%–95%).[12] Ultrasound typically exhibits a sensitivity of 60% to 94% and specificity of 88% to 95% for detecting liver steatosis. Sensitivity decreases with lower lipid content, reaching 80% above 30% fat content compared to 55% when the lipid content is below 20%.[13] The limitations of ultrasonography include its low diagnostic accuracy for the presence of mild steatosis (<30%), its low interobserver and intraobserver reproducibility, and its nonquantitative and subjective features.[12,14] Moreover, its diagnostic accuracy for detecting steatosis is lower in patients with obesity, with sensitivity and specificity dropping to 49% and 75% in this specific population, respectively.[15]

The controlled attenuation parameter (CAP) is the first method approved for liver fat quantification and remains one of the most widely validated noninvasive methods used so far. CAP measures ultrasound attenuation when as it travels through fatty liver tissue compared to healthy liver. A meta-analysis including 2735 patients reported that the clinical use of CAP provides a standardized and accurate noninvasive measure of hepatic steatosis with an area under the receiver operating characteristics curve (AUROC) score ranging between 0.82 and 0.86 (depending on steatosis grade) when liver biopsy was considered to be the reference standard.[16] However, in this meta-analysis, patients with ALD were underrepresented, as it included over 70% of patients with viral-associated liver disease and 20% with metabolic dysfunction-associated steatotic liver disease (MASLD). In a study involving 562 alcohol-overusing patients who underwent concomitant liver biopsy, CAP, and liver ultrasound, a CAP above 290 dB/m accurately identified any stage of steatosis with 88% specificity and a 92% positive predictive value, making it a suitable tool for ruling in steatosis.[17] Conversely, in this study, CAP exhibited a relatively poor negative predictive value (NPV), making it inadequate an adequate tool for ruling out steatosis in this specific population. Interestingly, it was found that CAP decreased rapidly after alcohol withdrawal, a trend observed only in non-obese patients. This suggests that the method may be suitable for monitoring patients during and after alcohol detoxification.

CAP has been shown to be superior to classical B-mode ultrasonography for diagnosing steatosis in ALD cohorts. An advantage of CAP is that it can be performed simultaneously during LS measurement with vibration-controlled transient elastography (TE) using the Fibroscan® platform. Other advantages include its noninvasiveness, nonionizing nature, ease of performance, and instant results at the bedside. The CAP value, however, is influenced by the presence of various conditions that can impair the diagnostic accuracy of steatosis, such as obesity, diabetes mellitus, MASLD, and patients with ALD. Optimal CAP thresholds for detecting steatosis in the latter conditions are likely much higher than the optimal thresholds obtained from meta-analyses encompassing multiple etiologies of liver disease. However, certain reliability criteria could enhance the diagnostic performance of CAP for identifying any stage of steatosis in clinical practice, including a CAP interquartile range/median less than 0.3.[18] CAP has been demonstrated to be independent of factors such as fibrosis, liver inflammation, lipid and glycemic profiles, hypertension, age, and gender when adjusted for steatosis.[19]

MRI

Magnetic resonance spectroscopy (MRS) is considered the gold standard method for noninvasive liver fat assessment. MRS outperforms other methods primarily because it is unaffected by factors such as fibrosis, iron deposition, or the presence of coexisting liver disease.[20] In contrast to other noninvasive methods, MRS has the distinct advantage of enabling the precise quantitative assessment of liver fat composition in vivo. Nevertheless, MRS faces limited availability in routine clinical practice and is still primarily employed in research settings.

Like MRS, MRI is a technique relying on the principles of nuclear magnetic resonance that allow for indirect liver fat quantification. MRI-proton density fat fraction (PDFF) is one of the most accurate and validated noninvasive measures to quantify liver fat content. MRI-PDFF is measured as the ratio between the density of mobile protons from triglycerides and the total density of protons from mobile triglycerides and mobile water.[21] Although MRI-PDFF estimates differ from triglyceride concentrations, several studies have demonstrated the association between the liver fat content estimated by MRI-PDFF and the steatosis severity estimated by liver histology assessment.[22] Recently, a meta-analysis including 1100 patients reported that the AUROC values for classifying liver steatosis grade 1, 2, and 3 were 0.98, 0.91, and 0.92, respectively, with histology as reference standard.[23] Moreover, several studies have highlighted the association between changes in MRI-PDFF values and improvements in liver biomarkers or changes in MASLD histologic features, including steatosis grade.[24,25] The limitations of MRI involve limited accessibility relative to other modalities, its high cost, extended durations, and potential limitations due to claustrophobia or the presence of metallic implants.

Diagnosis and Staging of Liver Fibrosis

The presence of liver cirrhosis is often asymptomatic, with laboratory tests appearing almost normal and ultrasound imaging lacking typical cirrhotic features. This has two major clinical implications: (1) the disease is often identified only at the decompensation stage and (2) its global prevalence is greatly underestimated. The hallmark of any form of chronic liver disease is the deposition of fibrosis in response to persistent liver injury. The liver fibrosis burden remains the key parameter associated with the development of liver-related events, including the development of hepatocellular carcinoma (HCC) or portal hypertension-related complications, the progression of the underlying liver disease, and liver-related mortality in patients with chronic liver disease. Its quantification and characterization are, therefore, critical parameters in the risk stratification of liver-related complications, impacting both primary and secondary prevention strategies, but also playing a role in monitoring the progression of the underlying liver disease. It is not surprising that over the last three decades, numerous invasive and noninvasive techniques have been developed to focus on liver fibrosis assessment. As mentioned earlier, liver biopsy remains the gold standard technique for assessing liver fibrosis. The fibrosis stage is histologically assessed through a semiquantitative scale comprising traditionally four stages initially described in the Metavir classification developed for populations with hepatitis C, ranging from F0 (no cirrhosis) to F3 (portal–portal and/or portal–central bridging) and F4 (cirrhosis).[6] Recently, an ALD-specific semiquantitative grading and staging system has been developed for ALD by an international group of pathologists (SALVE).[9] In this classification, fibrosis staging encompasses 7 main fibrosis stages, including three different cirrhosis stages defined by the septa diameter of the smallest nodule (SF4A-C). The current semiquantitative assessment of liver fibrosis, relying on histology, establishes the ground truth for evaluating the performance of noninvasive methods. Beyond the inherent biases related to interobserver variability and the potential non-representativeness of biopsy samples, this semiquantitative evaluation could lead to an inaccurate quantification of fibrosis burden, especially in cases situated at the boundaries between two fibrosis stages.[8] Moreover, despite the potential for NITs to offer a more accurate assessment of fibrosis burden, the current gold standard staging systems compel the discretization of these biomarkers, potentially leading to an erroneously evaluated accuracy.

Elastography

LS is defined as the degree to which the liver resists deformation in response to an applied force and is traditionally measured in Pascal (Pa).[19]

In 2003, TE was the first method introduced to evaluate LS. Since then, TE has been extensively evaluated and is now the most commonly used method of elastography worldwide. TE has proven to be a valuable tool for assessing liver fibrosis in at-risk patients for chronic liver disease, especially in those with harmful alcohol consumption. Globally, the evaluated predictive performance of TE in predicting alcohol-associated cirrhosis on liver biopsy consistently showed high accuracy, with the AUROC in the literature ranging between 0.87 and 0.97.[26–28] However, it has been observed that the cut-off values for diagnosing F3–F4 in patients with ALD span a broad range, from 11.5 to 25.8 kPa.[19] Interestingly, this variability in cut-off values is not described in other etiologies of chronic liver disease. It has been observed that the presence of coexisting steatohepatitis and lobular-associated liver inflammation markedly increased LS independently of liver fibrosis stage.[29] Moreover, the presence of underlying steatohepatitis strongly correlated with the level of aspartate transaminase (AST). These results were later confirmed in a meta-analysis including 1026 patients with ALD, liver biopsy, and TE, which established LS cut-offs of 12.1 kPa for F3 and 18.6 kPa for F4.[30] In this study, the presence of histologic features of asymptomatic and non-severe alcohol-associated hepatitis was associated with increased LS. In the multivariable analysis, AST, bilirubin, and prothrombin activity were independently associated with the presence of histologic features of asymptomatic and non-severe alcoholic hepatitis. Therefore, elevated LS values in patients with suspected ALD and AST serum levels greater than 100 U/L or elevated bilirubin levels should be interpreted with caution due to the possibility of falsely elevated LS as a result of superimposed alcohol-associated steatohepatitis.[31] In several studies, it has been shown that LS tends to decrease by 17% to 32% after 1 week in response to alcohol withdrawal.[29,32] Additional data could suggest that long-term abstinence is even more beneficial. This is why it is recommended to repeat TE 1 to 2 weeks after alcohol withdrawal, particularly in cases where LS was initially elevated (ref). In addition to liver inflammation, TE results could be artifactually elevated due to several confounders, including vascular congestion, cholestasis, and recent food intake. Although several confounders could increase LS, none has been associated with a decrease in TE. Consequently, it is reasonable to consider a normal LS of less than 8 kPa as ruling out significant fibrosis. Conversely, a threshold value of 15 kPa in patients with harmful alcohol use has a sensitivity and specificity of 86% and 94%, respectively, for advanced fibrosis.[30] All things considered, it is recommended to start primary prophylaxis for decompensation in patients with an LS measurement greater than 25 kPa, which serves as an indicative cut-off for the presence of clinically significant portal hypertension (CSPH).[33] In a recent cohort including 5,648 patients (17% with ALD), who underwent both liver biopsy and TE within 6 months, a dual cut-off of less than 8 kPa and greater than 12 kPa demonstrated improved diagnostic accuracy for advanced chronic liver disease ($\geq$F3).[34] In the later study, a subgroup analysis involving patients with MASLD and ALD confirmed that a cut-off less than 8 kPa can be employed to rule out advanced chronic liver disease in these populations with a sensitivity of 93%.

In addition to TE, which involves the external mechanical generation of shear waves, ultrasound-based shear wave elastography methods have been evaluated for their ability to noninvasively detect fibrosis. These methods include notably acoustic radiation force imaging (ARFI), point shear wave elastography (SWE), and two-dimensional (2D) SWE. Overall these acoustic radiation force methods are influenced by food intake and liver inflammation and have reported a failure rate lower of 2%–4%, which is lower than that of classical TE (3%–5%).[35] Nevertheless, they do not appear to be influenced by the presence of underlying obesity or the presence of ascites.

These methods seem to demonstrate similar accuracy for the detection of advanced fibrosis compared to TE.[36,37] However, there is a lack of large cohorts evaluating their prognostic performance specifically in ALD. A cohort study involving 112 patients with ALD, for whom liver biopsy and ARFI were available, demonstrated an AUROC of 0.875 for advanced fibrosis detection with ARFI. The study also reported a higher optimal cut-off for those patients with elevated AST.[38] In a prospective study of 462 patients with compensated ALD, it was revealed that both 2D-SWE and TE serve as highly accurate prognostic markers in predicting the first liver-related events (Harrell's C prognostic performance: TE: 0.876 vs 0.868 for 2D-SWE).[39]

Magnetic resonance elastography (MRE) is a phase-contrast-based MRI technique that was initially described at the Mayo Clinic in 1995.[40] The methodology involves 3 main phases: (1) generating low-frequency mechanical vibrations in the liver; (2) constructing a propagating shear wave map using a phase-contrast MRI technique that includes oscillating motion-sensitizing gradients; and (3) applying an inversion algorithm to convert the wave image into an elastogram.[41] In contrast to TE, MRE has the ability to generate a 3D elastography map by capturing the entire liver. Moreover, it maintains accuracy even in the context of obesity and in patients with ascites. However, MRE has limitations, including its limited utility in cases of iron overload, and it is a time-consuming, expensive method not routinely available in clinical practice. Moreover, only one study has explored the diagnostic accuracy of MRE in 90 patients with a history of excessive alcohol consumption. In this study, MRE demonstrated high diagnostic accuracy compared to TE, with an AUROC ranging from 0.937 for mild-to-moderate fibrosis ($\geq$F1) to 0.978 for advanced fibrosis ($\geq$F3). Notably, the various MRE parameter cutoffs remained unaffected by the presence of liver inflammation, as indicated by the level of aspartate transaminase (AST).[42] It should be acknowledged that there are currently limitations in the noninvasive assessment of fibrosis in patients with ALD, as it relies on the absence of MRE-based evaluation. Further research in this area is warranted to explore the potential utility of MRI techniques in managing patients in this specific population.

Blood-based fibrosis biomarkers

Over the past 2 decades, a wide spectrum of blood-based tests has been predominantly developed to indirectly assess the burden of liver fibrosis. Overall, these blood-based markers can be divided into 2 categories: indirect serum markers, which incorporate easily accessible biological parameters that reflect either indirectly either hepatic injury (eg, AST/alanine aminotransferase [ALT]), liver function, or portal hypertension (eg, prothrombin time, platelets).[8] The advantages of these indirect bio-markers lie in their high accuracy for ruling out the presence of advanced fibrosis, their reproducibility, their easy accessibility in daily clinical practice, and their afford-ability compared to patented markers. Their weaknesses include overall lower diag-nostic accuracy compared to direct blood-based biomarkers and TE. They may yield false positive results, particularly in populations over 65 years of age, and can be influenced by various extrahepatic clinical conditions (eg, inflammation). On the other hand, direct blood-based biomarkers, which are typically patented, focus on quanti-fying products released into the circulatory system during fibrogenesis or extracel-lular remodeling. The advantage of these biomarkers is their reproducibility and greater accuracy in detecting advanced fibrosis compared to indirect markers. Their drawback is that they have limited availability and are expensive. A common feature of these blood-based markers is their low accuracy in detecting early fibrosis stages and have not been validated to detect the presence of CSPH, particularly in patients with ALD.[43] Although they generally have a high diagnostic accuracy for ruling out advanced fibrosis, their overall accuracy to confirm advanced fibrosis is limited.

Direct serum biomarkers. The most commonly used single marker to directly discern the stage of fibrosis remains hyaluronic acid. A systematic review, including 15 studies, demonstrated a median AUROC of 0.79 (range: 0.69–0.93) for advanced fibrosis diagnosis in patients with ALD.[43] Other individual biomarkers, such as pro-collagen III, tissue inhibitor of metalloproteinase 1, or PRO-C3, have been evaluated. Nevertheless, the use of combined serum-based markers has been shown to be more accurate for detecting advanced fibrosis compared to the use of single markers alone.[8] FibroTest® was the first algorithm combining direct biomarkers to identify advanced fibrosis in patients with hepatitis C infection.[44] It relies on a calculation involving 6 serum markers, age, and gender. Subsequently, several direct tests have been developed, including the Enhanced Liver Fibrosis (ELF®) score, which measures three serum markers of the extracellular matrix, including hyaluronic acid, tissue inhibitor of metalloproteinase-1, and the N-terminal propeptide for collagen type III.[45] Other commonly mentioned direct blood-based tests included Fibrometer® and HepScore®.[46,47]

In a prospective cohort study comprising 289 patients recruited from primary and secondary care, FibroTest® and ELF® accurately discriminated advanced fibrosis (AUROC ELF: 0.92; FibroTest: 0.88) using biopsy as a reference.[48] In the same study, an ELF value below 10.5 or a FibroTest value below 0.58 can be employed to rule out advanced fibrosis in a primary health care setting, with NPVs of 98% and 97%, respectively. PRO-C3, a systemic marker indicating type III collagen formation and fibroblast activity, in combination with indirect biomarkers such as age, type 2 dia-betes status, and platelet count (ADAPT), has demonstrated promising efficacy in detecting fibrosis in MASLD but also in ALD populations. In a prospective biopsy-controlled study involving 426 patients with alcohol overuse, it exhibited an AUC of 0.88 for identifying advanced fibrosis.[49] Globally, direct blood-based tests for fibrosis appear to have a slightly better performance than indirect tests, with AUCs typically greater than 0.8 for advanced fibrosis and cirrhosis.[50] However, their limited availabil-ity and cost seem to constrain their utilization in daily clinical practice. Furthermore, it remains to be seen whether combining them with other noninvasive evaluation methods such as imaging-based approaches enhances detection accuracy. Nonethe-less, a study has highlighted that in a population of heavy drinkers, the combination of patented tests, such as FibroTest®, along with TE, does not improve the detection of advanced fibrosis.[51]

Indirect serum biomarkers. ALT and AST/ALT ratio (AAR), also called the De Ritis ratio, are simple blood-based serum tests that have been extensively evaluated for liver fibrosis assessment. Initially, an AST/ALT ratio of 1 or greater was identified as a fibrosis marker in patients with MASLD and chronic hepatitis C virus (HCV) infection; however, subsequent studies have not confirmed this association.[52,53] Interestingly, AST and ALT values, and consequently the AST/ALT ratio, do not behave similarly between ALD and other etiologies, including portal-related chronic liver diseases such as those associated with chronic HCV infection. It has been observed that AST levels tend to remain consistently elevated across various fibrosis stages among ALD patients, whereas these values tend to increase parallelly with fibrosis stages in HCV-associated liver disease. Moreover, ALT values exhibit an upward trend with the progression of fibrosis in viral-related liver diseases, contrasting with a tendency to decrease in ALD.[54] In ALD, AST/ALT ratio is higher than 2 in 70% of cases, with AST levels rarely higher than 300 UI/L. The elevation of AST over ALT has been attributed to the hepatic mitochondrial isoform of AST, which increases in the context of heavy alcohol consumption. However, recent data suggest that this increase could be likely due to hemolysis and enhanced red blood cell turnover.[55] Several models, integrating clinical and biological parameters, have been secondarily developed to enhance the diagnostic performance of primarily indirect blood-based biomarkers. The most widely used include the Fibrosis-4 index (FIB-4) and the AST to platelet ratio index (APRI). The FIB-4 was originally developed for hepatitis C/human immunodeficiency virus co-infected patients and was secondarily validated in patients with MASLD.[56,57] The score is based on biological and clinical variables including age, ALT, AST, and platelets. Since then, FIB-4 has undergone extensive validation in numerous studies across a wide spectrum of etiologies and is consistently regarded as one of the best performing non-patented blood tests. AUROC for detecting advanced fibrosis was classically reported as 0.80, with positive predictive values of 80% for a FIB-4 score of 2.67 (rule-in threshold) and negative predictive values of 90% for a FIB-4 score of 1.3 (rule-out threshold).[58,59] In this context, the current guidelines from the European Association for the Study of Liver (EASL) recommend screening patients with a history of excess drinking for liver disease using a simple and readily available liver blood test, preferably the FIB-4.[60] The FIB-4 cut-off at 1.3 can accurately exclude patients with advanced fibrosis, serving as a reliable rule-out threshold in primary care settings. If the FIB-4 value exceeds 1.3, the patient may be referred for LS measurement by TE. However, this recommendation has been recently challenged in several studies, including those involving patients with MASLD, revealing that up to half of patients with significantly elevated LS measurements have FIB-4 scores below 1.3.[61] Moreover, the performance of FIB-4 appears to demonstrate lower accuracy in detecting significant fibrosis, particularly in high-risk populations, such as patients with diabetes.[62] APRI has undergone validation for fibrosis assessment across various etiologies, demonstrating a performance accuracy of 0.80. The classical cut-offs for ruling in and ruling out advanced fibrosis are less than 0.5 and 1.5 or greater, respectively. However, in direct head-to-head comparisons, it has proven to be less accurate than FIB-4, specifically in patients with ALD.[59] **Table 1** summarizes the diagnostic performance of NITs for advanced fibrosis.

NONINVASIVE TESTS IN CLINICAL PRACTICE

The selected screening strategy to detect advanced fibrosis will be influenced by various parameters, including its cost, accessibility, and test performance, which is directly conditioned by the prevalence of the disease in the studied population.

Table 1
Performance of noninvasive tests for the diagnosis of liver fibrosis in alcohol-associated liver disease

Study, Year	NIT	Patients, N (ALD %)	Cut-offs	Fibrosis Stage	Sensitivity	Specificity	AUROC
Nguyen-Khac et al,[30] 2018	TE	1,026 (100%)	≥9.0 kPa	≥F2	78%	77%	0.86
			≥12.1 kPa	≥F3	81%	83%	0.90
			≥18.6 kPa	≥F4	84%	85%	0.91
Thiele et al,[48] 2018	TE	269 (100%)	≥15.0 kPa	≥F3	86%	94%	0.89
Papatheodoridi et al,[34] 2021	TE	5,483 (17%)	≥15.0 kPa	≥F3	48%	95%	
		932 (100%)	<8.0 kPa	≥F3	96.3%	60.9%	
			>12 kPa	≥F3	77.8%	88.8%	
Thiele et al,[48] 2018	2D-SWE	265 (100%)	≥16.4 kPa	≥F3	88%	95%	0.93
Zhang et al,[38] 2015	ARFI	112 (100%)	≥1.4(m/s)	≥F3	84%	82%	0.875
Madsen et al,[49] 2021	PRO-C3	426 (100%)	≥15.6	≥F3	81%	73%	0.85
Thiele et al,[48] 2018	ELF	289 (100%)	≥10.51	≥F3	79%	91%	0.92
Naveau et al,[63] 2009	FibroTest	218 (100%)	≥0.70	≥F2	42.9%	97%	0.83
Thiele et al,[48] 2018	FibroTest	285 (100%)	≥0.58	≥F3	67%	87%	0.88
Naveau et al,[63] 2009	APRI	218 (100%)		≥F2			0.59
Thiele et al,[48] 2018	APRI	289 (100%)	≥1.0	≥F3	38%	90%	0.80
Naveau et al,[63] 2009	FIB-4	218 (100%)		≥F2			0.70
Thiele et al,[48] 2018	FIB-4	289 (100%)	≥3.25	≥F3	58%	91%	0.84

Performance of all studies included in the table are defined with liver biopsy was considered as gold standard.

Abbreviations: 2D-SWE, 2D-shear wave elastography; ALD, alcohol-associated liver disease; APRI, AST to platelet ratio index; ARFI, acoustic radiation force imaging; FIB-4, Fibrosis-4 index; NITs, noninvasive test; TE, transient elastography.

Unfortunately, the majority of studies evaluating the performance of NITs to detect advanced fibrosis in patients with excessive alcohol consumption focus on populations recruited from secondary health care centers. Furthermore, most of these studies do not exclude cases of clinically evident cirrhosis, resulting in the assessment of NITs in populations with a high prevalence of advanced fibrosis. This potentially leads to an overestimation of diagnostic performances, notably their positive predictive value.[60] However, a study involving a cohort of patients recruited prospectively from an alcohol rehabilitation center suggests a high prevalence (29%) of clinically significant fibrosis (F$\geq$2), even in heavy drinkers recruited in a primary care setting.[48] The question is, therefore, who to select for screening to increase the pretest probability of disease. A cut-off of 30 g per day for a minimum of 1 to 5 years appears to be a sufficient threshold for performing a noninvasive screening test.[64] Most cases of ALD cirrhosis are diagnosed between the ages of 50 and 60 years; therefore, screening strategies could be reasonably initiated at the age of 30 to 40 years. In line with this, current guidelines from EASL recommend screening a patient with chronic harmful alcohol use with TE to rule out advanced fibrosis (**Fig. 1**).[60] Two metaanalyses reported sensitivities of 92% and 94% for detecting advanced fibrosis using cut-offs of 9.5 kPa and 8 kPa, respectively.[34,65] This allows considering a cut-off below 8 kPa as a rule-out for advanced fibrosis. Conversely, a threshold value of 15 kPa demonstrates a specificity for rule-in advanced fibrosis ranging between 92% and 94%.[30,34] In practice, TE is conducted immediately following abdominal ultrasound and serum blood tests. The ultrasound is performed to eliminate potential confounders for liver stiffness measurement (LSM) elevation, such as venous congestion and biliary dilatation, and to assess spleen/liver size, indirect stigmata of cirrhosis, or the presence of ascites. TE is primarily carried out with the M probe, switching to the XL probe after M probe failure, especially in cases of obvious obesity or in patients with ascites. A minimum fasting period of 3 hours is required, as meal

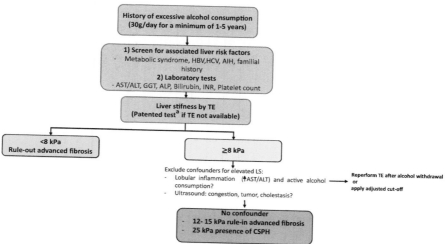

Fig. 1. A practical algorithm overview of patients with excessive alcohol consumption. [a]ELF® <9.8 or FibroTest® <0.48 to exclude advanced fibrosis. AIH, autoimmune hepatitis; ALP, alkaline phosphatase; ALT, alanine aminotransferase; AST, aspartate transaminase; CSHP, clinically significant portal hypertension; HBV, hepatitis B virus infection; HCV, hepatitis C virus infection; INR, international normalized ratio; TE, transient elastography.

ingestion is associated with LSM elevation regardless of the method used. Patients should maintain a horizontal position for a minimum of 5 minutes to stabilize hemo-dynamics.[50] As mentioned earlier, LSM may be elevated due to liver inflammation associated with chronic alcohol consumption. In accordance with this, EASL guide-lines recommend repeating LSM by TE after 1 week of alcohol abstinence in patients with elevated LS and biochemical evidence of liver inflammation (AST or gamma-glutamyl transferase >2X ULN).[60] In cases where abstinence is not possible, or if it is challenging to reschedule a TE, an AST-adapted cut-off value exists to directly assess LS, even in the context of pronounced liver inflammation.[50,54] If TE is not avail-able, patented (ELF® <9.8 or FibroTest® <0.48) or not patented test (FIB-4 <1.3) could be alternatively used to rule out advanced fibrosis. However, non-patented tests are not recommended for ruling in advanced fibrosis due to the high probability of misclassification. Patented markers are a reliable alternative when TE is not avail-able for evaluating advanced fibrosis, as they have demonstrated similar or close AUROC values. However, there appears to be high variability in the cut-offs and per-formance accuracy used across studies. Therefore, these markers should be more robustly validated and standardized. Liver biopsy should be reserved for cases of un-certain diagnosis, particularly in the context of potential alcohol-associated hepatitis, instances with indeterminate NITs, or in the setting of clinical trials.

DISCLOSURE

L. Otero Sanchez has nothing to disclose. C. Moreno was paid as speaker or adviser from Echosens, Surrozen, Intercept, and Gildead Sciences pharmaceutical com-panies. He is consultant for Julius clinical. He received research Grant from Gilead Sciences.

Authors' contributions: L. Otero Sanchez and C. Moreno designed and wrote the re-view. All authors critically revised the study and approved the final version to be published.

REFERENCES

1. Parker R, Aithal GP, Becker U, et al. Natural history of histologically proven alcohol-related liver disease: a systematic review. J Hepatol 2019;71(3):586–93.
2. Jepsen P, Ott P, Andersen PK, et al. Clinical course of alcoholic liver cirrhosis: a Danish population-based cohort study. Hepatol Baltim Md 2010;51(5):1675–82.
3. Lackner C, Spindelboeck W, Haybaeck J, et al. Histological parameters and alcohol abstinence determine long-term prognosis in patients with alcoholic liver disease. J Hepatol 2017;66(3):610–8.
4. Filingeri V, Francioso S, Sforza D, et al. A retrospective analysis of 1.011 percu-taneous liver biopsies performed in patients with liver transplantation or liver dis-ease: ultrasonography can reduce complications? Eur Rev Med Pharmacol Sci 2016;20(17):3609–17.
5. Tapper EB, Lok ASF. Use of liver imaging and biopsy in clinical practice. N Engl J Med 2017;377(8):756–68.
6. Poynard T, Bedossa P, Opolon P. Natural history of liver fibrosis progression in pa-tients with chronic hepatitis C. The OBSVIRC, METAVIR, CLINIVIR, and DOSVIRC groups. Lancet Lond Engl 1997;349(9055):825–32.
7. Oberti F, Valsesia E, Pilette C, et al. Noninvasive diagnosis of hepatic fibrosis or cirrhosis. Gastroenterology 1997;113(5):1609–16.
8. Anstee QM, Castera L, Loomba R. Impact of non-invasive biomarkers on hepa-tology practice: past, present and future. J Hepatol 2022;76(6):1362–78.

9. Lackner C, Stauber RE, Davies S, et al. Development and prognostic relevance of a histologic grading and staging system for alcohol-related liver disease. J Hepatol 2021;75(4):810–9.

10. T D, H G, H V, et al. Cirrhosis and mortality risks of biopsy-verified alcoholic pure steatosis and steatohepatitis: a nationwide registry-based study. Aliment Pharmacol Ther 2012;35(11).

11. Hagström H, Thiele M, Roelstraete B, et al. Mortality in biopsy-proven alcohol-related liver disease: a population-based nationwide cohort study of 3453 patients. Gut 2021;70(1):170–9.

12. Hernaez R, Lazo M, Bonekamp S, et al. Diagnostic accuracy and reliability of ultrasonography for the detection of fatty liver: a meta-analysis. Hepatol Baltim Md 2011;54(3):1082–90.

13. Platon ML, Stefanescu H, Muresan D, et al. Noninvasive assessment of liver steatosis using ultrasound methods. Med Ultrason 2014;16(3):236–45.

14. Dasarathy S, Dasarathy J, Khiyami A, et al. Validity of real time ultrasound in the diagnosis of hepatic steatosis: a prospective study. J Hepatol 2009;51(6):1061–7.

15. Bril F, Ortiz-Lopez C, Lomonaco R, et al. Clinical value of liver ultrasound for the diagnosis of nonalcoholic fatty liver disease in overweight and obese patients. Liver Int 2015;35(9):2139–46.

16. Karlas T, Petroff D, Sasso M, et al. Individual patient data meta-analysis of controlled attenuation parameter (CAP) technology for assessing steatosis. J Hepatol 2017;66(5):1022–30.

17. Thiele M, Rausch V, Fluhr G, et al. Controlled attenuation parameter and alcoholic hepatic steatosis: diagnostic accuracy and role of alcohol detoxification. J Hepatol 2018;68(5):1025–32.

18. Semmler G, Wöran K, Scheiner B, et al. Novel reliability criteria for controlled attenuation parameter assessments for non-invasive evaluation of hepatic steatosis. United Eur Gastroenterol J 2020;8(3):321–31.

19. Mueller S, Liver elastography. Clinical use and interpretation, 2020, Springer. Available at: https://link.springer.com/book/10.1007/978-3-030-40542-7.

20. Pasanta D, Htun KT, Pan J, et al. Magnetic resonance spectroscopy of hepatic fat from Fundamental to clinical applications. Diagnostics mai 2021;11(5):842.

21. Caussy C, Alquiraish MH, Nguyen P, et al. Optimal threshold of controlled attenuation parameter with MRI-PDFF as the gold standard for the detection of hepatic steatosis. Hepatol Baltim Md 2018;67(4):1348–59.

22. Permutt Z, Le TA, Peterson MR, et al. Correlation between liver histology and novel magnetic resonance imaging in adult patients with non-alcoholic fatty liver disease - MRI accurately quantifies hepatic steatosis in NAFLD. Aliment Pharmacol Ther 2012;36(1):22–9.

23. Qu Y, Li M, Hamilton G, et al. Diagnostic accuracy of hepatic proton density fat fraction measured by magnetic resonance imaging for the evaluation of liver steatosis with histology as reference standard: a meta-analysis. Eur Radiol 2019;29(10):5180–9.

24. Patel NS, Doycheva I, Peterson MR, et al. Effect of weight loss on magnetic resonance imaging estimation of liver fat and volume in patients with nonalcoholic steatohepatitis. Clin Gastroenterol Hepatol 2015;13(3):561–8.e1.

25. Middleton MS, Heba ER, Hooker CA, et al. Agreement between magnetic resonance imaging proton density fat fraction measurements and pathologist-assigned steatosis grades of liver biopsies from adults with nonalcoholic steatohepatitis. Gastroenterology 2017;153(3):753–61.

26. Nahon P, Kettaneh A, Tengher-Barna I, et al. Assessment of liver fibrosis using transient elastography in patients with alcoholic liver disease. J Hepatol 2008; 49(6):1062–8.

27. Kim SG, Kim YS, Jung SW, et al. [The usefulness of transient elastography to diagnose cirrhosis in patients with alcoholic liver disease]. Korean J Hepatol 2009; 15(1):42–51.

28. Janssens F, de Suray N, Piessevaux H, et al. Can transient elastography replace liver histology for determination of advanced fibrosis in alcoholic patients: a real-life study. J Clin Gastroenterol 2010;44(8):575.

29. Mueller S, Millonig G, Sarovska L, et al. Increased liver stiffness in alcoholic liver disease: differentiating fibrosis from steatohepatitis. World J Gastroenterol WJG 2010;16(8):966–72.

30. Nguyen-Khac E, Thiele M, Voican C, et al. Non-invasive diagnosis of liver fibrosis in patients with alcohol-related liver disease by transient elastography: an individual patient data meta-analysis. Lancet Gastroenterol Hepatol 2018;3(9):614–25.

31. Thursz M, Gual A, Lackner C, et al. EASL clinical practice guidelines: management of alcohol-related liver disease. J Hepatol 2018;69(1):154–81.

32. Gelsi E, Dainese R, Truchi R, et al. Effect of detoxification on liver stiffness assessed by Fibroscan® in alcoholic patients. Alcohol Clin Exp Res 2011;35(3): 566–70.

33. de Franchis R, Bosch J, Garcia-Tsao G, et al. Baveno VII – renewing consensus in portal hypertension. J Hepatol 2022;76(4):959–74.

34. Papatheodoridi M, Hiriart JB, Lupsor-Platon M, et al. Refining the Baveno VI elastography criteria for the definition of compensated advanced chronic liver disease. J Hepatol 2021;74(5):1109–16.

35. Juárez-Hernández E, Uribe-Ramos MH, Ramos-Ostos MH, et al. Factors associated with the quality of transient elastography. Dig Dis Sci 2015;60(7):2177–82.

36. Bota S, Herkner H, Sporea I, et al. Meta-analysis: ARFI elastography versus transient elastography for the evaluation of liver fibrosis. Liver Int 2013;33(8):1138–47.

37. Thiele M, Detlefsen S, Sevelsted Møller L, et al. Transient and 2-dimensional shear-wave elastography provide comparable assessment of alcoholic liver fibrosis and cirrhosis. Gastroenterology 2016;150(1):123–33.

38. Zhang D, Li P, Chen M, et al. Non-invasive assessment of liver fibrosis in patients with alcoholic liver disease using acoustic radiation force impulse elastography. Abdom Imaging 2015;40(4):723–9.

39. Rasmussen DN, Thiele M, Johansen S, et al. Prognostic performance of 7 biomarkers compared to liver biopsy in early alcohol-related liver disease. J Hepatol 2021;75(5):1017–25.

40. Muthupillai R, Lomas DJ, Rossman PJ, et al. Magnetic resonance elastography by direct visualization of propagating acoustic strain waves. Science 1995; 269(5232):1854–7.

41. Low G, Kruse SA, Lomas DJ. General review of magnetic resonance elastography. World J Radiol 2016;8(1):59–72.

42. Bensamoun SF, Leclerc GE, Debernard L, et al. Cutoff values for alcoholic liver fibrosis using magnetic resonance elastography technique. Alcohol Clin Exp Res 2013;37(5):811–7.

43. Parkes J, Guha IN, Harris S, et al. Systematic review of the diagnostic performance of serum markers of liver fibrosis in alcoholic liver disease. Comp Hepatol 2012;11(1):5.

44. Imbert-Bismut F, Ratziu V, Pieroni L, et al. Biochemical markers of liver fibrosis in patients with hepatitis C virus infection: a prospective study. Lancet 2001; 357(9262):1069–75.
45. Rosenberg WMC, Voelker M, Thiel R, et al. Serum markers detect the presence of liver fibrosis: a cohort study. Gastroenterology 2004;127(6):1704–13.
46. Calès P, Oberti F, Michalak S, et al. A novel panel of blood markers to assess the degree of liver fibrosis. Hepatology 2005;42(6):1373–81.
47. Adams LA, Bulsara M, Rossi E, et al. Hepascore: an accurate validated predictor of liver fibrosis in chronic hepatitis C infection. Clin Chem 2005;51(10):1867–73.
48. Thiele M, Madsen BS, Hansen JF, et al. Accuracy of the enhanced liver fibrosis test vs FibroTest, elastography, and indirect markers in detection of advanced fibrosis in patients with alcoholic liver disease. Gastroenterology 2018;154(5): 1369–79.
49. Madsen BS, Thiele M, Detlefsen S, et al. PRO-C3 and ADAPT algorithm accurately identify patients with advanced fibrosis due to alcohol-related liver disease. Aliment Pharmacol Ther 2021;54(5):699–708.
50. Moreno C, Mueller S, Szabo G. Non-invasive diagnosis and biomarkers in alcohol-related liver disease. J Hepatol 2019;70(2):273–83.
51. Voican CS, Louvet A, Trabut JB, et al. Transient elastography alone and in combination with FibroTest® for the diagnosis of hepatic fibrosis in alcoholic liver disease. Liver Int 2017;37(11):1697–705.
52. Sheth SG, Flamm SL, Gordon FD, et al. AST/ALT ratio predicts cirrhosis in patients with chronic hepatitis C virus infection. Am J Gastroenterol 1998;93(1):44–8.
53. Imperiale TF, Said AT, Cummings OW, et al. Need for validation of clinical decision aids: use of the AST/ALT ratio in predicting cirrhosis in chronic hepatitis C. Am J Gastroenterol 2000;95(9):2328–32.
54. Mueller S, Englert S, Seitz HK, et al. Inflammation-adapted liver stiffness values for improved fibrosis staging in patients with hepatitis C virus and alcoholic liver disease. Liver Int 2015;35(12):2514–21.
55. Mueller S. Evidence for red blood cell-derived aspartate aminotransferase in heavy drinkers. In: Mueller S, Heilig M, editors. Alcohol and Alcohol-related diseases. Cham: Springer International Publishing; 2023. p. 785–93.
56. Sterling RK, Lissen E, Clumeck N, et al. Development of a simple noninvasive index to predict significant fibrosis in patients with HIV/HCV coinfection. Hepatology 2006;43(6):1317–25.
57. Shah AG, Lydecker A, Murray K, et al. Comparison of noninvasive markers of fibrosis in patients with nonalcoholic fatty liver disease. Clin Gastroenterol Hepatol 2009;7(10):1104–12.
58. Piazzolla VA, Mangia A. Noninvasive diagnosis of NAFLD and NASH. Cells 2020; 9(4):1005.
59. Adler M, Gulbis B, Moreno C, et al. The predictive value of FIB-4 versus FibroTest, APRI, FibroIndex and Forns index to noninvasively estimate fibrosis in hepatitis C and nonhepatitis C liver diseases. Hepatology 2008;47(2):762.
60. Berzigotti A, Tsochatzis E, Boursier J, et al. EASL Clinical Practice Guidelines on non-invasive tests for evaluation of liver disease severity and prognosis – 2021 update. J Hepatol 2021;75(3):659–89.
61. Graupera I, Thiele M, Serra-Burriel M, et al. Low accuracy of FIB-4 and NAFLD fibrosis scores for screening for liver fibrosis in the population. Clin Gastroenterol Hepatol 2022;20(11):2567–76.e6.
62. Gracen L, Hayward KL, Irvine KM, et al. Low accuracy of FIB-4 test to identify people with diabetes at low risk of advanced fibrosis. J Hepatol 2022;77(4):1219–21.

63. Naveau S, Gaudé G, Asnacios A, et al. Diagnostic and prognostic values of noninvasive biomarkers of fibrosis in patients with alcoholic liver disease. Hepatology 2009;49(1):97–105.
64. Simpson RF, Hermon C, Liu B, et al. Alcohol drinking patterns and liver cirrhosis risk: analysis of the prospective UK Million Women Study. Lancet Public Health 2019;4(1):e41–8.
65. Pavlov CS, Casazza G, Nikolova D, et al. Transient elastography for diagnosis of stages of hepatic fibrosis and cirrhosis in people with alcoholic liver disease. Cochrane Database Syst Rev 2015;2015(1).

Current Pharmacotherapy and Nutrition Therapy of Alcohol-Associated Liver Disease

Josiah E. Hardesty, PhD[a,b], Craig J. McClain, MD[a,b,c,d,e],*

KEYWORDS

- Alcohol-associated liver disease • Alcohol associated hepatitis • Malnutrition
- Nutrition support corticosteroids • Non-responders

KEY POINTS

- Malnutrition is a frequently underdiagnosed complication of ALD that can influence outcomes ranging from quality of life to mortality.
- Corticosteroids should be considered the current standard-of-care for treatment of severe AH, and one recent study showed an impressive greater than 90% 90-day survival (needs to be validated).
- Corticosteroids are not always effective and the Lille Score should be used in all patients receiving corticosteroids.

INTRODUCTION

Alcohol-associated liver disease (ALD) spans a spectrum of severity ranging from simple steatosis to steatohepatitis to cirrhosis and potentially to hepatocellular carcinoma. Therapy for ALD also covers a wide range of modalities. Every patient with alcohol use disorder (AUD) should be encouraged to incorporate lifestyle modifications. Indeed, stopping or decreasing harmful drinking is a cornerstone of ALD therapy, and optimally a team approach is used. Some patients with AUD and most patients with ALD should receive nutritional counseling and potential nutritional intervention. Patients with more advanced ALD may require drug therapy and only a few

[a] Department of Pharmacology and Toxicology, University of Louisville School of Medicine, Louisville, KY, USA; [b] Division of Gastroenterology, Hepatology, and Nutrition, Department of Medicine, University of Louisville, Louisville, KY, USA; [c] University of Louisville Alcohol Center, University of Louisville School of Medicine, Louisville, KY, USA; [d] Robley Rex Veterans Medical Center, Louisville, KY, USA; [e] University of Louisville Hepatobiology & Toxicology Center, University of Louisville School of Medicine, Louisville, KY, USA
* Corresponding author. Division of Gastroenterology, Hepatology, and Nutrition, Department of Medicine, University of Louisville, 505 South Hancock Street CTR Building Room 501, Louisville, KY 40202.
E-mail address: Craig.mcclain@louisville.edu

Clin Liver Dis 28 (2024) 731–745
https://doi.org/10.1016/j.cld.2024.06.018
1089-3261/24/Published by Elsevier Inc.

liver.theclinics.com

patients with advanced ALD will receive liver transplantation. This article reviews the roles of nutrition and drug therapy in ALD. Thus, as shown in **Fig. 1**, this article pertains to the majority of individuals with ALD.

NUTRITION THERAPY
Malnutrition Overview

The 2020 to 2025 Dietary guidelines for Americans (United States [US] Department of Health and Human Services and US Department of Agriculture, 2020) put forward the concept of the standard drink and the fact that if alcohol is consumed, it should be in moderation; that is, up to one drink per day for women and 2 drinks per day for men in adults of legal drinking age (**Fig. 2**). The standard drink contains 14 g of alcohol.[1] People who misuse alcohol frequently consume large amounts of alcohol, which may contribute to the displacement of needed nutrients. Indeed, we and others have reported that patients in alcohol treatment programs or hospitalized with alcohol-associated hepatitis (AH) may be consuming 1000 to 20000 calories per day in "empty calories" (**Fig. 2**). Of interest, there were not major differences between alcohol intake in subjects hospitalized for severe AH compared to those with or without early liver disease in a treatment program (**Fig. 2**). Thus, these subjects are consuming large amounts of alcohol-containing beverages that lack critical macronutrients such as protein, lack fiber, which is a substrate for short-chain fatty acid production by gut bacteria, and lack critical micronutrients such as thiamin and zinc.[1,2]

"Malnutrition" is a broad term that includes a deficiency, excess or imbalance of nutrients that result in adverse consequences on clinical outcomes.[3] Most frequently, the term malnutrition is used in the context of deficiency of calories or proteins but can also be applied to over-nourished individuals. This concept is important because subjects with ALD are becoming increasingly overweight, similar to the general population. Several societies have agreed upon a new term—"Met-ALD"—to describe subjects who have components of the metabolic syndrome and who have greater than "moderate" alcohol consumption.[4] Malnourished patients may present with global malnutrition with frailty or sarcopenia. They may also present with individual nutrient deficiency (eg, zinc) and a functional manifestation (eg, poor wound healing or skin lesions). The most frequent phenotype of the "undernourished" patient is sarcopenia, and this term relates to the clinical consequences of muscle loss, and it is a more specific term and critical component of malnutrition. Importantly, malnutrition can markedly impact multiple outcomes in ALD, ranging from quality of life to mortality.

It should not be surprising that many subjects with ALD have some degree of malnutrition and that the causes of this malnutrition are multifactorial.[5] The previously noted empty calories in alcohol and poor quality of food intake play an important role. Protein intake decreases as the liver disease progresses. Hormones (eg, testosterone) and

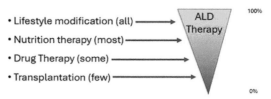

Fig. 1. Alcohol-associated Liver Disease (ALD) Therapy The majority of patients with ALD should receive nutrition therapy and some drug therapy.

Drinking Patterns/Amounts
Standard Drink = 14 grams alcohol

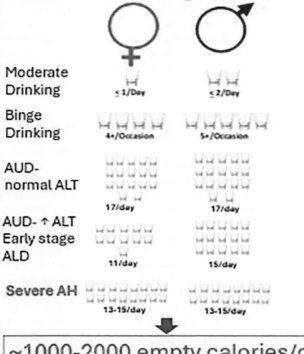

~1000-2000 empty calories/day

Fig. 2. Patients hospitalized in an alcohol treatment program were drinking between 11 and 17 drinks per day depending on presence or absence of liver injury and sex. Interestingly, those with early stage ALD (↑ALT) were drinking less than those with normal ALT. Patients hospitalized with severe AH were drinking ~13 to 15 drinks/day. All patients with AUD/ALD were consuming large amounts of "empty calories". *NIH website on drinking:* http://www.rethinkingdrinking.niaaa.nih.gov.

cytokines (eg, tumor necrosis factor) can have adverse and potentially beneficial effects. Complications of liver disease, such as ascites and encephalopathy, can also impair adequate dietary intake.[6] Patients with ALD frequently have dysbiosis, which can negatively impact nutritional status. Anorexia is common in ALD, and patients with ALD who have anorexia are at increased risk of malnutrition compared to patients with ALD without anorexia. Moreover, the incidence of anorexia increases with increasing severity of liver disease.[7,8]

Assessment of malnutrition in patients with liver disease can be challenging. Many of the tests commonly used to assess malnutrition can be influenced by the underlying liver disease. Anthropometry is influenced by factors such as edema and ascites. Even though the body mass index can be impacted by fluid status changes, we still routinely use this test because of its simplicity and availability. Visceral proteins, such as albumin and prealbumin are synthesized in the liver and can also be influenced by infection or inflammation. Bioelectrical impedance (BIA) is increasingly used for body composition analysis. The theory behind it is that each body tissue has a specific electrical conductivity that is directly related to the water and electrolyte content of that tissue. Pirlich and coworkers showed a strong correlation between BIA and the gold standard of total body potassium for assessing malnutrition.[9] Advances have made this method more accurate, even in patients with ascites, which was previously a limiting factor. This technology is simple to use and provides not only information on muscle mass but also on extracellular water, and we predict it will be increasingly used in liver clinics. Lastly, we routinely use assessment of muscle strength with a hand grip dynamometer as an inexpensive and easy marker of nutrition or muscle strength, and it is particularly good for serial evaluation.[10]

Outpatient Nutrition Support

Initial interest in nutrition therapy for ALD was stimulated in 1948 by Patek and colleagues, who demonstrated that a "nutritious diet" improved the 5-year outcome of patients with alcohol-associated cirrhosis (AC) compared with historic controls.[11] Subsequent outpatient studies showed that enteral nutrition EN supplements improved nutritional status and immune function in patients with AC and reduced hospitalization.[12,13] The role of a late evening snack (LES) before bedtime was established after altered energy metabolism was reported in patients with liver cirrhosis. Depleted hepatic glycogen stores led to catabolism in times of fasting. An early study demonstrated that patients with stable cirrhosis maintained a positive nitrogen balance when given 4 to 6 meals a day that included an LES as opposed to 3 equicaloric and equinitrogenous meals without an LES.[14] An elegant outpatient study by Plank and coworkers showed that provision of an LES to patients with cirrhosis resulted in body protein accrual equivalent to about 2 kg of lean tissue sustained over 12 months, and this benefit was not observed with daytime snacks. Thus, LESs are an important nutritional intervention in outpatients with cirrhosis.[14] A subsequent study from Japan showed that using a multidisciplinary nutrition support team with recommendations that included LES improved 5-year mortality in patients with cirrhosis.[15]

Deficiencies in individual micro-nutrients such as zinc, magnesium, thiamin, and so on also are frequent in ALD. Moreover, micronutrient deficiencies often occur in early stage liver disease before the occurrence of more global malnutrition. A good example of this is the high incidence of hypozincemia in early stage liver disease.[16] A discussion concerning micronutrient supplementation is beyond the scope of this article but has been reviewed by us previously.[17,18] **Table 1** lists selected micronutrient deficiencies in ALD and possible manifestations.

Zinc is an essential trace element required for normal cell growth, development, and differentiation. It is a critical component in many zinc protein enzymes, including critical zinc transcription factors for liver function such as 4HNFα.[19] Zinc deficiency or altered metabolism is often observed in ALD, even in early stage ALD. Some of the mechanisms for zinc deficiency or altered metabolism include decreased dietary intake, increased urinary excretion, activation of certain zinc transporters, and induction of hepatic metallothionein. Zinc deficiency may manifest itself in many ways in liver disease, including skin lesions, poor wound healing or liver regeneration, altered metal status, or altered immune function. Zinc supplementation has been documented to block or attenuate experimental ALD through multiple processes, including stabilization of gut-barrier function, reduced endotoxemia, decreased proinflammatory cytokine production, limited oxidative stress, and the attenuation of hepatocyte death. Only limited zinc supplementation studies have been performed in ALD, and several looked at the reversal of zinc deficiency manifestations such as skin lesions. An open label study showed improvement in muscle cramps.[20] The dose of zinc used

Table 1
Possible micronutrient deficiencies in alcohol-associated liver disease

Nutrient Deficiency	Possible Manifestations
Vitamin A	Night blindness, dry skin
Thiamine	Neurologic problems, Wernike's encephalopathy
Folate	Anemia, possible increased susceptibility to ALD, and altered methionine metabolism
Vitamin D	Bone disease altered immune function
Vitamin E	Possible increased susceptibility to liver injury, oxidative stress
Niacin	Pellegra dermatitis, neurologic alterations, and hallucinations
Pyridoxine	Hypochromic anemia
Zinc	Skin lesions, anorexia, depressed wound healing, hypogonadism, altered immune function, impaired night vision, depressed mental function, diarrhea, and increased susceptibility to liver injury
Magnesium	Muscle cramps, glucose intolerance
Selenium	Myopathy, cardiomyopathy, and oxidative stress

for the treatment of liver disease is usually 50 mg of elemental zinc taken with a meal to decrease the potential side effect of nausea. Higher doses should be avoided because of potential risks of copper deficiency or immune dysfunction.

Inpatient Nutrition Support

Nutritional supplementation for inpatients with ALD is also important. Early Veterans Administration (VA) Cooperative studies showed that inpatients with AH who consumed less protein and calories had greater mortality. Nutritional supplementation through a feeding tube was shown to improve liver function significantly in inpatients with ALD, as assessed by serum bilirubin levels and antipyrine clearance, compared with inpatients who ate a hospital diet.[21] A multicenter study by Cabré and colleagues randomized patients with severe AH to receive either prednisone, 40 mg daily, or a liver-specific formula containing 2000 calories per day through a feeding tube.[22] The 1-month mortality was the same in both groups, but the 1-year mortality was significantly lower in the enteral nutrition group compared with the glucocorticoid group, mainly because of fewer infectious complications. This study clearly documents the importance of enteral nutrition in severe AH. In a more recent multicenter trial, patients with severe AH were treated with either intensive EN plus methylprednisolone or convention nutrition plus methylprednisolone.[23] EN was given via feeding tube for 14 days. The 6-month mortality (primary endpoint) was numerically but not statistically lower in the EN group (44.4%) compared with the control group (52.1%). Importantly, patients from either group receiving less than 21.5 kcal per kg per day had significantly lower survival rates, as did those receiving less than 77.6 gm of protein per day. Thus, it is clear that meeting caloric, especially protein, requirements is important for optimal outcomes.

When the patient is hospitalized with ALD, it is critical to rapidly diagnose metabolic disturbances, including electrolyte disorders, and to monitor food consumption and use oral nutritional supplements, including a nighttime snack, in patients to ensure optimal protein or energy requirements by the oral route.[6] It is important to engage the subject early to gain early patient cooperation concerning the need for nutrition as a critical component of their treatment plan (**Box 1**). If the patient has inadequate

---

Box 1
Nutrition support goals for hospitalized patients with alcohol-associated hepatitis

- Early nutrition assessment and evaluation of serum electrolytes
- Aggressive replacement of electrolytes to prevent refeeding syndrome
- Formulate water and electrolyte intake to individual needs, renal function, and diuretic sensitivity
- Total energy intake goal: ~1.0 to 1.4 x resting energy expenditure or ~25 to 40 Kcal/kg body weight per day
- Protein: ~1.2 to 2.0 g/kg per day
- Fat: ~30 to 40% of nonprotein energy
- Replace vitamins and minerals as indicated and avoid excessive iron, copper, and vitamin A supplementation
- Supplement daily oral intake with enteral feedings (parenteral if enteral route otherwise contraindicated), if oral intake is insufficient
- Hypocaloric, high-protein diet for obese subjects
- Nutrition education with dietitian, including implementation of nighttime snacks

---

oral intake, initiation of early EN support is especially important because it has the potential to positively impact patient outcomes. EN is favored over parenteral nutrition because of the risk of infections, cost, and maintenance of the gut barrier function. EN support should be initiated within 24 to 48 hours following hospitalization in patients unable to maintain oral nutritional intake, with the aim to provide greater than 80% of estimated or calculated goal energy and protein within 48 to 72 hours. Concentrated formulas are preferable in patients with ascites to avoid positive fluid balance. Protein intake is usually recommended at 1.2 to 1.5 g per kg body weight per day (g/kg BW/d). A caloric target of 35 to 40 Kcal per kg body weight per day (cal/kg BW/d) is recommended in hospitalized nonobese patients.[24] Interrupting feeding for diagnostic tests or nurse procedures should be minimized. Obese patients with AH represent a nutrition challenge. Current guidelines recommend hypocaloric, high-protein nutrition therapy in an attempt to preserve lean body mass, to mobilize fat stores, and to minimize overfeeding complications in these at-risk obese patients with liver disease.[25]

PHARMACOTHERAPY
Overview of Medications for Alcohol-Related Liver Disease

Multiple drugs have been studied for the treatment of AC or AH, and all but one category, glucocorticoids, have generally failed. Some of the failures for the treatment of fibrosis or cirrhosis include colchicine and polyenylphosphatidylcholine, which were evaluated in large VA Cooperative Studies.[26–28] The trial on polyenylphosphatidylcholine is particularly instructive because patients with ALD were initially drinking about 16 drinks a day, but within 3 months they had decreased their intake to approximately 2 drinks a day (irrespective of treatment).[27] This marked change in drinking was presumed to be due to their close clinical follow-up. Thus, it was unlikely that any drug could have shown beneficial effect following this marked reduction in alcohol intake. On the other hand, this study was one of the first to show the positive impact of close patient follow-up ("brief interventions") in decreasing drinking. This highlights some of the difficulties in performing clinical trials in ALD. Several drugs have also been tried in

AH, and a list of recent failures is included in **Box 2**. Pentoxifylline (PTX) is the drug that was used by many physicians to treat AH, but whose efficacy has recently been called into question. PTX is a relatively weak nonspecific phosphodiesterase (PDE) inhibitor, which has been shown to attenuate liver injury and fibrosis in animal models of liver disease.[29,30] PDE inhibitors increase cyclic adenosine monophosphate levels, thereby inhibiting tumor necrosis factor production in vivo and in vitro.[31-35] Importantly, PDE4 inhibitors have also been demonstrated to upregulate the anti-inflammatory or antifibrotic cytokine interleukin 10.[34,36-40] PTX was initially reported to reduce mortality in patients with severe AH.[41] Subsequent larger trials reached similar conclusions.[42,43] Most of the reduction in mortality appeared to be related to a decrease in the frequency of hepatorenal syndrome in the survivors.[41] However, more recent trials and meta-analyses failed to show beneficial effects, and the large STOPAH trial showed no benefit of PTX.[44] A major disadvantage of PTX is that it is an oral drug that is taken 3 times a day. This is required for drug efficacy. Patients with AUD or ALD are well-known to be non-compliant with medications. In a recent study, the compliance with PTX in severe AH patients was only 49% over a 1-month treatment period.[45] Thus, while the concept of phosphodiesterase inhibition in AH is likely reasonable, better medications with longer durations of action are required. S-adenosyl methionine is another drug that showed favorable results in one large trial in AC, but also requires Strict three times a day (t.i.d.) therapy and there have been no major published follow-up studies.[46] Lastly, multiple studies have evaluated antioxidant cocktails and individual antioxidants in ALD or AH without benefit.[47,48] There are some data that intravenous n-acetylcysteine may be beneficial as an adjunct to corticosteroid therapy in AH. Indeed, this adjunct therapy was recommended in recent American College of Gastroenterology guidelines, but further trials are necessary.[48]

Glucocorticoids

Glucocorticoids are considered to be the standard-of-care for severe AH by many gastroenterologists or hepatologists and professional organizations. Glucocorticoids bind to receptors (GRs) in the cytoplasm. GRs subsequently translocate to the nucleus and bind to the glucocorticoid response elements in the promoter regions of glucocorticoid responsive genes to switch on expression of certain anti-inflammatory genes.[49] Glucocorticoids can also act indirectly to repress activity of a number of relevant transcription factors (eg, nuclear factor kappa B — NFκB), with subsequent downregulation of inflammatory genes. This process requires recruitment of corepressor molecules, particularly histone deacetylases-6 and -2.[50,51]

Importantly, corticosteroids should only be used in patients with severe AH, and the definition for AH has evolved over a half century. In 1977, Maddrey and colleagues used the serum bilirubin and prothrombin time to define a group of patients with AH

Box 2
Current status of other drugs for alcohol-associated hepatitis

Older Drugs with questionable efficacy
- SAMe
- Pentoxifylline
- N-acetylcysteine/antioxidants

Recent Negative Trials
- Amoxicillin + clavulinic acid
- Selonsertib (ASK-1 inhibitor)
- Anakinra (IL-1R antagonist)
- Canakinumab (IL-1 blocker)

who had a 28-day mortality rate above 50%.[52] This formula, known as the Maddrey Discriminant Function (MDF), was subsequently used to stratify subjects for inclusion into clinical trials. Early trials and a subsequent randomized multicenter trial indicated that only those patients with more severe manifestations of AH and MDF greater than 32 benefited from treatment with glucocorticoids.[52] The Model for End-Stage Liver Disease (MELD) score was also shown to predict 28-day and 90-day mortality. The age, bilirubin, international normalized ratio, and creatinine score (ABIC score) and the Glasgow AH Score also predict 90-day mortality, as do several other bio-markers.[53–55] All of these scoring systems have been validated to predict severe outcomes with a high degree of reliability, with MDF being the least reliable.[56]

Clinical trials and clinical practice have evolved greatly over the half century that glucocorticoids have been used for the treatment of severe AH. We now have a widely used definition for AH that was devised by National Institute on Alcohol Abuse and Alcoholism (NIAAA) consensus group, and criteria are mainly clinical and biochemical.[57] Liver biopsy is infrequently done in the US for the diagnosis of AH. Clinical trials initially used an endpoint of 30-day mortality, and this has now generally evolved to a primary endpoint of 90-day mortality.[58] The 90-day survival has slowly improved, probably in large part due to improvement in the standard-of-care. The survival endpoint results observed in the STOPAH trial at 30- and 90- days are generally considered optimal.[44] These results showed approximately 15% 30-day mortality and approximately 30% 90-day mortality, and these are now considered to be the current standard (**Fig. 3**). Unfortunately, the STOPAH trial and others report over 50% mortality at 1 year, and most of this later mortality relates to a return to drinking. Virtually all studies show that glucocorticoids modestly improve 1 month survival, but not at later time points. Basically, all of the published studies have treated patients for 30 days with approximately 40 mg of prednisone or prednisolone. Both the duration and dose are empiric. Importantly, none of the studies up to now had used the Lille Stopping Rule because of complexity of study design. However, a recent article in

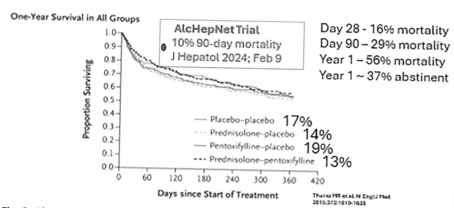

STOPAH Trial
Prednisolone or Pentoxifylline for AH

Fig. 3. The STOPAH Trial and many recent studies show a 90 day mortality of approximately 30%. The recent AlcHepNet Trial showed a 90 day mortality of only 10% with prednisolone therapy and use of Lille stopping rules.

the Journal of Hepatology that used the Lille Stopping Rule shows dramatic therapeutic effects with glucocorticoid therapy.[59] This study was halted mid-point because the prednisone group was outperforming the anakinra-plus-zinc group, with only 10% mortality at 90 days in the prednisone group (**Fig. 3**).[59] This trial was the first to show major effects on mortality at 90 days with prednisone, and these data clearly need to be repeated in a glucocorticoid study employing Lille stopping rule. However, there are very promising new data on the use of glucocorticoids in severe AH.

Importantly, it has been reported that up to 40% of AH patients do not respond to corticosteroids as assessed by the 7-day Lille Score.[60] If after 7 days of corticosteroid treatment the Lille Score is greater than 0.45, patients discontinue treatment and are characterized as non-responders. AH patients that respond to treatment as determined by a Lille Score less than 0.45, patients will remain on corticosteroids for up to 30 days. There have been clinical trials that have observed reduced efficacy of corticosteroids for the treatment of AH and have identified an increased risk of infection associated with corticosteroid treatment.[44,61] However, evidence has suggested that early response to corticosteroids is the determining factor of patient prognosis and not infection.[62] This prompted a recent clinical trial evaluating the combination of prophylactic antibiotics and corticosteroids as a treatment strategy for AH, but no added benefit regarding 60-day mortality was observed.[63] Our current standard-of-care for patients with severe AH is to determine whether they are candidates for glucocorticoid therapy. If they meet criteria for severe AH including a MELD greater than 20 and are steroid eligible, they are started on glucocorticoids and their progress is assessed by Lille score at 4 or 7 days. If their Lille score drops to less than 0.45, patients continue therapy for a total of 4 weeks and the drug is then discontinued. If patients are not responding by the Lille model, or if they are steroid ineligible, they are referred to transplant centers or considered for clinical trials (**Fig. 4**).

There is considerable ongoing research attempting to predict who will respond to steroids and why some patients do not respond to steroids. As noted previously, the Lille score is increasingly used clinically to predict steroid non-response. This is a dynamic test in which biochemical parameters (with bilirubin the dominant test) are evaluated at baseline and either 4 or 7 days later.[64,65] A decrease in the score (<.45) indicates patients are responding to steroids and should continue therapy. An elevated score (≥.45) indicates the subset of patients who did not respond to therapy,

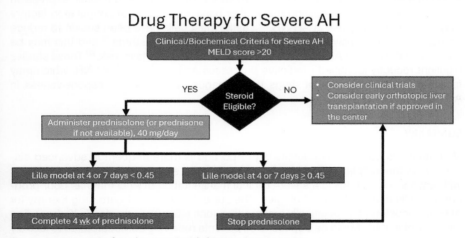

Fig. 4. Decision tree for glucocorticoid therapy in severe AH.

and steroids should be stopped. A goal is to prevent ongoing steroid use in patients who will not benefit from steroids but will incur their side effects. The K18 is a biomarker of cell death, and the data from the STOPAH trial showed that patients with a very high level of greater than or equal to 5000 were those who would respond to steroids and were the subgroup of patients who should receive steroid therapy.[66,67]

Other studies are evaluating biochemical or immunologic mechanisms of steroid non-responsiveness. Recently, many multi-omic approaches have been used to characterize differences between AH-R (responder) and AH-NR (non-responder) to corticosteroid therapies. For example, transcriptomic analysis of AH patient peripheral blood mononuclear cells (PBMCs) acquired from AH-R and AH-NR demonstrated that gene modules related to lymphoid lineage including cell division and mitochondria respiration were upregulated in AH-NR at baseline.[68] After 7 days of treatment with corticosteroids, AH-R PBMCs had reduced expression of genes involved in innate and adaptive immunity whereas AH-NR had no significant changes.[68] Corticosteroids are widely regarded as immunomodulatory drugs that are anti-inflammatory.[69] This study demonstrated distinct effects on the respective PBMC transcriptome between AH-R and AH-NR at baseline and 7 days post treatment demonstrating multiple immune cell processes are changed at baseline in AH-NR and in response to treatment in AH-R.

A recent hepatic proteomic study using liver biopsy samples acquired prior to corticosteroid treatment identified predictive markers of corticosteroid non-responsiveness in AH patients.[70] Notably, AH-NR had reduced expression of hepatic glucocorticoid receptor,[70] which intuitively could contribute to a lack of therapeutic response to corticosteroids. In fact, this has been documented in clinical and pre-clinical models of sepsis and associated with exacerbated liver injury, inflammation, and compromised liver function.[71] In addition, hepatic markers that predicted AH-NR mortality were identified. These included reduced hepatic protein expression of acute phase proteins (APPs) and coagulation factors but elevated expression of mast cell markers.[72] Many APPs are upregulated in response to corticosteroids during inflammation and in AH-NR patients that survived higher expression of APPs prior to treatment may contribute to their reduced mortality risk.[73] Previously, corticosteroids have been shown to improve blood coagulation in AH patients and this recent study found that AH-NR survivors versus AH-NR survivors had elevated hepatic expression of coagulation factor suggesting that higher basal expression of coagulation factors may reduce mortality risk in AH-NR.[74] Lastly, mast cells have been shown to reduce corticosteroid responsiveness in experimental models of asthma[75] and this may be the case in the liver for AH-NR contributing to increased mortality risk.[70] These studies highlight recently identified predictive processes and markers of AH-NR, which may facilitate the development of drugs that enhance corticosteroid responsiveness in AH patients.

SUMMARY

Malnutrition is common in patients with ALD and is more frequent in advanced disease. A nutrition "plan" including late night snacks should be provided to patients with advanced ALD. AH is a severe clinical manifestation of ALD that has poor prognosis and limited treatment strategies. The current standard-of-care drug therapy for AH is corticosteroids, specifically oral prednisolone (40 mg per day for 7–30 days). The Lille stopping rule should be applied to all patients receiving corticosteroids to identify non-responders, and research is ongoing to identify mechanisms of non-response.

FUTURE OUTLOOK OF CORTICOSTEROID TREATMENT FOR PATIENTS WITH ALCOHOL-ASSOCIATED HEPATITIS

While corticosteroids remain the current standard for treatment of AH, treatment efficacy, improved patient outcomes, and the development of shorter prognostic tests can be improved upon. Novel therapies used in tandem with corticosteroids may increase patient responsiveness to treatment reducing the percentage of AH-NR. In addition, novel therapies used concurrently with corticosteroids may also improve long-term prognosis as opposed to only short-term mortality as currently shown with corticosteroids alone. Further, novel prognostic tests that can be used the day of hospitalization may be useful for identifying an AH-NR prior to day 4[65] or day 7[60] of corticosteroid treatment shortening the unnecessary exposure to corticosteroids in AH-NR patients.

CLINICS CARE POINTS

- Patients with ALD are frequently malnourished, especially those with more advanced disease.
- Patients with advanced ALD should consume nighttime snacks to prevent muscle loss.
- Corticosteroids are the current standard-of-care drug treatment for severe AH, but patients receiving corticosteroids should be evaluated with the Lille score to determine continuation of therapy

DISCLOSURE

The authors have no conflicts of interest to disclose as it pertains to this work.

Financial support: This work was supported by the following grants: National Institutes of Health, United States grants R00AA030627 (J.E. Hardesty), U01AA026934 (C.J. McClain), U01AA026926 (C.J. McClain), and U01AA026980 (C.J. McClain) and the VA: 2I01CX002219-05A2 (C.J. McClain). This work was also supported by an Institutional Development Award (IDeA), United States from the National Institute of General Medical Sciences, United States of the National Institutes of Health under grant number P20GM113226 (C.J. McClain), and the National Institute on Alcohol Abuse and Alcoholism, United States of the National Institutes of Health under Award Number P50AA024337 (C.J. McClain). The content is solely the responsibility of the authors and does not necessarily represent the official views of the National Institutes of Health.

REFERENCES

1. Vatsalya V, Royer AJ, Jha SK, et al. Drinking and laboratory biomarkers, and nutritional status characterize the clinical presentation of early-stage alcohol-associated liver disease. Adv Clin Chem 2023;114:83–108.
2. Hariri Z, Hekmatdoost A, Pashayee-Khamene F, et al. Dietary fiber intake and mortality among survivors of liver cirrhosis: a prospective cohort study. Heliyon 2023;9(6):e16170.
3. Saunders J, Smith T. Malnutrition: causes and consequences. Clin Med 2010; 10(6):624–7.
4. Rinella ME, Lazarus JV, Ratziu V, et al. A multisociety Delphi consensus statement on new fatty liver disease nomenclature. J Hepatol 2023;79(6):1542–56.

5. Periyalwar P, Dasarathy S. Malnutrition in cirrhosis: contribution and consequences of sarcopenia on metabolic and clinical responses. Clin Liver Dis 2012;16(1):95–131.

6. McClain CJ, Rios CD, Condon S, et al. Malnutrition and alcohol-associated hepatitis. Clin Liver Dis 2021;25(3):557–70.

7. Mendenhall CL, Anderson S, Weesner RE, et al. Protein-calorie malnutrition associated with alcoholic hepatitis. Veterans administration cooperative study group on alcoholic hepatitis. Am J Med 1984;76(2):211–22.

8. Mendenhall C, Roselle GA, Gartside P, et al. Relationship of protein calorie malnutrition to alcoholic liver disease: a reexamination of data from two Veterans Administration Cooperative Studies. Alcohol Clin Exp Res 1995;19(3):635–41.

9. Pirlich M, Schütz T, Spachos T, et al. Bioelectrical impedance analysis is a useful bedside technique to assess malnutrition in cirrhotic patients with and without ascites. Hepatology 2000;32(6):1208–15.

10. Gaikwad NR, Gupta SJ, Samarth AR, et al. Handgrip dynamometry: a surrogate marker of malnutrition to predict the prognosis in alcoholic liver disease. Ann Gastroenterol 2016;29(4):509–14.

11. Patek AJ Jr, Post J, et al. Dietary treatment of cirrhosis of the liver; results in 124 patients observed during a 10 year period. J Am Med Assoc 1948;138(8):543–9.

12. Hirsch S, Bunout D, de la Maza P, et al. Controlled trial on nutrition supplementation in outpatients with symptomatic alcoholic cirrhosis. JPEN J Parenter Enteral Nutr 1993;17(2):119–24.

13. Hirsch S, de la Maza MP, Gattás V, et al. Nutritional support in alcoholic cirrhotic patients improves host defenses. J Am Coll Nutr 1999;18(5):434–41.

14. Swart GR, Zillikens MC, van Vuure JK, et al. Effect of a late evening meal on nitrogen balance in patients with cirrhosis of the liver. BMJ 1989;299(6709):1202–3.

15. Iwasa M, Iwata K, Hara N, et al. Nutrition therapy using a multidisciplinary team improves survival rates in patients with liver cirrhosis. Nutrition 2013;29(11–12): 1418–21.

16. Vatsalya V, Kong M, Cave MC, et al. Association of serum zinc with markers of liver injury in very heavy drinking alcohol-dependent patients. J Nutr Biochem 2018;59:49–55.

17. Hanje AJ, Fortune B, Song M, et al. The use of selected nutrition supplements and complementary and alternative medicine in liver disease. Nutr Clin Pract 2006;21(3):255–72.

18. Zhou Z SZ, Pigneri D, McClain M, et al. Longterm management of alcoholic liver disease. In: Preedy VR, Lakshman R, Srirajaskanthan R, et al, editors. Nutrition, diet therapy, and the liver. 1st edition. Boca Raton, FL: CRC Press; 2010. p. 1–373.

19. McClain C, Vatsalya V, Cave M. Role of zinc in the development/progression of alcoholic liver disease. Curr Treat Options Gastroenterol 2017;15(2):285–95.

20. Kugelmas M. Preliminary observation: oral zinc sulfate replacement is effective in treating muscle cramps in cirrhotic patients. J Am Coll Nutr 2000;19(1):13–5.

21. Kearns PJ, Young H, Garcia G, et al. Accelerated improvement of alcoholic liver disease with enteral nutrition. Gastroenterology 1992;102(1):200–5.

22. Cabre E, Rodríguez-Iglesias P, Caballería J, et al. Short- and long-term outcome of severe alcohol-induced hepatitis treated with steroids or enteral nutrition: a multicenter randomized trial. Hepatology 2000;32(1):36–42.

23. Moreno C, et al. Intensive enteral nutrition is ineffective for patients with severe alcoholic hepatitis treated with corticosteroids. Gastroenterology 2016;150(4): 903–910 e8.

24. Plauth M, Cabré E, Riggio O, et al. ESPEN guidelines on enteral nutrition: liver disease. Clin Nutr 2006;25(2):285–94.
25. McClave SA, Taylor BE, Martindale RG, et al. Guidelines for the provision and assessment of nutrition support therapy in the adult critically ill patient: society of critical care medicine (SCCM) and American society for parenteral and enteral nutrition (A.S.P.E.N.). JPEN J Parenter Enteral Nutr 2016;40(2):159–211.
26. Morgan TR, Weiss DG, Nemchausky B, et al. Colchicine treatment of alcoholic cirrhosis: a randomized, placebo-controlled clinical trial of patient survival. Gastroenterology 2005;128(4):882–90.
27. Lieber CS, Weiss DG, Groszmann R, et al. I. Veterans Affairs Cooperative Study of polyenylphosphatidylcholine in alcoholic liver disease: effects on drinking behavior by nurse/physician teams. Alcohol Clin Exp Res 2003;27(11):1757–64.
28. Lieber CS, Weiss DG, Groszmann R, et al. II. Veterans Affairs Cooperative Study of polyenylphosphatidylcholine in alcoholic liver disease. Alcohol Clin Exp Res 2003;27(11):1765–72.
29. Kucuktulu U, Alhan E, Tekelioglu Y, et al. The effects of pentoxifylline on liver regeneration after portal vein ligation in rats. Liver Int 2007;27(2):274–9.
30. Raetsch C, Jia JD, Boigk G, et al. Pentoxifylline downregulates profibrogenic cytokines and procollagen I expression in rat secondary biliary fibrosis. Gut 2002; 50(2):241–7.
31. Spina D. PDE4 inhibitors: current status. Br J Pharmacol 2008;155(3):308–15.
32. Gobejishvili L, Barve S, Joshi-Barve S, et al. Chronic ethanol-mediated decrease in cAMP primes macrophages to enhanced LPS-inducible NF-kappaB activity and TNF expression: relevance to alcoholic liver disease. Am J Physiol Gastrointest Liver Physiol 2006;291(4):G681–8.
33. Essayan DM. Cyclic nucleotide phosphodiesterases. J Allergy Clin Immunol 2001;108(5):671–80.
34. Kwak HJ, Song JS, No ZS, et al. The inhibitory effects of roflumilast on lipopolysaccharide-induced nitric oxide production in RAW264.7 cells are mediated by heme oxygenase-1 and its product carbon monoxide. Inflamm Res 2005; 54(12):508–13.
35. Ouagued M, Martin-Chouly CAE, Brinchault G, et al. The novel phosphodiesterase 4 inhibitor, CI-1044, inhibits LPS-induced TNF-alpha production in whole blood from COPD patients. Pulm Pharmacol Ther 2005;18(1):49–54.
36. Le Moine O, Marchant A, De Groote D, et al. Role of defective monocyte interleukin-10 release in tumor necrosis factor-alpha overproduction in alcoholics cirrhosis. Hepatology 1995;22(5):1436–9.
37. Platzer C, Fritsch E, Elsner T, et al. Cyclic adenosine monophosphate-responsive elements are involved in the transcriptional activation of the human IL-10 gene in monocytic cells. Eur J Immunol 1999;29(10):3098–104.
38. Eigler A, Siegmund B, Emmerich U, et al. Anti-inflammatory activities of cAMP-elevating agents: enhancement of IL-10 synthesis and concurrent suppression of TNF production. J Leukoc Biol 1998;63(1):101–7.
39. Verghese MW, McConnell RT, Strickland AB, et al. Differential regulation of human monocyte-derived TNF alpha and IL-1 beta by type IV cAMP-phosphodiesterase (cAMP-PDE) inhibitors. J Pharmacol Exp Ther 1995;272(3):1313–20.
40. Kambayashi T, Jacob CO, Zhou D, et al. Cyclic nucleotide phosphodiesterase type IV participates in the regulation of IL-10 and in the subsequent inhibition of TNF-alpha and IL-6 release by endotoxin-stimulated macrophages. J Immunol 1995;155(10):4909–16.

41. Akriviadis E, Botla R, Briggs W, et al. Pentoxifylline improves short-term survival in severe acute alcoholic hepatitis: a double-blind, placebo-controlled trial. Gastroenterology 2000;119(6):1637–48.

42. Sidhu SS, Goyal O, Singla M, et al. Pentoxifylline in severe alcoholic hepatitis: a prospective, randomised trial. J Assoc Physicians India 2012;60:20–2.

43. De BK, Gangopadhyay S, Dutta D, et al. Pentoxifylline versus prednisolone for severe alcoholic hepatitis: a randomized controlled trial. World J Gastroenterol 2009;15(13):1613–9.

44. Thursz MR, Richardson P, Allison M, et al. Prednisolone or pentoxifylline for alcoholic hepatitis. N Engl J Med 2015;372(17):1619–28.

45. Szabo G, Mitchell M, McClain CJ, et al. IL-1 receptor antagonist plus pentoxifylline and zinc for severe alcohol-associated hepatitis. Hepatology 2022;76(4): 1058–68.

46. Mato JM, Cámara J, Fernández de Paz J, et al. S-adenosylmethionine in alcoholic liver cirrhosis: a randomized, placebo-controlled, double-blind, multicenter clinical trial. J Hepatol 1999;30(6):1081–9.

47. Mezey E, Potter JJ, Rennie-Tankersley L, et al. A randomized placebo controlled trial of vitamin E for alcoholic hepatitis. J Hepatol 2004;40(1):40–6.

48. Jophlin LL, Singal AK, Bataller R, et al. ACG clinical guideline: alcohol-associated liver disease. Am J Gastroenterol 2024;119(1):30–54.

49. Smart L, Gobejishvili L, Crittenden N, et al. Alcoholic hepatitis: steroids vs. Pentoxifylline. Curr Hepat Rep 2013;12(1):59–65.

50. De Bosscher K, Haegeman G. Minireview: latest perspectives on antiinflammatory actions of glucocorticoids. Mol Endocrinol 2009;23(3):281–91.

51. Barnes PJ, Adcock IM. Glucocorticoid resistance in inflammatory diseases. Lancet 2009;373(9678):1905–17.

52. Maddrey WC, Boitnott JK, Bedine MS, et al. Corticosteroid therapy of alcoholic hepatitis. Gastroenterology 1978;75(2):193–9.

53. Dunn W, Jamil LH, Brown LS, et al. MELD accurately predicts mortality in patients with alcoholic hepatitis. Hepatology 2005;41(2):353–8.

54. Dominguez M, Rincón D, Abraldes JG, et al. A new scoring system for prognostic stratification of patients with alcoholic hepatitis. Am J Gastroenterol 2008;103(11): 2747–56.

55. Forrest EH, Morris AJ, Stewart S, et al. The Glasgow alcoholic hepatitis score identifies patients who may benefit from corticosteroids. Gut 2007;56(12):1743–6.

56. Bissonnette J, Altamirano J, Devue C, et al. A prospective study of the utility of plasma biomarkers to diagnose alcoholic hepatitis. Hepatology 2017;66(2): 555–63.

57. Crabb DW, Bataller R, Chalasani NP, et al. Standard definitions and common data elements for clinical trials in patients with alcoholic hepatitis: recommendation from the NIAAA alcoholic hepatitis consortia. Gastroenterology 2016;150(4): 785–90.

58. Dasarathy S, Mitchell MC, Barton B, et al. Design and rationale of a multicenter defeat alcoholic steatohepatitis trial: (DASH) randomized clinical trial to treat alcohol-associated hepatitis. Contemp Clin Trials 2020;96:106094.

59. Gawrieh S, Dasarathy S, Tu W, et al. Randomized trial of anakinra plus zinc vs. prednisone for severe alcohol-associated hepatitis. J Hepatol 2024;80(5):684–93.

60. Louvet A, Naveau S, Abdelnour M, et al. The Lille model: a new tool for therapeutic strategy in patients with severe alcoholic hepatitis treated with steroids. Hepatology 2007;45(6):1348–54.

61. Vergis N, Atkinson SR, Knapp S, et al. Patients with severe alcoholic hepatitis, prednisolone increases susceptibility to infection and infection-related mortality, and is associated with high circulating levels of bacterial DNA. Gastroenterology 2017;152(5):1068–1077 e4.
62. Louvet A, Wartel F, Castel H, et al. Infection in patients with severe alcoholic hepatitis treated with steroids: early response to therapy is the key factor. Gastroenterology 2009;137(2):541–8.
63. Louvet A, Labreuche J, Dao T, et al. Effect of prophylactic antibiotics on mortality in severe alcohol-related hepatitis: a randomized clinical trial. JAMA 2023; 329(18):1558–66.
64. Mehta H, Dunn W. Determining prognosis of ALD and alcohol-associated hepatitis. J Clin Exp Hepatol 2023;13(3):479–88.
65. Garcia-Saenz-de-Sicilia M, Duvoor C, Altamirano J, et al. A day-4 Lille model predicts response to corticosteroids and mortality in severe alcoholic hepatitis. Am J Gastroenterol 2017;112(2):306–15.
66. McClain CJ, Vatsalya V, Mitchell MC. Keratin-18: diagnostic, prognostic, and theragnostic for alcohol-associated hepatitis. Am J Gastroenterol 2021;116(1):77–9.
67. Atkinson SR, Grove JI, Liebig S, et al. Severe alcoholic hepatitis, serum keratin-18 fragments are diagnostic, prognostic, and theragnostic biomarkers. Am J Gastroenterol 2020;115(11):1857–68.
68. Sharma S, Baweja S, Maras JS, et al. Differential blood transcriptome modules predict response to corticosteroid therapy in alcoholic hepatitis. JHEP Rep 2021;3(3):100283.
69. Pavlov CS, Varganova DL, Casazza G, et al. Glucocorticosteroids for people with alcoholic hepatitis. Cochrane Database Syst Rev 2017;11(11):Cd001511.
70. Hardesty J, Hawthorne M, Day L, et al. Steroid responsiveness in alcohol-associated hepatitis is linked to glucocorticoid metabolism, mitochondrial repair, and heat shock proteins. Hepatol Commun 2024;8(3):1–20.
71. Jenniskens M, Weckx R, Dufour T, et al. The hepatic glucocorticoid receptor is crucial for cortisol homeostasis and sepsis survival in humans and male mice. Endocrinology 2018;159(7):2790–802.
72. Josiah Hardesty MH, Day Le, Warner J, et al. Steroid responsiveness in alcohol-associated hepatitis is linked to glucocorticoid metabolism, mitochondrial repair, and heatshock proteins. Hepatology Communications 2024;8(3):e0393.
73. Baumann H, Richards C, Gauldie J. Interaction among hepatocyte-stimulating factors, interleukin 1, and glucocorticoids for regulation of acute phase plasma proteins in human hepatoma (HepG2) cells. J Immunol 1987;139(12):4122–8.
74. Ramond MJ, Poynard T, Rueff B, et al. A randomized trial of prednisolone in patients with severe alcoholic hepatitis. N Engl J Med 1992;326(8):507–12.
75. Alzahrani A, Hakeem J, Biddle M, et al. Human lung mast cells impair corticosteroid responsiveness in human airway smooth muscle cells. Front Allergy 2021;2: 785100.

Emerging Pharmacologic Treatments for Alcohol-Associated Hepatitis
Current Status and Future Landscape

Timothy R. Morgan, MD[a,b],*

KEYWORDS

- Alcohol-associated hepatitis • Interleukin-22 • Fecal microbiota transfer
- Larsucosterol • Rifaximin • Phage therapy

KEY POINTS

- Prednisolone is the only available medication and approved by organizations (American College of Gastroenterology, American Association for the Study of Liver Diseases, American Gastroenterological Association, Asociacion Lationamericana para Estudio del Higado [Latin American Associaton for the Study of the Liver] [ALEH], and European Association for the Study of the Liver).
- Although there have been multiple negative trials of alcohol-associated hepatitis (AH) in the past decade, several treatments have shown promise for improving outcomes in AH and are currently being evaluated in clinical trials.
- Potential treatments address different pathophysiologic pathways of liver injury, including hepatocyte regeneration, microbiome, and oxidative stress; several treatments may reduce the risk of infection and have fewer complications than corticosteroids.
- Management of alcohol use disorder is required for improving long-term outcomes.

INTRODUCTION

Alcohol-associated hepatitis (AH) is an inflammatory liver injury that occurs in a minority of patients who have a long history of heavy alcohol use. The cardinal clinical sign is jaundice. Other signs and symptoms can include fever, elevated white blood cell, aspartate transaminase, and alanine transaminase, and prolonged international normalized ratio. The disease spectrum runs from mild to severe, with severe often defined as having a Maddrey Discriminate Function (mDF) score greater than or equal to 32 or a Model for End-Stage Liver Disease (MELD) score greater than 20. Patients

a Medical Service/Gastroenterology, VA Long Beach Healthcare System, 5901 East Seventh Street, Long Beach, CA 90822, USA; b Department of Medicine, University of California, Irvine, CA, USA
* Corresponding author. Medical Service (Gastro), VA Long Beach Healthcare System, 5901 East Seventh Street, Long Beach, CA 90822.
E-mail address: timothy.morgan@va.gov

Clin Liver Dis 28 (2024) 747–760
https://doi.org/10.1016/j.cld.2024.06.014
1089-3261/24/Published by Elsevier Inc.

liver.theclinics.com

with mild AH usually recover spontaneously with alcohol abstinence and are not candidates for pharmacotherapy. Patients with severe AH have an estimated 20% mortality at 90-days, which can increase to greater than 50% among patients who fail to respond to corticosteroids.

The pathophysiology of AH is complex and incompletely understood.[1] Reported abnormal pathophysiology include oxidative stress, zone 3 hypoxia, hepatocyte death (apoptosis/necrosis/necroptosis), impaired hepatocyte regeneration or proliferation, intestinal dysbiosis, increased intestinal permeability, endotoxemia, and hepatic and systemic inflammation, which underlie the clinical manifestations of increased infections (spontaneous bacterial peritonitis, pneumonia, etc.), acute kidney injury, hepatic encephalopathy, and malnutrition. It is unclear whether DNA polymorphisms that increase the risk of developing alcohol-associated cirrhosis (ALC), such as PNPLA3, TM6SF2, MBOAT7, HSD17B13, serpin A1 (alpha-1 antitrypsin), also increase the risk of developing AH.

The American Association for the Study of Liver Diseasesand European Association for the Study of the Liverrecommend corticosteroids (eg, prednisone, prednisone) for 28 days among patients with severe AH.[2–4] Corticosteroid treatment modestly reduces mortality at 30 days; corticosteroids have not been shown to reduce mortality at 90 days or thereafter. Multiple other treatments have been evaluated during the past 50 years with none of them being accepted as effective. Treatments that are generally considered to be ineffective based on clinical trials conducted in the United States (US) or Europe, include nutritional supplementation (to address severe malnutrition), pentoxifylline, prophylactic antibiotics (to treat/prevent bacterial infections), anti-cytokine treatments (eg, anti-TNF-alpha, anakinra, selonsertib, CCR2-CCR5 blockers), anti-cell death treatments (eg, caspase inhibitors, anti-apoptosis), and extracorporeal liver support systems. Other treatments, such as oxandrolone and propylthiouracil, have shown limited efficacy but are not being considered for future trials. However, multiple other treatments have shown efficacy in pre-clinical models and potential efficacy in humans with AH and may be reasonable to test in the future (**Fig. 1**).

Interleukin-22

Interleukin-22 (IL-22) is member of the IL-10 cytokine family that produces TH17, TH22, and other immune cells.[5] IL-22 binds to a heterodimer receptor on the cell surface composed of IL-22R1 and IL-10R2. Although IL-10R2 is expressed on multiple cell types, expression IL-22R1 is limited to epithelial cells (eg, hepatocytes, skin, lungs, and intestines), thereby limiting the number of tissues or cells that are activated by IL-22. Binding to the receptor on hepatocytes activates the Jak1/Tyk2-STAT3 pathway, leading to transcription of genes involved in promoting the acute phase response, hepatocyte survival, liver regeneration, and antibacterial responses. Hepatic stellate cells also express IL22R1 receptors. In these cells, IL22 induces expression genes associated with senescence, which should decrease liver fibrogenesis. Hepatocellular carcinoma (HCC) cells also express high levels of IL-22R1 and IL-10R, although IL-22 has not been shown to initiate HCC transformation it may promote HCC growth.[6]

In pre-clinical models, IL-22 protected against multiple types of liver injury.[5] In a chronic-plus-binge ethanol-induced liver injury model, IL-22 activated STAT3 and reduced liver injury and oxidative stress.[7] In a model of acute-on-chronic liver failure (ACLF) using carbon tetrachloride for 8 weeks followed by a double dose of carbon tetrachloride and subsequent injection of *Klebsiella pneumonia*, Xiang and colleagues demonstrated lack of hepatocyte proliferation, likely caused by interferon-gamma-induced activation of STAT1.[8] IL-22 injection activated STAT3 leading to

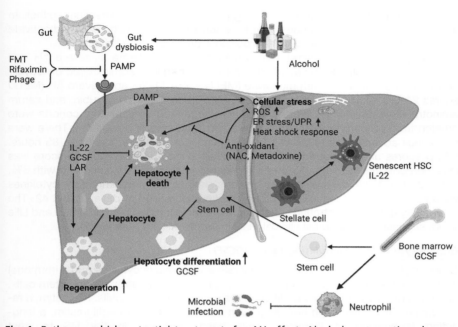

Fig. 1. Pathways which potential treatments for AH affect. Alcohol consumption changes the microbiome, with an increase in "harmful" bacteria and a decrease in "beneficial" bacterial species. FMT from a healthy donor can replenish beneficial bacteria. Rifaximin may decrease bacterial growth while phage therapy against *E. faecalis* may selectively decrease cytotoxic *E. faecalis*. All of these treatments may decrease delivery of DAMPs to the liver. Hepatic alcohol metabolism increases oxidative stress and endoplasmic reticulum stress, which can lead to hepatocyte death. Anti-oxidants (eg, NAC, metadoxine) reduce oxidant injury and decrease hepatocyte death. IL-22 and larsucosterol (LAR) may also reduce hepatocyte death. AH is characterized by decreased hepatocyte regeneration. GCSF, IL-22, and LAR stimulate hepatocyte regeneration. GCSF's effects on the bone marrow include release and maturation of neutrophils, which can protect against infections. GCSF also releases pluripotent stem cells from the bone marrow, some of which engraft in the liver and differentiate into hepatocyte precursors, contributing to increased hepatocyte mass.

improved survival, reduced bacterial load, decreased hepatocyte injury, and increased hepatocyte regeneration. Overall, multiple pre-clinical studies demonstrate a beneficial effect of IL-22 on reducing hepatocellular injury and improving hepatocyte regeneration, both of which would be beneficial in humans with alcoholic hepatitis.

IL-22 derivatives have been administered to healthy subjects in Phase I trials. IL22Fc (F-652, manufactured by Generon Corporation [Shanghai], Ltd.) is a dimer of 2 IL-22 molecules linked to an immunoglobulin (Ig) constant region (IgG$_2$-Fc), which has a longer half-life and longer activation of STAT-3. Intravenous injection of F-652 into healthy males had a half-life of 40 to 209 hours and induced dose-dependent increases in serum amyloid A, C-reactive protein, and fibrinogen but did not alter the levels of 36 other common pro-inflammatory cytokines or chemokines.[9] In another Phase I trial with healthy volunteers, UTTR1147 A (human IL-22 Fc [IgG-4] fusion protein; Genentech) was well-tolerated and had a half-life of approximately 1 week. UTTR1147 A led to dose-dependent increases in serum amyloid AA and C-reactive protein, consistent with hepatocyte stimulation, as well as increases in regenerating islet-derived protein 3 alpha (REG3A) suggesting pancreatic or intestinal epithelium activation.[10] Both studies suggest that IL22 administration may be safe and activate pro-survival genes in hepatocytes and possibly intestinal epithelial cells.

F-652 (IL-22Fc) was administered to subjects with moderate or severe AH in a phase 2 clinical trial.[11] F-652 at 10, 30, or 45 ug per kg was administered on Days 1 and 7 to 3 patients each with moderate (MELD score 11–20) and severe AH (MELD scores 21–28). Outcomes were change in MELD score, serum bilirubin, and serum aminotransferases at days 28 and 42. Three separated comparators cohorts were created from propensity matched patients with moderate or severe AH. There were no serious adverse events leading to discontinuation. Half-life was 61 to 85 hours. MELD scores and aminotransferases improved at days 28 and 42. Lille score was less than or equal to 0.45 in 83% of patients receiving F-652 as compared with 6%, 12%, and 56% of the comparator cohorts, respectively. Inflammatory cytokines were decreased, and regeneration markers were increased at days 28 and 42. The preliminary data demonstrating safety and more rapid improvement in MELD and Lille score suggest that additional clinical trials in severe AH are reasonable.

Granulocyte Colony Stimulating Factor (GCSF)

Granulocyte colony stimulating factor (GCSF) is a protein (a cytokine and a hormone) that stimulates the bone marrow to produce and release neutrophils and stem cells, and for immature neutrophils to differentiate into mature neutrophils. Filgrastim, a re-combinant GCSF with high homology with native GCSF, and pegfilgrastim, a long-acting formulation of filgrastim, have been approved in the US to treat chemotherapy-induce neutropenia for decades, with minimal adverse effects.

GCSF has at least 2 mechanisms of action that could be beneficial in alcoholic hep-atitis. First, GCSF can promote hepatocyte regeneration. Bone marrow derived stem cells, released in response to GCSF, can engraft in the liver and differentiate into he-patocytes. Also, hepatocytes have GCSF receptors, so GCSF could have a direct ef-fect on stimulating hepatocyte differentiation. The second mechanism of action is to reduce infections. Infections are frequent among patients with AH, and infections are a common cause of death or of worsening of ACLF. GCSF may decrease infec-tions by increasing the release of neutrophils from the bone marrow, increasing their differentiation into mature neutrophils, and increasing their function.

In a rat model of thioacetamide-induced fulminant hepatic failure, GCSF reduced hepatocyte injury, enhanced proliferation of hepatocytes, and improved survival.[12] In a carbon tetrachloride model of ACLF in mice, GCSF reduced liver injury and increased hepatocyte regeneration.[13] Although bone marrow-derived cells were observed in the liver, the primary effect of GCSF appeared to be increasing prolifera-tion of hepatocytes.

GCSF has been used to treat patients with AH and patients with ACLF (approxi-mately half of whom had AH). The results are conflicting. In a meta-analysis of 7 trials published prior to 2020, GCSF decreased 90-day mortality (Odds Ratio [OR] 0.28; 95% confidence interval [CI] 0.09–0.88; $P = .03$) and reduced the risk of infection.[14] However, there was heterogeneity between the studies. Among the 5 trials performed in India, GCSF was associated with a significantly reduced risk of death at 90 days (OR 0.15; 95% confidence interval [CI] 0.08–0.28; $P<.001$) and reduced occurrence of infection (OR 0.12; 95% CI 0.06–0.23; $P<.001$). The 2 studies performed in Europe did not demonstrate improvement with GCSF treatment. In the European studies, GCSF treatment non-significantly increased 90-day mortality (OR 1.89; 95% CI 0.90–3.98; $P = .09$), while the occurrence of infections was similar in the GCSF and control groups (OR 0.92; 95% CI 0.50–1.69; $P = .78$). A subsequent trial from the

US reported similar survival and infections among patients with AH who received GCSF + corticosteroids versus corticosteroids alone.[15] The reasons for the difference in survival among trials performed in India as compared with trials performed in the West are not known. In general, patients in India with AH had higher MELD scores than patients enrolled in the West. However, it is unclear how this difference could explain the marked difference in results in the 2 continents.

The future of GCSF as a treatment for AH is uncertain. In Europe or US, the preliminary data would make future trials unlikely unless a subset of patients who were likely to benefit could be identified based on analyses of existing trials. GCSF improved survival among patients in India with AH and future trials are reasonable. The trials from India include a mixture of AH patients (initial treatment for AH, ACLF [with subset having AH], corticosteroid non-responders) and a variety of control treatments (placebo, pentoxifylline). A multicenter trial of GCSF versus a standard-of-care (SOC) (either pentoxifylline or placebo) as an initial treatment for AH would be helpful to resolve whether GCSF benefits AH in India. A clinical trial of GCSF in another Asian country might also assist with an assessment of GCSF as a treatment for AH.

Larsucosterol (25HC3S)

Larsucosterol is an endogenous derivative of cholesterol that modifies hepatic lipid synthesis, inflammatory response, and cell survival. Larsucosterol, also known as 25-hydroxycholesterol 3-sulfate (25HC3S), is an oxidized form of cholesterol (oxysterol) in which the 25-position has been hydroxylated ($H \rightarrow OH$) (25HC) and 3-position of the first ring has been sulfated ($H \rightarrow SO_3H$). Larsucosterol is found in the nucleus, where it binds to, and inhibits the enzymatic activity of DNA methyltransferases. This reduces DNA methylation of cytosines, de-repressing DNA enhancer areas on multiple genes. In human hepatocyte cell culture, 25HC3S increased expression of more than 1000 genes, including genes involved in lipid metabolism, anti-inflammatory response, and cell survival.[16]

In pre-clinical studies, 25HC3S decreased lipid accumulation, inflammatory responses, and liver fibrosis in a mouse model of non-alcoholic fatty liver disease[17] and reduced liver injury and inflammatory responses in a lipopolysaccharide model of liver injury in mice.[18] DUR-928 (Durect Corporation; www.durect.com) is a pharmaceutic formulation of 25HC3S that has been administered acutely and repeatedly to animals (mice, rats, rabbits, dogs, and primates) orally and parenterally for up to 28 days without observable drug-related adverse events.

In Phase Ia trials, DUR-928 was administered orally and parenterally to healthy volunteers as a single dose or repeated dose for up to 5 days without observable toxicity. Oral DUR-928 has been tested in a phase Ib trial of clinically diagnosed non-alcoholic steatohepatits, with demonstration of safety and drug tolerability. The trial was not designed to assess efficacy although significant decreases were reported in M65 and M30 cytokeratin 18 and high-sensitivity C-reactive protein, suggesting a decrease in cell death markers and inflammation (Kemp International liver congress, Amsterdam 2017 and Wang 2021).

In a phase 2a trial, 19 patients with moderate (MELD 11–20, n = 7) or severe (MELD 21–30; N = 12) received 30, 90, or 150 mg of DUR-928 intravenous initially, respectively and again 72 hours later if the patient remained in the hospital.[19] Patients tolerated the intravenous infusions without significant adverse events. The patients were compared with AH patients receiving SOC in a contemporaneous AH clinical trial. Although MELD improvement was similar among patients receiving SOC and DUR-928, the percent of patients with Lille score less than0.45 was greater for patients receiving DUR-928 (10 of 12) as compared with patients receiving SOC (~50% with Lille score <0.45).

The top-line results of an international, multicenter, placebo-controlled trial of DUR-928 versus SOC among patients with clinically diagnosed AH has been reported.[20] Three hundred and seven patients with mDF score greater than or equal to 32 and MELD score 21 to 30 were randomized to SOC, larsucosterol 30 mg, or larsucosterol 90 mg, with the larsucosterol given intravenously initially and again in 72 hours if the patient remained in hospital. SOC was determined by the perfusion index. Primary outcome was death or liver transplant at 90 days, with liver transplant evaluated in a hierarchical outcome as less desirable than survival but more desirable than death. There were no serious adverse events attributable to larsucosterol. Both doses of larsucosterol led to a non-significant reduction in death or liver transplant at 90 days compared with SOC. When considering death as the outcome (ie, excluding liver transplant), larsucosterol reduced mortality by 35% to 41%, which approached statistical significance. There were no serious adverse events attributable to larsucosterol. For reasons that are not yet understood, larsucosterol was more effective at reducing mortality among subjects enrolled in the US. Given the potential improvement overall and the considerable reduction in mortality among US subjects with AH, future trials should be considered.

Microbiome

The gut microbiota consists of bacteria, fungi, viruses (including phages), and archaea. More than 100 trillion organisms live in the gut, and they contain, in total, greater than 100 times more genes than are present in the human genome.[21] The gut microbiota contributes to energy production (5%–10% of daily energy production comes from gut microbiota), production of several vitamins (B-vitamins), and beneficial metabolites (eg, short chain fatty acids, long chain fatty acids, indol-3-acetic acid, and tryptophan metabolites), maintenance of the intestinal barrier integrity, production of mucins, and synthesis of antimicrobial peptides. Microbiome research often uses polymerase chain reaction amplicon-based sequencing of 16S ribosomal ribonucleic acid or DNA-based metagenomic sequencing or RNA-based transcriptomic sequencing. Bioinformatic analysis of the raw sequencing data produces taxonomic and microbial community analyses that can be compared between different disease conditions.[21]

Alcohol use, ALC, and AH are associated with multiple changes in the gut microbiome (ie, dysbiosis). In broad strokes, there is a decrease in "beneficial" bacterial species such as Clostridiales (produce butyrate) and an increase in "harmful" bacterial species in ALC, and particularly AH. Among the harmful bacterial species are Streptococcaceae, Enterobacteriaceae (pro-inflammatory), and Enterococcus faecalis. There is also a change in the fungal species, with an increase in Candida species in ALC and in AH. The diversity of the intestinal virome is increased in alcoholic liver disease, including an increase in Escherichia-, Enterobacteria-, and Enterococcus phages, as well an increase in mammalian viruses such as Parvoviridae and Herpesviridae.[21]

Preclinical (mouse) models have shown that various prebiotics reduce inflammation, steatosis, and oxidative stress, and reduces liver injury. Importantly, transplantation of the microbiota from patients with AH into germ-free mice that have been fed alcohol caused significant liver injury in the mouse[22] demonstrating that susceptibility to alcohol-related liver injury could be transmitted from one host (human) to another (mouse) and, theoretically, from human to another human.

Fecal Microbiota Transfer

Fecal microbiota transfer (FMT) refers to changing the microbiota of a patient by administration of the fecal microbiota from a healthy donor. Typically, stool from a donor is administered to a recipient through a nasogastric (NG) tube, often daily for several consecutive days. Several trials in India have reported benefit among patients with AH who receiving FMT from a healthy donor. The initial trial administered FMT obtained from consenting family members to 8 patients with steroid-ineligible AH due to recent upper gastrointestinal bleeding or sepsis and compared outcomes with 18 matched historic patients with AH.[23] The 8 patients receiving FMT had severe AH, with an average MELD-sodium of 33.6 and computed tomography perfusion of 14. FMT was administered by NG tube daily for 7 days. One of the 8 patients died within the first 30 days; the remaining 7 survived for 1 year (87.5% survival). Eight of the historic controls died within the first 30 days and another 3 died within 6 months, for a 33.3% survival at 1 year. The relative abundance of K. pneumonia (a pathogenic species) decreased at 1 year along while several non-pathogenic species decreased at 6 months (Enterococcus illorum, Bifidobcterium longum) or 12 months (Megasphaera elsdenii). Metabolic pathways for methane metabolism, fluorobenzoate acid degradation, and bacterial invasion of epithelial cells were downregulated at 1 year relative to baseline.

The same institution subsequently conducted a prospective randomized clinical trial comparing FMT (n = 60) with prednisolone therapy (n = 60) in steroid-eligible patients with AH.[24] Primary outcome was survival at 90 days. FMT was obtained from a healthy donor and administered daily for 7 days by NG tube. At baseline, mDF score was approximately 65 and MELD was approximately 17. There were no serious complications of FMT treatment. Ninety-day survival was 75% in the FMT group as compared with 56.6% in the prednisolone group (P = .044; FMT hazard ratio = 0.53; 95% CI: 0.279–0.998). Infections accounted for 3.6% of deaths in the FMT group as compared with 19.3% in the prednisolone group. Microbiota analyses showed a reduction in pathogenic taxa (19-fold reduction in Campylobacter) and anaerobes (Parcubacteria, Weisella, and Leuconostocaceae), and an increase in Alphaproteobacteria and Thaumarcheota.

Two other institutions in India have conducted trials of FMT in severe AH. In one institution, an open-label study compared 90-day survival among 13 patients receiving a single administration FMT from a healthy family member with SOC among patients with AH and ACLF.[25] There were no serious adverse events related to FMT administration. Survival at 90 days was 54% among patients receiving FMT versus 25% in the SOC arm (P = .02). Hepatic encephalopathy and ascites resolved in significantly more patients receiving FMT versus SOC, while spontaneous bacterial peritonitis and gastrointestinal bleeding were similar in both groups.

Philips and colleagues retrospectively evaluated 6-month survival among 47 patients with AH who received FMT daily for 7 days with 25 matched patients who received pentoxifylline.[26] Primary outcome was survival at 6 months. Adverse events were minimal. Survival at 6 months was 83% among patients receiving FMT and 56% among patients receiving pentoxifylline (P = .012). At 6 months, fewer patients receiving FMT had ascites (25.5% vs 56%) or hepatic encephalopathy (10.6% vs 40%). During the 6 months of follow-up, fewer patients receiving FMT had infections requiring hospital admission (14.9% vs 52%) or non-critical infections requiring outpatient antibiotic treatment (17% vs 40%). There was no difference in the development of acute kidney injury.

Several studies have evaluated the long-term outcome of patients with AH who received FMT. A retrospective study evaluated survival at 1.5 years among patients with AH + ACLF who received FMT because they were ineligible for corticosteroids.[27] Eighty-eight patients underwent FMT treatment, 72 of them completed treatment. Thirty-eight patients completed the 1.5 year follow-up, of whom 15 were excluded for alcohol relapse (n = 9) or other reasons. Of the remaining 23 patients, 18 (78%) had Grade 2 or Grade 3 ACLF at entry into the trial. After 1.5 years, 15 patients survived (65%), with infections being the most common cause of death. The same investigators reported improved survival at 3 years among patients receiving FMT in a similar, non-randomized trial of FMT versus SOC (65.7% with FMT vs 38.5% with SOC; P = .052).[28] The incidences of ascites, hepatic encephalopathy, infections, and major hospitalizations were lower among subjects receiving FMT (P<.05 for each adverse event).

In summary, one prospective randomized controlled trial and several non-randomized prospective and retrospective studies reported improved survival at 3 months among patients receiving FMT as compared with similar patients with AH who received SOC. Complications of liver disease, such as ascites, hepatic encephalopathy, and infections, were lower among patients receiving FMT in several retrospective trials. Adverse events related to FMT were minimal. Several studies reported a change in the gut bacteria over time consisting of a decrease in toxic species and an increase in potentially beneficial species, as well as a mixture of the original bacteria and the donor bacteria. Given the improvement in survival reported in these trials, it is reasonable test FMT in clinical trials performed outside of India.

Cytolytic Enterococcus faecalis

A more precise modification of the gut microbiome may improve outcome select among patients with AH. As compared with non-drinking patients or drinking patients without liver disease, patients with AH have increased number of fecal *Enterococcus faecalis*. Some strains of *E faecalis* produce cytolysin, a 2-subunit endotoxin that causes hepatocyte death and liver injury. The presence of cytolysin-producing *E. faecalis* in the stool of patients with AH is associated with increased liver disease severity at presentation and with decreased survival during follow-up. Using humanized mice colonized with bacteria from the feces of patients with AH, the investigators studied bacteriophage targeting of cytolytic *E faecalis*. Bacteriophage treatment reduced cytolysin in the liver and reduced alcohol-induced liver disease in the mice suggesting the cytolysin-positive *E faecalis* is a driver of more severe liver disease and higher mortality in AH.[29] This proof-of-concept study showing that precision therapy using bacteriophages to target cytolytic *E faecalis* might improve outcomes in AH is being tested in a phase II clinical trial in patients with AH.

Rifaximin

Rifaximin is a poorly absorbed oral antibiotic with a broad spectrum of activity against gram-negative and gram-positive bacteria. It is used to treat hepatic encephalopathy and has been studied as a treatment to prevent recurrent spontaneous bacterial peritonitis. The proposed mechanism of action is by decreasing bacterial growth in the intestines, with resulting decreased systemic absorption of bacterial products (eg, endotoxin, ammonia, etc.).

In a retrospective study, rifaximin in combination with corticosteroids improved outcome when compared with a matched cohort of patients with AH who received corticosteroids alone.[30] Twenty-one patients with biopsy-proven AH and mDF greater than or equal to 32 or MELD greater than or equal to 21 received rifaximin 400 mg every 8 hours for 90 days as add on to standard medical therapy (SMT), which included corticosteroids for patients without contraindications. Primary outcome was the number of infections during the 90 days. Secondary outcome included liver-related complications, mortality, and improvements in bilirubin, MELD, and Lille score. The comparison group consisted of patients receiving corticosteroids for severe biopsy-proven AH enrolled in another multi-center clinical trial. Baseline clinical data were similar between the groups, including age ($\sim$54), gender (predominately male), mDF (48), and MELD ($\sim$22). There were 11 serious adverse events in the rifaximin cohort, none of which were related to rifaximin use; rifaximin was not discontinued due to adverse events. The average number of infections was 0.29 per patient among the rifaximin group and 0.62 per patient among the SMT group ($P = .049$). Only one patient receiving rifaximin developed sepsis, which did not lead to the patient's death. Twenty-six infections were reported among the 18 patients in the control group, and 8 of the 26 progressed to sepsis, with 6 developing ACLF. Three of the 21 patients receiving rifaximin died during the 90 days (14.2%), one each from ACLF, intracerebral hemorrhage related to lymphoma, and suicide. Thirteen of the 42 patients in the SMT group (30.9%) died within the first 90 days, 11 of whom developed ACLF. Liver-related mortality through 90 days was considerably lower among patients receiving rifaximin than those receiving SMT (30.9% vs 9.5%). Rifaximin improved outcomes in 2 other studies of patients with alcoholic liver disease (but without AH). Vlachogiannakos and colleagues reported rifaximin for 30 days decreased hepatic vein pressure gradient from 18 mm Hg to 14.7 mm Hg on day 30, associated with an approximately 50% decrease in endotoxin level in the systemic and splanchnic circulation.[31] Israelsen and co-workers conducted a prospective, randomized, double-blind trial of daily rifaximin (n = 68) versus placebo (n = 68) for 18 months among patients with biopsy proven alcoholic liver fibrosis without a prior decompensation event.[32] The primary outcome was the proportion of patients with regression (improvement) in liver fibrosis with secondary outcome being the percent of patients with progression of liver fibrosis. Rifaximin did not result in greater regression of liver fibrosis although it did lead to significantly less progression of liver fibrosis and greater regression of lobular inflammation. Most patients continued to drink alcohol during the trial, with the median daily alcohol consumption for active drinkers being 51 g per day.

A single-center exploratory trial of SMT (n = 16) or SMT (n = 16) + rifaximin 550 mg 3 times a day for 28 days.[33] SMT consisted of pentoxifylline 400 mg 3 times a day or prednisolone 40 mg per day, depending on the attending physician's choice. Primary outcome was change in inflammatory (eg, endotoxin, IL-10, IL-6, IL-8) and metabolic markers (eg, amino acids, etc.). Secondary outcomes included changes in portal pressure wedged hepatic vein pressure (WHVP), kidney function, and neurocognitive function. There were no significant adverse events related to rifaximin. At baseline, mDF was significantly higher in the SMT + rifaximin group (60.1 vs 97.8; $P = .049$); MELD was also higher (28.9 vs 24.9; $P = .18$), with nonsignificantly higher bilirubin (21.6 vs 17.4 mg/dL) and creatinine (0.92 vs 0.76 mg/dL) among patients receiving SMT + rifaximin. Inflammatory markers were elevated at baseline and at Day 28. Levels of inflammatory markers improved after 1 month, without a significant difference in improvement among patients receiving SMT vs. patients receiving SMT + rifaximin. Wedged hepatic vein pressure gradient (WHPG) improved similarly in both groups; creatinine improved in the SMT group and worsened in the SMT + rifaximin (not significantly different between groups). Four patients in SMT and 5 patients in SMT + rifaximin group died within 90 days; all deaths were due to liver failure.

In summary, study by Jimenez and colleagues, in combination with the trials of rifaximin in decompensated cirrhosis and alcoholic fibrosis suggest that rifaximin might benefit patients with AH. Although the study by Kimer did not demonstrate an improvement with rifaximin treatment, the trial was small and should not be accepted as the definitive trial of rifaximin for AH.

Antioxidants

N-acetylcysteine

The rationale for using antioxidants to treat AH is based in increased oxidative stress because of metabolism of ethanol, increased activity of cytochrome P450 2E1, and decreased mitochondrial glutathione content with resultant sensitivity of mitochondria damage by reactive oxygen species. In addition, hepatocytes are more sensitive to damage by TNF-alpha when their antioxidant reserves are depleted. N-acetylcysteine has been proposed as a treatment because of its antioxidant properties and its effectiveness in the treatment of acetaminophen overdose, another liver disease with increased oxidative stress.

Several studies have evaluated N-acetylcysteine (NAC) as a treatment for AH. Nguyen-Khac and colleagues conducted a prospective, randomized, multi-center French study of prednisolone alone versus prednisolone + NAC among patients with biopsy proven AH.[34] Eighty-nine patients received prednisolone for 28 days while 85 patients received prednisolone plus NAC. NAC was given intravenously for 5 days, at a dose of 300 mg per kg the first day and 100 mg per kg on days 2 through 5. The primary outcome was survival at 6 months. Secondary outcomes included survival at 1 and 3 months, change in bilirubin at 7 and 14 days, and rates of complications of AH (eg, hepatorenal syndrome, HRS, infections, variceal bleeding, etc.). At enrollment, the average mDF (54–58) and an average bilirubin (14–15 mg/dL) were similar in the 2 groups. There were no serious adverse events related to the use of NAC. Treatment with prednisolone + NAC led to a non-significant decreased mortality at 6 months (27% vs 38%, $P = .07$) and at 3 months (22% vs 34%, $P = .06$). Mortality was significantly lower at 1 month among subjects receiving prednisolone + NAC (8% vs 24%, $P = .006$). The incidence of hepatorenal syndrome was lower among patients receiving prednisolone + NAC (12% vs 25%; OR 0.41, $P = .02$) as was the incidence of infections (19% vs 42%; OR 0.33, $P = .001$). The 2 groups did not differ significantly in other complications of liver disease nor in relapse to alcohol use (17%–18%). Although this trial did not demonstrate statistical improvement in survival at 6 months among subjects receiving prednisolone + NAC (the primary outcome), the difference in survival at 6 months and 3 months approached statistical significance, and there was a significant improvement in survival at 1 month.

Other trials of NAC should be considered when evaluating potential efficacy of NAC in AH. Two other clinical trials of prednisolone + NAC (with other antioxidants) failed to demonstrate improvement in survival.[35,36] Another clinical trial of NAC + enteral nutrition failed to demonstrate improved survival or reduction in liver-related complications when compared with enteral nutrition alone.[37] Finally, in a clinical trial from India, combination treatment of pentoxifylline + GCSF + NAC had slightly worse 90-day survival (68.4%) than treatment with pentoxifylline + GCSF (88.9%), both of which were better than pentoxifylline alone (30%; $P<.05$ vs both comparison groups).[38]

In summary, one large prospective, randomized trial of prednisolone + NAC versus prednisolone reported "borderline significant" improvement in survival at 6 months while several smaller trials of prednisolone + NAC failed to demonstrate improved survival at any timepoint. Given the relative safety of NAC and the short duration of treatment (5 days), it is reasonable to consider NAC + corticosteroids as a potential future trial among patients with AH.

Metadoxine

Metadoxine is an oral antioxidant that was used in combination with prednisone or with pentoxifylline to treat patients with AH.[39] The single center clinical trial from Mexico City randomized 135 patients with a clinical diagnosis of AH to: (1) prednisone

Table 1
3-month and 6-month survival among patients with severe alcohol-associated hepatitis receiving treatment with prednisone, prednisone + metadoxine, pentoxifylline, or pentoxifylline + metadoxine

Treatment	n	3-Month Survival	P-Value	6-Month Survival	P-Value
Prednisone	35	20%	P = .0001	20%	P = .003
Prednisone + MTD	35	68.6%		48.6%	
Pentoxifylline	33	33%	P = .04	18.2%	P = .01
Pentoxifylline + MTD	32	59.4%		50%	

40 mg per day (n = 35), (2) prednisone + metadoxine [MTD] 500 mg TID (n = 35), (3) pentoxifylline 400 mg TID (n = 33), and (4) pentoxifylline + MTD TID (n = 32). All treatment was for 30 days. The primary outcome was survival at 3 and 6 months. Patients had severe AH, with average mDF of 67 to 93, MELD of 28 to 31, creatinine of 1.5 to 1.9 mg per dL, and bilirubin of ~24 mg per dL. Survival rates at 3 and 6 months were significantly higher among subjects receiving MTD for both prednisone and pentoxifylline, with no significant difference neither in survival between the prednisone and pentoxifylline monotherapy groups at 3 or 6 months nor between the MTD groups at 3 or 6 months (**Table 1**).

There was significantly less development of hepatic encephalopathy and hepatorenal syndrome among patients who received prednisone + MTD versus prednisone alone, although there was no difference in these outcomes between patients receiving pentoxifylline + MTD as compared with pentoxifylline alone. Adverse events were similar in all groups and consisted mostly of epigastric symptoms, nausea, and vomiting. Approximately 74% of patients receiving MTD maintained abstinence for 6 months compared with approximately 59% of patients receiving monotherapy. In multivariate analysis, metadoxine treatment and relapse to alcohol consumption were independent factors associated with mortality. Overall, this study demonstrated clinically important improvement in 3- and 6-month survival among patients severe AH who receive metadoxine orally 3 times per day for 30 days in combination with either prednisone or pentoxifylline. Given the safety and ease of administration it is reasonable to consider metadoxine as a potential future treatment for AH.

SUMMARY

Multiple treatments have shown preliminary efficacy for the treatment of alcoholic hepatitis. These treatments address different pathophysiologic pathways, including hepatocyte regeneration, changing the microbiome, and antioxidants. Many of these approaches use relatively inexpensive treatments that are currently available, although not for alcoholic hepatitis. Other treatments would require support from pharmaceutic companies. Given the burden of AH in many countries, the potential adverse events with corticosteroid treatment (or contraindications to corticosteroids), and the positive preliminary data with several agents, trials of new agents for the treatment of AH are reasonable.

DISCLOSURE

This manuscript was supported by NIAAA, United States grant U01AA021886. The author has no conflicts of interest. This article discusses non-FDA-approved treatments for alcohol-associated hepatitis.

REFERENCES

1. Mandrekar P. Pathogenesis of alcohol-associated liver disease. Clin Liver Dis 2024.
2. Crabb DW, Im GY, Szabo G, et al. Diagnosis and treatment of alcohol-associated liver diseases: 2019 practice guidance from the American association for the study of liver diseases. Hepatology (Baltimore, MD) 2020;71(1):306–33.
3. European Association for the Study of the Liver. Electronic address eee, European association for the study of the L. EASL clinical practice guidelines: management of alcohol-related liver disease. J Hepatol 2018;69(1):154–81.
4. McClain CJ. Current medical treatment of alcohool-associated liver disease: pharmacological and nutrition. Clin Liver Dis 2024.
5. Xiang X, Hwang S, Feng D, et al. Interleukin-22 in alcoholic hepatitis and beyond. Hepatology International 2020;14(5):667–76.
6. Park O, Wang H, Weng H, et al. In vivo consequences of liver-specific interleukin-22 expression in mice: implications for human liver disease progression. Hepatology (Baltimore, Md) 2011;54(1):252–61.
7. Ki SH, Park O, Zheng M, et al. Interleukin-22 treatment ameliorates alcoholic liver injury in a murine model of chronic-binge ethanol feeding: role of signal transducer and activator of transcription 3. Hepatology (Baltimore, Md) 2010;52(4): 1291–300.
8. Xiang X, Feng D, Hwang S, et al. Interleukin-22 ameliorates acute-on-chronic liver failure by reprogramming impaired regeneration pathways in mice. J Hepatol 2020;72(4):736–45.
9. Tang KY, Lickliter J, Huang ZH, et al. Safety, pharmacokinetics, and biomarkers of F-652, a recombinant human interleukin-22 dimer, in healthy subjects. Cell Mol Immunol 2019;16(5):473–82.
10. Rothenberg ME, Wang Y, Lekkerkerker A, et al. Randomized phase I healthy volunteer study of UTTR1147A (IL-22Fc): a potential therapy for epithelial injury. Clin Pharmacol Ther 2019;105(1):177–89.
11. Arab JP, Sehrawat TS, Simonetto DA, et al. An open-label, dose-escalation study to assess the safety and efficacy of IL-22 agonist F-652 in patients with alcohol-associated hepatitis. Hepatology (Baltimore, Md) 2020;72(2):441–53.
12. Theocharis SE, Papadimitriou LJ, Retsou ZP, et al. Granulocyte-colony stimulating factor administration ameliorates liver regeneration in animal model of fulminant hepatic failure and encephalopathy. Dig Dis Sci 2003;48(9):1797–803.
13. Yannaki E, Athanasiou E, Xagorari A, et al. G-CSF-primed hematopoietic stem cells or G-CSF per se accelerate recovery and improve survival after liver injury, predominantly by promoting endogenous repair programs. Exp Hematol 2005; 33(1):108–19.
14. Marot A, Singal AK, Moreno C, et al. Granulocyte colony-stimulating factor for alcoholic hepatitis: a systematic review and meta-analysis of randomised controlled trials. JHEP Rep 2020;2(5):100139.
15. Tayek JA, Stolz AA, Nguyen DV, et al. A phase II, multicenter, open-label, randomized trial of pegfilgrastim for patients with alcohol-associated hepatitis. EClinical-Medicine 2022;54:101689.
16. Wang Y, Lin W, Brown JE, et al. 25-Hydroxycholesterol 3-sulfate is an endogenous ligand of DNA methyltransferases in hepatocytes. J Lipid Res 2021;62: 100063.

17. Xu L, Kim JK, Bai Q, et al. 5-cholesten-3beta,25-diol 3-sulfate decreases lipid accumulation in diet-induced nonalcoholic fatty liver disease mouse model. Mol Pharmacol 2013;83(3):648–58.
18. Ning Y, Kim JK, Min HK, et al. Cholesterol metabolites alleviate injured liver function and decrease mortality in an LPS-induced mouse model. Metabolism 2017; 71:83–93.
19. Hassanein T, McClain CJ, Vatsalya V, et al. Safety, pharmacokinetics, and efficacy signals of larsucosterol (DUR-928) in alcohol-associated hepatitis. Am J Gastroenterol 2024;119(1):107–15.
20. Corporation D. DURECT corporation announces topline results from phase 2b AHFIRM trial of larsucosterol in alcohol-associated hepatitis with promising effect on mortality. 2023. Available at: https://wwwdurectcom/2023/11/durect-corporation-announces-topline-results-from-phase-2b-ahfirm-trial-of-larsucosterol-in-alcohol-associated-hepatitis-with-promising-effect-on-mortality/.
21. Fairfield B, Schnabl B. Gut dysbiosis as a driver in alcohol-induced liver injury. JHEP Rep 2021;3(2):100220.
22. Llopis M, Cassard AM, Wrzosek L, et al. Intestinal microbiota contributes to individual susceptibility to alcoholic liver disease. Gut 2016;65(5):830–9.
23. Philips CA, Pande A, Shasthry SM, et al. Healthy donor fecal microbiota transplantation in steroid-ineligible severe alcoholic hepatitis: a pilot study. Clin Gastroenterol Hepatol 2017;15(4):600–2.
24. Pande A, Sharma S, Khillan V, et al. Fecal microbiota transplantation compared with prednisolone in severe alcoholic hepatitis patients: a randomized trial. Hepatology International 2023;17(1):249–61.
25. Sharma A, Roy A, Premkumar M, et al. Fecal microbiota transplantation in alcohol-associated acute-on-chronic liver failure: an open-label clinical trial. Hepatology International 2022;16(2):433–46.
26. Philips CA, Ahamed R, Rajesh S, et al. Clinical outcomes and gut microbiota analysis of severe alcohol-associated hepatitis patients undergoing healthy donor fecal transplant or pentoxifylline therapy: single-center experience from Kerala. Gastroenterol Rep (Oxf) 2022;10:goac074.
27. Philips CA, Augustine P, Padsalgi G, et al. Only in the darkness can you see the stars: severe alcoholic hepatitis and higher grades of acute-on-chronic liver failure. J Hepatol 2019;70(3):550–1.
28. Philips C, Abduljaleel J, Zulfikar R, et al. Three-year follow-up of alcohol-related hepatitis patients undergoing healthy donor fecal transplant: analysis of clinical outcomes, relapse, gut microbiota and comparisons with standard care. Hepatology (Baltimore, Md) 2021;74:8A.
29. Duan Y, Llorente C, Lang S, et al. Bacteriophage targeting of gut bacterium attenuates alcoholic liver disease. Nature 2019;575(7783):505–11.
30. Jimenez C, Ventura-Cots M, Sala M, et al. Effect of rifaximin on infections, acute-on-chronic liver failure and mortality in alcoholic hepatitis: a pilot study (RIFA-AH). Liver Int 2022;42(5):1109–20.
31. Vlachogiannakos J, Saveriadis AS, Viazis N, et al. Intestinal decontamination improves liver haemodynamics in patients with alcohol-related decompensated cirrhosis. Aliment Pharmacol Ther 2009;29(9):992–9.
32. Israelsen M, Madsen BS, Torp N, et al. Rifaximin-alpha for liver fibrosis in patients with alcohol-related liver disease (GALA-RIF): a randomised, double-blind, placebo-controlled, phase 2 trial. Lancet Gastroenterol Hepatol 2023;8(6):523–32.

33. Kimer N, Meldgaard M, Hamberg O, et al. The impact of rifaximin on inflammation and metabolism in alcoholic hepatitis: a randomized clinical trial. PLoS One 2022; 17(3):e0264278.
34. Nguyen-Khac E, Thevenot T, Piquet MA, et al. Glucocorticoids plus N-acetylcysteine in severe alcoholic hepatitis. N Engl J Med 2011;365(19):1781–9.
35. Phillips M, Curtis H, Portmann B, et al. Antioxidants versus corticosteroids in the treatment of severe alcoholic hepatitis–a randomised clinical trial. J Hepatol 2006;44(4):784–90.
36. Stewart S, Prince M, Bassendine M, et al. A randomized trial of antioxidant therapy alone or with corticosteroids in acute alcoholic hepatitis. J Hepatol 2007; 47(2):277–83.
37. Moreno C, Langlet P, Hittelet A, et al. Enteral nutrition with or without N-acetylcysteine in the treatment of severe acute alcoholic hepatitis: a randomized multicenter controlled trial. J Hepatol 2010;53(6):1117–22.
38. Singh V, Keisham A, Bhalla A, et al. Efficacy of granulocyte colony stimulating factor and N-acetyl cysteine therpies in patients with severe alcoholic hepatitis. Clin Gastroenterol Hepatol 2018;16(10):1650–6.e2.
39. Higuera-de la Tijera F, Servin-Caamano AI, Serralde-Zuniga AE, et al. Metadoxine improves the three- and six-month survival rates in patients with severe alcoholic hepatitis. World J Gastroenterol : WJG 2015;21(16):4975–85.

Treatment of Alcohol Use Disorder
Behavioral and Pharmacologic Therapies

Kinza Tareen, MD[a],*, Erin G. Clifton, PhD[a],
Ponni Perumalswami, MD[b,c], Jessica L. Mellinger, MD, MSc[a,c],
Gerald Scott Winder, MD, MSc[a,d,e]

KEYWORDS

- Alcohol liver disease • Alcohol use disorder • Alcohol use disorder psychotherapy
- Alcohol use disorder pharmacotherapies • Psychiatric comorbidities

KEY POINTS

- The prevalence of alcohol use disorder (AUD) has significantly increased over the last decade, leading to a rise in alcohol-associated liver disease (ALD) rates worldwide.
- Despite this prominence, AUD in ALD remains under-treated and carries significant implications in the progression to end-stage ALD and increased mortality.
- Interprofessional and integrated AUD treatment is necessary for patients with ALD to ensure early detection and an appropriately targeted level of care. While pharmacotherapy, psychotherapy, and psychosocial interventions independently play a role in treating AUD, a combination of these evidence-based modalities often results in lasting change.
- Hepatologists and mental health providers alike should bolster their therapeutic alliance with brief interventions promoting intrinsic motivation for behavior change and, where appropriate, make referrals for cognitive behavioral and motivational enhancement therapy and encourage engagement in mutual aid societies.
- Psychopharmacologic interventions should take into account the medical complexity and hepatic limitations and be directed at both relapse prevention and management of common psychiatric comorbidities.

Financial support: J.L. Mellinger is supported by NIAAA, United States (AA R01 030748, AA R01 030969, AA R01 030470).

[a] Department of Psychiatry, University of Michigan, Ann Arbor, MI, USA; [b] Gastroenterology Section, Veterans Affairs, Ann Arbor Healthcare System, Ann Arbor, MI, USA; [c] Department of Internal Medicine, University of Michigan, Ann Arbor, MI, USA; [d] Department of Surgery, University of Michigan, Ann Arbor, MI, USA; [e] Department of Neurology, University of Michigan, Ann Arbor, MI, USA

* Corresponding author. 9814 University Hospital, 1500 East Medical Center Drive, Ann Arbor, MI 48109.

E-mail address: tkinza@med.umich.edu

Clin Liver Dis 28 (2024) 761–778
https://doi.org/10.1016/j.cld.2024.06.011

INTRODUCTION

Alcohol use disorder (AUD) treatment is increasingly relevant to hepatologists as the hazards of alcohol-related liver disease (ALD) continue to increase in the liver disease population,[1] and alcohol's substantial negative contributions to other liver nonalcohol-associated diseases are better quantified.[2] Early detection and treatment of hazardous drinking and AUD in this population are essential given the risk associated with liver decompensation, including cirrhosis, ascites, hepatic encephalopathy (HE), and variceal bleeds; higher mortality; and greater health care costs than patients with nonalcohol-related cirrhosis causes.[3,4] The landscape of AUD treatment within hepatology has changed dramatically in recent years. In this review, the authors aim to equip hepatologists with an understanding of multidisciplinary approaches to AUD treatment, outline varied models of care, and highlight evidence-based psychotherapies, behavioral strategies, and pharmacotherapies in promoting sobriety, preventing relapse, and managing comorbid psychiatric conditions in ALD.

INTERPROFESSIONAL EDUCATION AND PRACTICE

Although hepatologists often recognize psychiatric and substance use disorders (SUD) contributing to liver pathologic condition, the ability to adequately evaluate and treat both ALD and AUD varies across clinicians and practice settings.[5,6] Consequently, the treatment of AUD in ALD by a single medical specialty is often incomplete. Collaborative care (CC) is an integration strategy that integrates mental health (MH) services into medical settings and requires substantial interprofessional collaboration, including strong professional relationships, shared goals, efficient communication, and robust coordination. CC is cost-effective, improves access, and demonstrates greater abstinence from alcohol at 6 months when compared with usual care.[7] This care method may also reduce clinician burnout and promote shared decision making in AUD treatment.[8,9] Although sometimes limited by logistical and financial constraints, early care integration can significantly improve patient outcomes and limit disease progression.[10]

ALCOHOL USE DISORDER PSYCHOTHERAPIES

The influence of alcohol on neurobiology and behavior is multifaceted. AUD, like other addictions, is characterized by physiologic and behavioral responses rooted in alcohol's effects on varied neural circuits, neurotransmitters systems, and brain plasticity. The intoxicating effects of alcohol are mediated by its influence on dopamine, γ-amino butyric acid (GABA), glutamate, serotonin, and opioid neurotransmitter systems, which modulate various aspects of addiction, including reward processing, impulse control, and emotional regulation.[11] These neurotransmitter effects reflect opportunities for pharmacologic interventions for AUD, which will be discussed in detail later. The mesolimbic reward pathway is a key mediator of positive and negative reinforcement systems, as alcohol activates dopaminergic neurons projecting to the ventral tegmental area and nucleus acumens.[11] Behavioral interventions, on the other hand, are centered on an understanding of alcohol's influence on the complexities of these reinforcement systems, learning, and memory deficits associated with resilience and problem-solving capacity, and assessment of the hypothalamic-pituitary-adrenal axis stress response and capacity to regulate reactions to triggers and cravings.[11]

Although pharmacology may receive more attention among medically oriented clinicians, psychotherapy is equally critical in creating lasting change and is far more prevalent in AUD treatment. Psychotherapy uses therapeutic alliances and a supportive environment as patients discover the underlying causes of and triggers to their substance use, develop coping strategies, effect lifestyle changes, and implement changes to their behavioral patterns. Evidence suggests roles of brief interventions, cognitive behavioral therapy (CBT), motivational interviewing (MI), motivational enhancement therapy (MET), and contingency management (CM) in the ALD population. No individual psychotherapeutic intervention is consistently successful in maintaining abstinence alone; instead, integrated psychotherapies alongside other medical care and lifestyle changes appear to be most effective in reducing relapse risk.[12]

Brief Interventions

Screening, Brief Intervention, and Referral to Treatment (SBIRT) involves elements of MI in brief patient-centered discussions focused on alcohol education, behavior change, and referrals to treatment when needed. Although SBIRT is insufficient for patients with severe AUD, meta-analysis shows that SBIRT reduces alcohol use in patients with mild to moderate AUD.[13,14] SBIRT is an important early intervention. Encouraging screening allows for early identification of severe AUD, and referral for treatment is a crucial component of SBIRT. Its brevity (10–15 minutes) allows for easy adoption in medical clinics, and standardized tools allow hepatologists to engage in psychologically minded discussions. The FRAMES model is an example of a classic framework for SBIRT to provide personalized Feedback, encourage individual Responsibility, provide valuable Advice for change, and share a Menu of options in an Empathic manner to promote Self-Efficacy.[15]

Motivational Interviewing and Motivational Enhancement Therapy

MI is a patient-centered, goal-oriented therapeutic approach that rejects the punitive language and paternalism that can affect communication surrounding alcohol use. As a collaborative communication style that enhances patients' intrinsic motivation and self-efficacy, focuses a person on their goals, and lowers ambivalence about behavior change, MI is an effective SUD treatment.[16–18] MI is a generalizable tool for any clinician discussing change with patients, and MET is a structured therapy implementing MI over several sessions.[19] The literature on the specific role of MET and MI in the ALD population is sparse. There are mixed results regarding sustained abstinence when MET is used as the sole treatment intervention.[20–23] A randomized control trial (RCT) study evaluated the experiences of patients with severe AUD and ALD who had previously been unsuccessful in alcohol treatment and participated in integrated CBT and MET (24–48 sessions) alongside comprehensive medical care over 2 years as compared with standard AUD care (referrals to inpatient and outpatient treatment services). Integrated CBT and MET resulted in significantly greater abstinence rates than controls (74% vs 48%, respectively).[23] In an RCT of patients with ALD undergoing LT evaluation and who had consumed alcohol at least once during the past 2 years, Weinrieb and colleagues[22] evaluated the efficacy of MET with the encouragement of Alcoholics Anonymous (AA) and case management support over 6 months to standard treatment (referral to intensive outpatient program [IOP] and AA). Although there were similar proportions of relapse noted between both study arms (MET, 26%; control, 24%; $P = .95$), those who engaged in MET had fewer total number of drinks (95% CI $= [-4.14, -0.87]$; $P = .003$), and significantly fewer drinking days (95% CI $= [-4.40, -0.83]$; $P = .004$). Kuchipudi and colleagues[20] evaluated the efficacy of MI in an RCT of medically admitted patients actively using alcohol who also had a broader range of gastrointestinal pathologic conditions (ulcers, cirrhosis, or pancreatitis) and found no significant difference in self-reported sobriety at 10 to 16 weeks' follow-up between those exposed to a 2-hour MI session and those receiving standard care.

Cognitive Behavioral Therapy

CBT is a structured therapeutic approach to understanding and changing negative thought patterns and adjusting unhelpful behaviors to alleviate emotional distress. Relapse prevention therapy is a form of CBT used in patients with ALD that focuses on bolstering healthy coping strategies, building tools to recognize cues and triggers for relapse, encouraging assertiveness in refusal of substances (eg, self-directed cravings, peer pressure), and promoting a problem-solving approach to coping with high-risk situations and cravings.[24,25] As previously discussed, integrated CBT and MET-based therapies in AUD management have demonstrated increased sobriety in ALD.[23] Regarding abstinence maintenance, another nonrandomized study found that patients who received integrated CBT and psychiatric management before liver transplantation (LT) had lower rates of relapse and lower mortality after LT than those receiving only pre-LT supportive therapy.[21]

Contingency Management

CM strategies are rooted in operant conditioning. Targeted behavioral changes are reinforced by incentives (ie, vouchers, prizes, clinic privileges) to encourage further engagement with the desired behavior.[26,27] CM has yet to be universally adopted owing to barriers in training and perceptions about the modality simulating bribery.[28] To date, CM has not been studied in the ALD population. However, considerable literature supports its role as a cost-effective intervention in promoting treatment adherence and abstinence.[27–30] Notably, the incentives of qualifying for LT listing and successfully receiving a donor organ involve CM principles.

Family Therapy

AUD has the potential for a tremendous negative interpersonal and financial impact on the family unit.[31] Family therapy uses family systems theory and CBT in efforts to strengthen relationships and encourage individuals with AUD to engage in treatment. To date, there are limited community-based or RCTs that support the integration of family members in alcohol recovery; however, several small clinical samples support family inclusion in motivating persons with AUD to recognize the need to change, building tools for supportive therapy, and suggest long-AUD abstinence has positive effects for the family unit as a whole.[31]

Social Behavior and Network Therapy

The attitude toward drinking and AUD treatment shared among a social network has a significant impact on AUD treatment outcomes. Social behavior and network therapy allow for individuals to work with an individual therapist or in group settings to change aspects of their social environment that contribute to drinking. The positive influence of a social network supportive of sobriety is greater than that of concurrent engagement in AA.[32] In an RCT, network support treatment was superior to CBT in proportion of days abstinent and consequences related to drinking; however, the traditional psychotherapy treatment and social network support were equivalent in measures of 90-day abstinence, heavy drinking days, and drinks per drinking day.[32]

Digital Platforms

In contrast to psychotherapist-driven interventions, emerging online platforms offer increased access to addiction-based psychoeducation, behavior tracking, and motivation to maintain abstinence.[33,34] *Take Control* is one such computerized self-guided bibliotherapy platform developed by the National Institute on Alcohol Abuse and Alcoholism, which delivers structured educational modules through a lens of MI and encourages identification of addiction, strategies to meet goals, and an overview of treatment options.[33]

ALCOHOL USE DISORDER PHARMACOTHERAPIES

Medications for alcohol use disorder (MAUD) are severely underused in patients with ALD. Nevertheless, a recent retrospective review revealed that MAUD use in patients with hazardous alcohol use and alcohol-associated cirrhosis was associated with significantly improved survival, even after adjusting for the severity of liver disease.[35,36] Liver and MH clinicians alike would benefit from further education regarding MAUD use in ALD to bolster prescribing to this population. **Table 1** summarizes the utility and dose ranges of such medications.

Naltrexone

Naltrexone is a mu-opioid receptor antagonist approved for AUD and opioid use disorder (OUD) treatment in the United States in 1984. It can be administered as a daily oral tablet or monthly intramuscular (IM) injection. Avoiding first-pass metabolism with an IM injection might improve naltrexone's side-effect risk profile in liver disease.[37] AUD therapeutic effects are higher for IM administration, given lower levels of drug adherence for the oral formulation.[37] Naltrexone interacts with opioid medications, which should be discontinued 7 to 14 days before naltrexone initiation (longer periods are required for longer-acting opioids like methadone and buprenorphine). Oral Naltrexone should be stopped at least 3 days before opioid administration, and the IM formulation should be stopped at least 30 days prior. Although naltrexone metabolites accumulate in hepatic insufficiency,[38] it has not been linked to liver injury and has been deemed safe to use in patients with compensated cirrhosis; although more safety data are needed for decompensated patients, it no longer carries a black-box warning for use in liver disease.[39] Naltrexone is used in patients with liver disease for other indications, including pruritis[40] and, combined with bupropion in fixed ratios, as a weight loss medication. Nalmefene is a structurally similar medication not commonly used in the United States. It can be administered orally, IM, and intravenous (IV) and is not known to cause serum enzyme elevations or liver injury.

Acamprosate

Acamprosate is a Food and Drug Administration (FDA) -approved medication for relapse prevention in those who are abstinent (at least 1–2 weeks) at initiation. It primarily exerts its effects as a glutamatergic antagonist and partial GABA agonist.[41] Available only in oral formulations and requiring split dosing (3 times daily with meals), there is substantial evidence in the general AUD population of reducing high-risk drinking and increasing cumulative abstinence duration at doses ranging from 333 to 666 mg 3 times daily.[41,42] Although not widely studied in ALD, phase II results suggest both safety and efficacy of acamprosate in the ALD population.[43] Acamprosate is not hepatically metabolized, and with no reported hepatotoxicity, there is no need for dose adjustment in patients with Child-Pugh class C. In efforts to reduce risk of multiorgan failure and risk of hepatorenal syndrome, acamprosate, which is

Table 1
Summary of medications for alcohol use disorder and potential use in liver disease patients

Medication	AUD Indication or Endorsement	Metabolism and Excretion	Dose Range	Liver Disease Considerations
Disulfiram	FDA approved	M: hepatic E: 70% renal	250–500 mg daily	Not recommended for use in liver disease
Naltrexone	FDA approved	M: hepatic E: majority renal	Start: 25 mg daily Effective dose: 50 mg po daily, 480 mg IM every month	• Rare potential for hepatotoxicity; black box warning for liver disease removed • PO formulation preferred over IM in cirrhosis • Be mindful of naltrexone's interactions with opioids when starting; discontinue as appropriate in LT
Acamprosate	FDA approved	M: no hepatic E: renal	Start: 333 mg tid Effective dose: 666 mg tid	• No evidence of hepatotoxicity • Phase II studies support efficacy in AUD treatment and safety in ALD • Reduce dose in renal insufficiency; avoid if CrCl < 30 mL/min
Gabapentin	APA Guidelines—2nd-line treatment	M: no hepatic E: 75% renal, 25% fecal	Start: 300 mg qd Effective dose: 900–1800 mg tid	• No evidence of hepatotoxicity • Use with caution in hepatic encephalopathy • Reduce dose in renal failure
Topiramate	APA Guidelines—2nd-line treatment	M: limited hepatic E: renal	Start: 25–50 mg daily Effective dose: 300 mg daily	• No evidence of direct hepatotoxicity • Use with caution in hepatic encephalopathy • May exacerbate pruritus and anorexia • Reduce dose in advanced liver and kidney disease

Baclofen	No	M: limited hepatic E: renal	Start: 5 mg tid Effective dose: 10–20 mg tid	• RCT support its use as a MAUD in ALD • Reduce dose in renal insufficiency, avoid in end-stage renal disease
Varenicline	No	M: limited hepatic E: renal	Start: 0.5 mg daily Effective dose: unclear; some studies suggest 1–2 mg daily	• No evidence of hepatotoxicity • Emerging evidence as MAUD, not studied in ALD • Reduce dose in renal insufficiency, avoid in end-stage renal disease
N-Acetylcysteine	No	M: limited hepatic E: renal	Start: 600 mg twice daily Effective dose: unclear; 1200–3600 mg daily suggested in other SUD	• No evidence of hepatotoxicity • Glutathione deficiency is characteristic of ALD, and balancing this deficiency has been postulated to improve liver damage in ALD patients
Ondansetron	No	M: hepatic E: renal, 25% feces	Start: unclear Effective dose: unclear; some studies suggest 4 µg/kg twice daily	• No literature to support its use in ALD or as an effective MAUD independently • Consider in combination with naltrexone or CBT • Avoid in advanced liver disease, maximum dose 8 mg/d in Child-Pugh class C

Adapted from Mellinger JL, Fernandez AC, Winder GS. Management of alcohol use disorder in patients with chronic liver disease. Hepatology Communications. 2023 Jul 1;7(7):e00145. Copyright 2023 by Wolters Kluwer Health, Inc. on behalf of the American Association for the Study of Liver Diseases.

renally metabolized, should be reduced when glomerular filtration is less than 60 mL/min and avoided if less than 30 mL/min.[42]

Disulfiram

Disulfiram is FDA-approved as a psychological deterrent to alcohol by interrupting its metabolism, yielding an accumulation of serum acetaldehyde, a metabolite, which causes a highly unpleasant physiologic reaction. Disulfiram is known to increase aminotransferases and has been linked to acute liver injury and organ failure. It should not be used in patients with liver disease.

Gabapentin

Gabapentin is recommended by the American Psychiatric Association (APA) to reduce alcohol consumption and achieve abstinence, but is not FDA-approved.[44] It can be initiated in the detoxification phase as an adjunct for withdrawal management and acts as a GABA modulator by indirectly interacting with voltage-gated calcium channels.[45,46] Although not well studied in the ALD population, trials in the general population have demonstrated efficacy in reducing the percentage of heavy drinking days and drinks per day and increasing the rate of abstinent days.[47] Only available in oral formulations and better tolerated from a sedation standpoint with split (3 times daily) dosing, gabapentin is effective at doses ranging from 900 to 1800 mg/d.[46] Although a few case reports suggest a risk for a mild to moderate reversible cholestatic liver injury with gabapentin initiation, a causal relationship has not been defined, and gabapentin is generally safe in liver disease.[48] For this reason, gabapentin is reasonable for patients with ALD, particularly for those with comorbid diabetic neuropathy, and as an adjunct for multimodal pain management. Notably, gabapentin should be used with caution in patients with HE, as one of its most common adverse effects is somnolence. It carries the potential for misuse in at-risk individuals.[46] Like acamprosate, gabapentin is renally eliminated and requires dose adjustment in patients with impaired renal function.[46]

Topiramate

Although not FDA-approved for the disorder, the use of topiramate is recommended by both the US Department of Veterans Affairs and the APA for moderate to severe AUD.[44,49] The exact mechanism of action remains unclear, but it is thought to attenuate dopaminergic activity and, in turn, reduce alcohol cravings by inhibition of glutamate α-amino 3-hydroxy-5-methyl-4-isoxazoleproprionic acid and kainite receptors, influence L-type calcium channels, and enhance the inhibitory activity of GABA.[50] Topiramate is available only in oral formulations and titrated in 25- to 50-mg increments up to 300 mg daily for the management of AUD. It is not known to be hepatotoxic, but clearance may be reduced in both hepatic and renal insufficiency.[51] Although there is little ALD-specific literature regarding topiramate use, several characteristic side effects, including pruritis, anorexia, and cognitive impairment, might make its use less desirable in patients with certain liver diseases. However, patients seeking weight loss as part of their liver care may benefit from the side effect of decreased appetite. The cognitive impairments present as dose-associated deficits in working memory, verbal fluency, and generalized cognitive slowing, which could complicate or exacerbate HE.[52]

Baclofen

Baclofen has been used as MAUD for decades in Europe. However, its use has not been widely adopted in the United States because of inconsistent findings regarding abstinence rates, craving attenuation, and heavy drinking reduction.[53] Nonetheless, baclofen is one of the few agents that has been studied explicitly in the ALD population, including in those with advanced cirrhosis. In patients with ALD and AUD, baclofen has been used between 30 and 75 mg daily, with varying efficacy and dose-related side-effect profiles (ie, sedation at higher doses).[54–56] One study of patients with cirrhosis, which excluded those with HE, demonstrated increased abstinence at 12 weeks with the use of baclofen 10 mg 3 times daily over the control group.[54] Conversely, an RCT of veterans with chronic hepatitis C and active alcohol use determined that a 12-week course of baclofen (30 mg daily) did not differ from a placebo in abstinence rates.[55] These inconsistencies may be due to baclofen's inherent pharmacokinetic variability in patients with AUD.[57] Baclofen acts as a GABA-B receptor agonist, has no reported hepatoxicity, and is largely renally metabolized. As such, it requires dose reduction in patients with renal insufficiency and should be avoided in end-stage renal disease.[58]

Varenicline

Varenicline is a nicotinic acetylcholine receptor agonist that is FDA-approved for tobacco cessation and has emerging evidence for use in AUD. An RCT demonstrated that varenicline reduced the percentage of drinking days, drinks per day, and alcohol cravings over placebo.[51] Although not explicitly studied in the ALD population, varenicline represents a promising treatment given the cooccurrence of nicotine and alcohol use. Varenicline is not known to cause hepatoxicity. It is largely excreted unchanged in urine and requires dose adjustment with renal impairment; the maximum dose with creatinine clearance less than 30 mL/min or in dialysis-dependent patients is 0.5 mg daily.[59] Although postmarketing cases initially raised concerns of significant neuropsychiatric events (including suicidal ideation and behavior) in patients with no prior psychiatric history, subsequent controlled trials in patients with and without preexisting psychiatric disease did not bear this out when the varenicline group was compared with other tobacco cessation treatments (bupropion, nicotine replacement, and placebo).[60]

N-Acetylcysteine

N-acetylcysteine (NAC) is a low-cost antioxidant and cysteine prodrug used by hepatologists to reverse oxidative stress in acetaminophen-induced acute liver failure. NAC has been shown to be protective against liver injury and, in the absence of alcohol, improves serum lipids and hepatic antioxidant deficiencies.[61] A growing body of evidence suggests NAC's utility in treating SUD by restoring glutamatergic tone in reward circuitry.[51,61] Although further research is required to determine any role of NAC in ALD, promising evidence supports off-label use in the general AUD population. A secondary analysis of multisite RCT of NAC to treat cannabis use disorder revealed a 30% reduction in alcohol consumption as determined by drinks per day and drinking days per week.[57] Glutathione deficiency is characteristic of ALD, and balancing this deficiency has been postulated to improve liver damage in patients with ALD. NAC has the potential to treat both AUD and ALD and represents a promising treatment option.[61] NAC is available in oral, IV, and inhalation formulations, undergoes extensive first-pass metabolism, and requires dose adjustments in renal failure.

Ondansetron

Ondansetron is a 5-HT3 receptor antagonist that is primarily used in the treatment of nausea and vomiting but has been investigated as an MAUD given its role in modulating the function of 5-HT transporters and subsequently down-regulating dopaminergic neurons and decreasing alcohol-driven rewards.[57] There is no literature to support its use in ALD or as an effective MAUD treatment independently, but ondansetron (up to 8 μg/kg daily) used in combination with naltrexone or CBT has been associated with fewer drinks per day than placebo.[51,62] Ondansetron is available in IV and oral formulations and is extensively hepatically metabolized. Given current guidelines of a maximum 8 mg oral/IV daily in Child-Pugh class C, would be mindful of ondansetron dosing in severe hepatic impairment.[63] This limits its use potential in the ALD population, but further research is necessary to clarify effective doses of ondansetron for AUD.

Emerging Pharmacotherapies

Evolving research suggests potential for other AUD pharmacotherapies, including oxytocin, aldosterone antagonists, and GLP-1 agonists.[62–64] However, more studies are required to characterize their use in managing AUD and ALD. Although more robust studies are required, GLP-1 agonist in particular may have potential for those with overlapping metabolic dysfunction–associated steatotic liver disease and ALD, as there is some evidence to support its role in reducing steatosis.[64]

ALCOHOL USE DISORDER COMORBIDITIES PHARMACOTHERAPIES

Genetic predisposition, environmental factors, and bidirectional effects of alcohol use and psychiatric disorders contribute to psychiatric comorbidities in the AUD population.[65] With abstinence, psychiatric symptoms, including depression, anxiety, and insomnia, often diminish. If persistent or left untreated, these symptoms may impact the outcomes of AUD treatment in ALD. For instance, dysregulated mood and poor sleep can interfere with the ability to maintain sobriety by increasing cravings and reducing motivation to engage in treatment. Although the management of psychotropic medications is best done by specialists, hepatologists' awareness of psychiatric comorbidities in ALD is an important element of their clinical care and a foundation upon which to establish integrated treatments.

Selective Serotonin Reuptake Inhibitors

Selective serotonin reuptake inhibitors (SSRIs) represent the foundation of pharmacologic depression and anxiety treatment in liver disease. Although generally considered safe, pharmacokinetic changes associated with liver disease (ie, prolonged half-life and reduced drug elimination) mean that SSRIs should be dosed cautiously with maintenance doses of approximately 50% of those used in healthy individuals. SSRIs with a lower risk of liver injury include fluoxetine, paroxetine, citalopram, and escitalopram.[66] SSRIs have antiplatelet effects and increase gastric acid secretion, which may result in an increased risk of gastrointestinal bleeding. However, in patients with liver disease, the absolute risk of SSRI-related bleeding is relatively low, whereas adverse effects are reported when coadministered with antiplatelet agents.[66,67]

Serotonin Norepinephrine Reuptake Inhibitors

Serotonin norepinephrine reuptake inhibitors are used in the treatment of anxiety and depression and are particularly helpful for those with comorbid chronic pain syndromes. Venlafaxine has been rarely associated with hepatocellular and cholestatic drug-induced liver injury (DILI).[66] Duloxetine has been associated with severe DILI marked by hepatocellular, cholestatic, and mixed injury resulting in acute liver failure; it is not recommended for use in advanced liver disease.[66,68]

Other Antidepressants

Tricyclic antidepressants (TCAs) have a role in managing anxiety and depression. Their strong anticholinergic effects can be used in treating insomnia. In liver disease, reduced TCA clearance and subsequent risks of anticholinergic side effects and arrhythmias limit their utility in ALD.

Mirtazapine is a noradrenergic and specific serotonergic antidepressant that promotes sleep and appetite in addition to managing anxiety and depression. In a large-scale retrospective study of antidepressants in patients with ALD, mirtazapine monotherapy was associated with increased mortality (adjusted HR: 1.85; 95% CI: 1.08–3.16) and worse decompensated cirrhosis-free survival (adjusted HR: 2.18 [1.30–3.65]), a finding not seen when mirtazapine was used in combination with other antidepressants.[69] Although further prospective studies are warranted to address this correlation, mirtazapine should be used cautiously in ALD.

Bupropion is a dual reuptake inhibitor of dopamine and norepinephrine indicated for the treatment of depression and smoking cessation. As an activating agent that targets fatigue, apathy, and inattention, bupropion is often ideal for patients with ALD. Bupropion has a dose-dependent influence on lowering seizure threshold; because of its extensive hepatic metabolism to active metabolites, it should be used with caution in patients at risk of alcohol withdrawal and advanced liver disease.[70]

Anxiolytics

Benzodiazepines are often the first line for acute anxiety management; however, as discussed above, they should be used with caution in ALD and generally avoided in HE. Buspirone is a common anxiolytic and is used to augment the treatment of depression primarily by agonism of $5-HT_{1A}$ receptors. Animal studies suggest that buspirone may be an antioxidant that decreases liver oxidative stress.[71] Although safe in mild to moderate hepatic impairment, buspirone should be used with caution in advanced disease.[70]

Sleep Aids

Trazodone is an antidepressant that is commonly used for the management of insomnia at low doses (25–100 mg). Although it is generally safe, rare hepatocellular and cholestatic DILIs have been reported.[70] Doxepin, a TCA commonly used for sleep maintenance insomnia, should be used with caution in liver disease. Quetiapine is another psychotropic used off-label for insomnia at low doses. Of note, it is associated with mild, transient, and asymptomatic transaminitis; although rare, acute liver injury with quetiapine has been reported.[72] Z-drugs, including zaleplon (for sleep onset insomnia) and zolpidem (both sleep onset and maintenance), are hepatically metabolized and should be used with caution in ALD, as they have the propensity to cause oversedation and worsen mentation in HE, similar to benzodiazepines.[66] In addition to its use in AUD, gabapentin has sedative properties that can be leveraged for patients with ALD with insomnia. Polysomnogram evidence demonstrates gabapentin's role in enhancing slow-wave sleep and decreasing spontaneous arousal.[73]

TIERS AND VENUES OF CARE

AUD management is less algorithmic than other medical conditions. Treatment planning and level of care designation depend on the patient clinical status, preferences, insight, and motivation. Furthermore, the various challenges to accessing MH services for publicly and privately insured persons (eg, clinician shortages, visit limits, benefit carve-outs, and so forth) must be considered. According to the National Survey on Drug Use and Health data, many people with SUD do not receive any treatment,

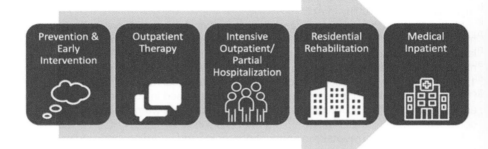

Fig. 1. Ascending levels of AUD treatment in terms of clinical urgency and treatment intensity. (*From* Winder GS, Clifton EG. Alcohol use disorder treatment delivered outside hepatology clinic. Clinical Liver Disease. 2023 May 1;21(5):134-7. Copyright 2023 by American Association for the Study of Liver Diseases.)

even when they desire it.[74] Stigma and low motivation to abstain and engage in treatment are more common barriers among insured persons, whereas financial barriers (ie, inability to afford treatment) are more prominent obstacles among the uninsured.[74] The American Society of Addiction Medicine describes SUD tiers of care ranging from early intervention, outpatient, IOPs, partial hospitalization programs (PHP), residential, and inpatient services that provide a framework for clinicians, payers, and managed care organizations. **Fig. 1** details the ascending levels of care; the goal is to match patients with the least intensive care that is safe and effective for patient needs.[75]

Early Intervention

Early intervention is predicated on screening individuals at risk for developing an SUD. Hepatologists have a critical window of opportunity to screen for AUD, as hepatic steatosis occurs in up to 95% of patients with chronic heavy alcohol use.[76] Percentages of 20% to 40% of patients who develop steatohepatitis progress to liver fibrosis, and 8% to 20% go on to develop cirrhosis.[76] Alcohol-associated hepatitis may occur anywhere along the spectrum of ALD. Therefore, early detection of AUD and intervention are vital. Differentiating uncomplicated "social drinking" from hazardous drinking patterns is an important skill set for all clinicians to develop. Validated screening surveys (that is, Alcohol Use Disorders Identification Test) and monitoring alcohol biomarkers, including urinary ethyl glucuronide, ethyl sulfate, hair ethyl glucuronide, and serum phosphatidyl ethanol, are valuable tools.[77,78] Of note, liver chemistry alone leads to ALD misdiagnoses in up to 41% to 75% of cases.[79] As such, clinicians must implement an SBIRT approach, discussed in detail above.

Outpatient Treatment

Outpatient services include individual and group counseling, mutual aid societies, monitoring laboratory tests/toxicology, and psychotropic medication management.

As discussed above, integrated models in ALD can bolster access to these services as part of routine ALD care.

Mutual aid societies are an important element of outpatient care. These organizations have varying philosophies but are rooted in peer support for those who seek to abstain from alcohol. AA uses a 12-step approach, which can be effective in improving abstinence rates compared with other interventions like CBT and MET.[80] Although AA remains ubiquitous, recent studies support the efficacy of secular alternatives to the 12-step method, such as Women for Sobriety and Self-Management and Recovery Training.[81] Regardless of the choice of a mutual aid group, 1-year engagement has been associated with better substance use outcomes than nonengagement in mutual aid societies.[81]

Intensive Outpatient and Partial Hospitalization Programs

IOP and PHP are beneficial for patients with ALD who require higher-intensity treatment and closer monitoring, given the elevated risk of continued use, relapse, or worsening psychiatric symptoms. These structured programs involve substantial time commitment over 2 to 4 weeks with a minimum of 9 hours per week in IOP and 20 hours per week in PHP. Patients participate in in-person or virtual individual and group therapies to manage AUD and psychiatric comorbidities. Patients often receive regular CBT, work to improve coping skills, and undergo medication management.[75]

Residential Treatment

Residential programs assist patients with ALD facing severe medical and psychosocial problems related to their SUD. These programs vary in duration, ranging from weeks to years, and provide stable housing, a drug and alcohol–free environment, and intensive treatment, often involving peer and professional support, cognitive behavioral strategies, and 12-step work.[75] An RCT comparing patients enrolled in a 24-month residential treatment to standard outpatient care found lower rates of relapse, higher monthly salaries, and lower incarceration rates.[82] Unfortunately, many patients with ALD cannot fully participate in long-term residential community programs given decompensation, which requires regular medical care and/or hospitalization.

Inpatient Treatment

Severe alcohol withdrawal management requires hospitalization and often relies on benzodiazepines as first-line agents. Lorazepam and oxazepam have no active metabolites and stable half-lives and are preferred in ALD. Benzodiazepines should be used judiciously in ALD, as they may precipitate HE, cause excessive sedation, or present risks for misuse.[83] A benzodiazepine-sparing protocol that enlists gabapentin and alpha-agonists can be considered in patients with ALD with no history of complicated withdrawals presenting with mild withdrawal symptoms.[45]

SUMMARY

AUD management in ALD requires the integration of diverse clinical perspectives and expertise in innovative ways to ensure early diagnosis of hazardous alcohol use, determine the appropriate venue of care, and effectively connect patients with treatment. In order to improve the known underutilization of MAUD in liver disease and address the substantial disease burden of ALD, liver and MH clinicians alike must improve their understanding of AUD treatment and its psychiatric comorbidities in the context of liver disease.

CLINICS CARE POINTS

- MAUDs are under utilized in the ALD population. Several medications are utilized in relapse prevention and safe to use in those with overt liver disease.
- Dysregulated mood and poor sleep can interfere with the ability to maintain sobriety by increasing cravings and reducing motivation to engage in AUD treatment, as such regular screening for psychiatric symptoms and early psychiatric treatment is important in overall AUD care.

DISCLOSURE

None of the authors report any conflicts of interest.

REFERENCES

1. Deutsch-Link S, Jiang Y, Peery AF, et al. Alcohol-associated liver disease mortality increased from 2017 to 2020 and accelerated during the COVID-19 pandemic. Clin Gastroenterol Hepatol 2022;20(9):2142–4. e2.
2. Staufer K, Huber-Schönauer U, Strebinger G, et al. Ethyl glucuronide in hair detects a high rate of harmful alcohol consumption in presumed non-alcoholic fatty liver disease. J Hepatol 2022;77(4):918–30.
3. Bouttell J, Lewsey J, Geue C, et al. The SCottish alcoholic liver disease evaluation: a population-level matched cohort study of hospital-based costs, 1991-2011. PLoS One 2016;11(10):e0162980.
4. Roerecke M, Vafaei A, Hasan OSM, et al. Alcohol consumption and risk of liver cirrhosis: a systematic review and meta-analysis. Am J Gastroenterol 2019; 114(10):1574–86.
5. Im GY, Mellinger JL, Winters A, et al. Provider attitudes and practices for alcohol screening, treatment, and education in patients with liver disease: a survey from the American association for the study of liver diseases alcohol-associated liver disease special interest group. Clin Gastroenterol Hepatol 2021;19(11): 2407–24016 e8.
6. Elfeki MA, Abdallah MA, Leggio L, et al. Simultaneous management of alcohol use disorder and liver disease: a systematic review and meta-analysis. J Addict Med 2023;17(2):e119–28.
7. Watkins KE, Ober AJ, Lamp K, et al. Collaborative care for opioid and alcohol use disorders in primary care: the SUMMIT randomized clinical trial. JAMA Intern Med 2017;177(10):1480–8.
8. Pourmand K, Schiano TD, Motwani Y, et al. Burnout among transplant hepatologists in the United States. Liver Transpl 2022;28(5):867–75.
9. Winder GS. Interprofessional teams are crucial to reduce transplantation hepatology burnout. Liver Transpl 2022;28(7):1264–5.
10. Winder GS, Fernandez AC, Klevering K, et al. Confronting the crisis of comorbid alcohol use disorder and alcohol-related liver disease with a novel multidisciplinary clinic. Psychosomatics 2020;61(3):238–53.
11. Diaz LA, Winder GS, Leggio L, et al. New insights into the molecular basis of alcohol abstinence and relapse in alcohol-associated liver disease. Hepatology 2023.
12. Khan A, Tansel A, White DL, et al. Efficacy of psychosocial interventions in inducing and maintaining alcohol abstinence in patients with chronic liver disease: a systematic review. Clin Gastroenterol Hepatol 2016;14(2):191–202, e1-4;quiz e20.

13. Glass JE, Hamilton AM, Powell BJ, et al. Specialty substance use disorder services following brief alcohol intervention: a meta-analysis of randomized controlled trials. Addiction 2015;110(9):1404–15.
14. O'Donnell A, Anderson P, Newbury-Birch D, et al. The impact of brief alcohol interventions in primary healthcare: a systematic review of reviews. Alcohol Alcohol 2014;49(1):66–78.
15. Mattoo SK, Prasad S, Ghosh A. Brief intervention in substance use disorders. Indian J Psychiatry 2018;60(Suppl 4):S466–72.
16. Frost H, Campbell P, Maxwell M, et al. Effectiveness of Motivational Interviewing on adult behaviour change in health and social care settings: a systematic review of reviews. PLoS One 2018;13(10):e0204890.
17. Klimas J, Fairgrieve C, Tobin H, et al. Psychosocial interventions to reduce alcohol consumption in concurrent problem alcohol and illicit drug users. Cochrane Database Syst Rev 2018;12(12):CD009269.
18. Kohler S, Hofmann A. Can motivational interviewing in emergency care reduce alcohol consumption in young people? A systematic review and meta-analysis. Alcohol Alcohol 2015;50(2):107–17.
19. Wu SS, Schoenfelder E, Hsiao RC. Cognitive behavioral therapy and motivational enhancement therapy. Child Adolesc Psychiatr Clin N Am 2016;25(4):629–43.
20. Kuchipudi V, Hobein K, Flickinger A, et al. Failure of a 2-hour motivational intervention to alter recurrent drinking behavior in alcoholics with gastrointestinal disease. J Stud Alcohol 1990;51(4):356–60.
21. Proeschold-Bell RJ, Evon DM, Yao J, et al. A randomized controlled trial of an integrated alcohol reduction intervention in patients with hepatitis C infection. Hepatology 2020;71(6):1894–909.
22. Weinrieb RM, Van Horn DH, Lynch KG, et al. A randomized, controlled study of treatment for alcohol dependence in patients awaiting liver transplantation. Liver Transpl 2011;17(5):539–47.
23. Willenbring ML, Olson DH. A randomized trial of integrated outpatient treatment for medically ill alcoholic men. Arch Intern Med 1999;159(16):1946–52.
24. Carroll KM, Kiluk BD. Cognitive behavioral interventions for alcohol and drug use disorders: through the stage model and back again. Psychol Addict Behav 2017; 31(8):847–61.
25. Mehta K, Hoadley A, Ray LA, et al. Cognitive-behavioral interventions targeting alcohol or other drug use and Co-occurring mental health disorders: a meta-analysis. Alcohol Alcohol 2021;56(5):535–44.
26. Benishek LA, Dugosh KL, Kirby KC, et al. Prize-based contingency management for the treatment of substance abusers: a meta-analysis. Addiction 2014;109(9): 1426–36.
27. Cowie ME, Hodgins DC. Contingency management in Canadian addiction treatment: provider attitudes and use. J Stud Alcohol Drugs 2023;84(1):89–96.
28. Donoghue K, Boniface S, Brobbin E, et al. Adjunctive Medication Management and Contingency Management to enhance adherence to acamprosate for alcohol dependence: the ADAM trial RCT. Health Technol Assess 2023; 27(22):1–88.
29. Bolivar HA, Klemperer EM, Coleman SRM, et al. Contingency management for patients receiving medication for opioid use disorder: a systematic review and meta-analysis. JAMA Psychiatr 2021;78(10):1092–102.
30. Rash CJ, Stitzer M, Weinstock J. Contingency management: new directions and remaining challenges for an evidence-based intervention. J Subst Abuse Treat 2017;72:10–8.

31. McCrady BS, Flanagan JC. The role of the family in alcohol use disorder recovery for adults. Alcohol Res 2021;41(1):06.
32. Litt MD, Kadden RM, Tennen H, et al. Network Support II: randomized controlled trial of Network Support treatment and cognitive behavioral therapy for alcohol use disorder. Drug Alcohol Depend 2016;165:203–12.
33. Devine EG, Ryan ML, Falk DE, et al. An exploratory evaluation of Take Control: a novel computer-delivered behavioral platform for placebo-controlled pharmacotherapy trials for alcohol use disorder. Contemp Clin Trials 2016;50:178–85.
34. Park LS, Kornfield R, Yezihalem M, et al. Testing a digital health app for patients with alcohol-associated liver disease: mixed methods usability study. JMIR Form Res 2023;7:e47404.
35. Rabiee A, Mahmud N, Falker C, et al. Medications for alcohol use disorder improve survival in patients with hazardous drinking and alcohol-associated cirrhosis. Hepatol Commun 2023;7(4):e0093.
36. Mellinger JL, Fernandez A, Shedden K, et al. Gender disparities in alcohol use disorder treatment among privately insured patients with alcohol-associated cirrhosis. Alcohol Clin Exp Res 2019;43(2):334–41.
37. Johnson BA. Naltrexone long-acting formulation in the treatment of alcohol dependence. Therapeut Clin Risk Manag 2007;3(5):741–9.
38. Bertolotti M, Ferrari A, Vitale G, et al. Effect of liver cirrhosis on the systemic availability of naltrexone in humans. J Hepatol 1997;27(3):505–11.
39. Ayyala D, Bottyan T, Tien C, et al. Naltrexone for alcohol use disorder: hepatic safety in patients with and without liver disease. Hepatology Communications 2022;6(12):3433–42.
40. Lindor KD, Bowlus CL, Boyer J, et al. Primary biliary cholangitis: 2018 practice guidance from the American association for the study of liver diseases. Hepatology 2019;69(1):394–419.
41. Rosner S, Hackl-Herrwerth A, Leucht S, et al. Acamprosate for alcohol dependence. Cochrane Database Syst Rev 2010;9:CD004332.
42. Mason BJ, Heyser CJ. Acamprosate: a prototypic neuromodulator in the treatment of alcohol dependence. CNS Neurol Disord: Drug Targets 2010;9(1):23–32.
43. Witkiewitz K, Saville K, Hamreus K. Acamprosate for treatment of alcohol dependence: mechanisms, efficacy, and clinical utility. Ther Clin Risk Manag 2012;8: 45–53.
44. Reus VI, Fochtmann LJ, Bukstein O, et al. The American Psychiatric Association practice guideline for the pharmacological treatment of patients with alcohol use disorder. Focus (Am Psychiatr Publ) 2019;17(2):158–62.
45. Maldonado JR. Novel algorithms for the prophylaxis and management of alcohol withdrawal syndromes-beyond benzodiazepines. Crit Care Clin 2017;33(3): 559–99.
46. Mason BJ, Quello S, Shadan F. Gabapentin for the treatment of alcohol use disorder. Expert Opin Investig Drugs 2018;27(1):113–24.
47. Furieri FA, Nakamura-Palacios EM. Gabapentin reduces alcohol consumption and craving: a randomized, double-blind, placebo-controlled trial. J Clin Psychiatry 2007;68(11):1691–700.
48. Arab JP, Izzy M, Leggio L, et al. Management of alcohol use disorder in patients with cirrhosis in the setting of liver transplantation. Nat Rev Gastroenterol Hepatol 2022;19(1):45–59.
49. Perry C, Liberto J, Milliken C, et al. The management of substance use disorders: synopsis of the 2021 U.S. Department of veterans Affairs and U.S. Department of defense clinical practice guideline. Ann Intern Med 2022;175(5):720–31.

50. Kranzler HR, Soyka M. Diagnosis and pharmacotherapy of alcohol use disorder: a review. JAMA 2018;320(8):815–24.
51. Burnette EM, Nieto SJ, Grodin EN, et al. Novel agents for the pharmacological treatment of alcohol use disorder. Drugs 2022;82(3):251–74.
52. Knapp CM, Ciraulo DA, Sarid-Segal O, et al. Zonisamide, topiramate, and levetiracetam: efficacy and neuropsychological effects in alcohol use disorders. J Clin Psychopharmacol 2015;35(1):34–42.
53. Rose AK, Jones A. Baclofen: its effectiveness in reducing harmful drinking, craving, and negative mood. A meta-analysis. Addiction 2018;113(8):1396–406.
54. Addolorato G, Leggio L, Ferrulli A, et al. Effectiveness and safety of baclofen for maintenance of alcohol abstinence in alcohol-dependent patients with liver cirrhosis: randomised, double-blind controlled study. Lancet 2007;370(9603):1915–22.
55. Hauser P, Fuller B, Ho SB, et al. The safety and efficacy of baclofen to reduce alcohol use in veterans with chronic hepatitis C: a randomized controlled trial. Addiction 2017;112(7):1173–83.
56. Morley KC, Baillie A, Fraser I, et al. Baclofen in the treatment of alcohol dependence with or without liver disease: multisite, randomised, double-blind, placebo-controlled trial. Br J Psychiatry 2018;212(6):362–9.
57. Farokhnia M, Deschaine SL, Sadighi A, et al. A deeper insight into how GABA-B receptor agonism via baclofen may affect alcohol seeking and consumption: lessons learned from a human laboratory investigation. Mol Psychiatry 2021;26(2):545–55.
58. Vlavonou R, Perreault MM, Barriere O, et al. Pharmacokinetic characterization of baclofen in patients with chronic kidney disease: dose adjustment recommendations. J Clin Pharmacol 2014;54(5):584–92.
59. Formanek P, Salisbury-Afshar E, Afshar M. Helping patients with ESRD and earlier stages of CKD to quit smoking. Am J Kidney Dis 2018;72(2):255–66.
60. Anthenelli RM, Benowitz NL, West R, et al. Neuropsychiatric safety and efficacy of varenicline, bupropion, and nicotine patch in smokers with and without psychiatric disorders (EAGLES): a double-blind, randomised, placebo-controlled clinical trial. Lancet 2016;387(10037):2507–20.
61. Morley KC, Baillie A, Van Den Brink W, et al. N-acetyl cysteine in the treatment of alcohol use disorder in patients with liver disease: rationale for further research. Expert Opin Investig Drugs 2018;27(8):667–75.
62. Kranzler HR, Pierucci-Lagha A, Feinn R, et al. Effects of ondansetron in early-versus late-onset alcoholics: a prospective, open-label study. Alcohol Clin Exp Res 2003;27(7):1150–5.
63. Figg WD, Dukes GE, Pritchard JF, et al. Pharmacokinetics of ondansetron in patients with hepatic insufficiency. J Clin Pharmacol 1996;36(3):206–15.
64. Nevola R, Epifani R, Imbriani S, et al. GLP-1 receptor agonists in non-alcoholic fatty liver disease: current evidence and future perspectives. Int J Mol Sci 2023;24(2):1703.
65. Castillo-Carniglia A, Keyes KM, Hasin DS, et al. Psychiatric comorbidities in alcohol use disorder. Lancet Psychiatr 2019;6(12):1068–80.
66. Menon V, Ransing R, Praharaj SK. Management of psychiatric disorders in patients with hepatic and gastrointestinal diseases. Indian J Psychiatry 2022;64(Suppl 2):S379–93.
67. Andrade C, Sandarsh S, Chethan KB, et al. Serotonin reuptake inhibitor antidepressants and abnormal bleeding: a review for clinicians and a reconsideration of mechanisms. J Clin Psychiatry 2010;71(12):1565–75.

68. Kang SG, Park YM, Lee HJ, et al. Duloxetine-induced liver injury in patients with major depressive disorder. Psychiatry Investig 2011;8(3):269–71.

69. Shaheen AA, Kaplan GG, Sharkey KA, et al. Impact of major depression and antidepressant use on alcoholic and non-alcoholic fatty liver disease: a population-based study. Liver Int 2021;41(10):2308–17.

70. Chen M, Suzuki A, Thakkar S, et al. DILIrank: the largest reference drug list ranked by the risk for developing drug-induced liver injury in humans. Drug Discov Today 2016;21(4):648–53.

71. Abdel-Salam NMS OME, Mohammed NA, Youness ER, et al. The 5-ht1a agonist buspirone decreases liver oxidative stress and exerts protective effect against CCl4– toxicity. Journal of Experimental and Clinical Toxicology 2017;1(1):13–26.

72. Gunther M, Dopheide JA. Antipsychotic safety in liver disease: a narrative review and practical guide for the clinician. J Acad Consult Liaison Psychiatry 2023; 64(1):73–82.

73. Lo HS, Yang CM, Lo HG, et al. Treatment effects of gabapentin for primary insomnia. Clin Neuropharmacol 2010;33(2):84–90.

74. Ali MM, Teich JL, Mutter R. Reasons for not seeking substance use disorder treatment: variations by health insurance coverage. J Behav Health Serv Res 2017; 44(1):63–74.

75. Mee-Lee DG. The ASAM criteria and matching patients to treatment. In: Ries RR R, Miller SC, Saitz R, et al, editors. The ASAM principles of addiction medicine 5th. Edition: Wolters Kluwer Health/Lippincott Williams & Wilkins; 2015. p. 428–41.

76. Ramkissoon R, Shah VH. Alcohol use disorder and alcohol-associated liver disease. Alcohol Res 2022;42(1):13.

77. Knox J, Hasin DS, Larson FRR, et al. Prevention, screening, and treatment for heavy drinking and alcohol use disorder. Lancet Psychiatr 2019;6(12):1054–67.

78. Mellinger JL, Fernandez AC, Winder GS. Management of alcohol use disorder in patients with chronic liver disease. Hepatol Commun 2023;7(7):e00145.

79. Simonetto DA, Shah VH, Kamath PS. Outpatient management of alcohol-related liver disease. Lancet Gastroenterol Hepatol 2020;5(5):485–93.

80. Kelly JF, Humphreys K, Ferri M. Alcoholics Anonymous and other 12-step programs for alcohol use disorder. Cochrane Database Syst Rev 2020;3(3): CD012880.

81. Zemore SE, Kaskutas LA, Mericle A, et al. Comparison of 12-step groups to mutual help alternatives for AUD in a large, national study: differences in membership characteristics and group participation, cohesion, and satisfaction. J Subst Abuse Treat 2017;73:16–26.

82. Jason LA, Olson BD, Ferrari JR, et al. An examination of main and interactive effects of substance abuse recovery housing on multiple indicators of adjustment. Addiction 2007;102(7):1114–21.

83. Chand PK, Panda U, Mahadevan J, et al. Management of alcohol withdrawal syndrome in patients with alcoholic liver disease. J Clin Exp Hepatol 2022;12(6): 1527–34.

Barriers to Alcohol Use Disorder Treatment in Patients with Alcohol-Associated Liver Disease

András H. Lékó, MD, PhD[a,b], Lorenzo Leggio, MD, PhD[a,c,d,e],*

KEYWORDS

- Treatment barriers • Alcohol use disorder • Stigma • Addiction
- Alcohol-associated liver disease • Integrated care

KEY POINTS

- Patients with alcohol-associated liver disease (ALD) have alcohol use disorder (AUD), which is the underlying reason for the development of ALD.
- There are patient-level, clinician-level, and organization-level barriers that prevent the effective development of hepatology/addiction multidisciplinary integrated care approaches to treat these patients with dual pathology (ALD and AUD).
- Stigma around AUD is clearly the chief challenge across all barriers summarized here; stigma affects the ability to screen, diagnose, treat, and manage AUD.
- Investments aimed at developing effective and sustainable multidisciplinary integrated approaches are much needed for patients with AUD and ALD.

INTRODUCTION

Prolonged abstinence is critically important, and the ideal goal is to decrease mortality in alcohol-associated liver disease (ALD). Historically, total abstinence has been a

[a] Clinical Psychoneuroendocrinology and Neuropsychopharmacology Section, Translational Addiction Medicine Branch, National Institute on Drug Abuse Intramural Research Program and National Institute on Alcohol Abuse and Alcoholism Division of Intramural Clinical and Biological Research, National Institutes of Health, 251 Bayview Boulevard, Baltimore, MD 21224, USA; [b] Department of Psychiatry and Psychotherapy, Semmelweis University, Balassa utca 6, 1083, Budapest, Hungary; [c] Department of Behavioral and Social Sciences, Center for Alcohol and Addiction Studies, School of Public Health, Brown University, 121 South Main Street, Providence, RI 02903, USA; [d] Division of Addiction Medicine, Department of Medicine, School of Medicine, Johns Hopkins University, 4940 Eastern Avenue, Baltimore, MD 21224, USA; [e] Department of Neuroscience, Georgetown University Medical Center, 3970 Reservoir Road Northwest, NRB, EP04, Washington, DC, USA
* Corresponding author. NIDA and NIAAA, National Institutes of Health, Biomedical Research Center, 251 Bayview Boulevard, Baltimore, MD 21224.
E-mail address: lorenzo.leggio@nih.gov

Clin Liver Dis 28 (2024) 779–791
https://doi.org/10.1016/j.cld.2024.06.012
1089-3261/24/Published by Elsevier Inc.

requirement to be eligible for liver transplantation (LT),[1,2] although a significant shift in paradigm has taken place in the last decade.[3] Any alcohol consumption in patients with liver-related decompensation and/or alcohol-associated hepatitis and even in patients with compensated cirrhosis is not advisable.[4] After the first ALD-related hospitalization, rates of returning to alcohol use are 40% to 70%.[5–8] After LT, in a mean follow-up period of 48.4 ± 24.7 months, rates of alcohol relapse and heavy alcohol relapse were 22% and 14%, respectively.[9] Mortality is 3 fold higher during a 10 year follow-up in those patients who relapse into alcohol drinking.[10] Still, only a very small portion of patients with ALD receive any therapeutic intervention for alcohol use disorder (AUD). For example, in a retrospective cohort study among veterans with liver cirrhosis and comorbid AUD, only 14% received AUD treatment, including 12% receiving solely behavioral therapy, 0.4% receiving pharmacotherapy, and 1% receiving combined therapy.[11] The same study showed the benefits of receiving AUD therapy as it resulted in lower risk of hepatic decompensation (adjusted odds ratio [AOR] 0.63) and reduced long-term mortality (AOR 0.87).[11] Integrative care models, like multidisciplinary ALD clinics, are critical for patients with ALD. In such clinics, hepatology and addiction teams work jointly to treat ALD and AUD simultaneously.[12,13] These multidisciplinary approaches allow a holistic and unified management of patients with AUD/ALD and facilitate an earlier diagnosis of relapse, hence allowing for timely interventions and reduced mortality.[13–16] Nevertheless, implementing this approach in clinical practice is challenging, and widespread adoption of these recommended models is poor.[1,11,17–19]

In this article, we outline the barriers to AUD treatment in patients with ALD. Consistent with DiMartini and colleagues,[20] we categorize them into 3 groups: patient-level, clinician-level, and system-level barriers. Furthermore, we discuss strategies to overcome these obstacles. We summarized this information in **Table 1**.

DISCUSSION
Patient-Level Barriers

Lack of insight of alcohol use disorder diagnosis and inaccurate information about alcohol use disorder

At the time of the initial visit with a hepatologist, a patient with ALD may not be aware of having an AUD, and an AUD diagnosis could come as a surprise. Facing the information that AUD and the related problematic/hazardous alcohol consumption is the cause of their liver disease may lead to denial of the AUD diagnosis in the first place.[20] Awareness of having a drinking problem is a crucial step toward readiness to change and accept any AUD treatment. As shown by a study, in more than half of individuals with AUD, lack of insight of drinking problems was the reason for not seeking treatment.[21] In patients with ALD, Younger age, higher drinking severity, and higher self-stigma predict stronger self-awareness of the individual's drinking problems.[22] Many of them do not believe that alcohol consumption is a significant problem for themselves; therefore, they refuse having a diagnosis.[23] Even if a patient accepts the diagnosis, they may not understand that it is a chronic medical disease with a high potential to relapse. They may think that if they reach abstinence once, then no more sustained treatment is necessary, and there is no risk of relapse.[20,23–26] Furthermore, patients also tend to prioritize ALD treatment and decline simultaneous AUD treatment because they feel liver problems are more important and a higher priority than AUD,[23,25] hence not appreciating that in actuality AUD is the underlying cause of ALD. Of note, a recent study showed some gender disparity in some of these misconceptions, for example, more women (18% of women vs 10% of men) think incorrectly that women have to drink

Table 1
Barriers to alcohol use disorder treatment in individuals with alcohol-associated liver disease and possible strategies to overcome these challenges

Identified Barriers	Strategies to Overcome
Patient-level barriers	
Misconceptions about the chronicity of AUD and the risk of relapse	Patient education
Stigmatization	Educational campaigns from the appropriate organizations to overcome stigma Avoid using stigmatizing language by health care providers
Underreporting alcohol consumption	Using direct or indirect biomarkers of alcohol consumption Revise the 6 mo abstinence criterion for LT
Lack of information and discomfort about AUD treatment options	Provide information about treatment options Integrated care with addiction and hepatology specialists Collaborative attitude toward the patient
Insufficient motivation to reduce or stop alcohol consumption	Motivational interviewing
Lack of social/family support	Include social workers and case managers in the medical team Family therapy and psychoeducation of the family
Clinician-level barriers	
Inadequate identification of AUD	Education about useful screening/diagnostic tools (eg, AUDIT) Consensus about the definition of relapse
Imprecise quantification of alcohol use	Reduce stigmatization of individuals with AUD Provide additional time for patient history taking
Lack of knowledge about AUD treatment options	Educational symposia and campaigns by addiction experts
Choosing inappropriate treatments for AUD	Distribute propagable, concise educational materials among health care providers
Discomfort in AUD treatment	Incorporating addiction medicine training in the hepatology fellowship curriculum
System-level barriers	
Geographically separated addiction medicine and hepatology units	Facilitate funding for integrated care Increase communication between clinicians from different units (eg, hepatology, internal medicine, addiction medicine, and psychiatry) Facilitate the use of telehealth
Insufficient human and technical resources	Increase funding for mental health staff and clinics
Private health insurances do not facilitate integrated care	Increase federal and state-level funding for integrated care models

(continued on next page)

Table 1 (continued)	
Identified Barriers	Strategies to Overcome
Difficulties in combined billing, separate administrative systems	Develop integrated care models
Gender, racial/ethnic, and socioeconomic inequities	Uniform protocols, screening, and monitoring Increase availability of mental health care in marginalized and socially deprived communities

more alcohol than men to get ALD, and approximately 20% of women (8% of men) believe that women, in general, do not have to worry about having AUD.[24]

Tendency to minimize/underestimate the use of alcohol
A remarkable group of patients underreport their actual alcohol consumption or belittle their alcohol use.[27] An important reason for this behavior is that they may feel discomforted discussing their illness with health care providers as well as feeling that their condition "disappoints" them.[24] Some people may also be afraid of AUD inpatient care, should they be honest about their actual alcohol use.[28] For patients with AUD and ALD requiring LT, some of them may conceal their relapse because they fear a penalty or being removed from the waiting list.[29] Patients may perceive stigma not only about having AUD but also about having liver disease. The association between alcohol and liver disease is so strong that in a survey study, 82% of patients with liver disease perceived stigma from society, health care providers, and family for being an "alcoholic"; however, only 12% of them had ALD.[30] Society often blames patients with ALD for their behavior leading to the illness, which prevents them from accurately self-reporting the actual alcohol consumption.[31,32]

Lack of information, misconceptions, and discomfort about alcohol use disorder treatment options
Even if a patient accepts the diagnosis of AUD and accurately reports their alcohol consumption, they may be reluctant against AUD treatment. Numerous patients feel they do not need therapy because, in their opinion, it is ineffective and a waste of time.[24] Pharmacotherapy is the least well-known type of AUD treatment, and there is a lack of knowledge about its side effects and benefits as well.[28,29] Patients may not appreciate that AUD treatment may also improve their mental/emotional health and social relationships. They think that it is too late to treat AUD when symptoms of advanced liver disease are present, which is also a frequent misconception. Receiving AUD treatment is perceived to be stigmatizing because of its associations with character weakness, personal failure, or signs of poor commitment to abstinence.[29] In addition, there is a solid perception of the "ideal ALD transplant patient" who is invincible and able to avoid any relapse without getting help.[29] Many patients prefer to deal with a relapse themselves before involving any staff because they think that they "should be strong enough to handle it alone."[28] There is also a reluctance to group therapy, mainly due to social anxiety, concerns about the perceived negative influence of groups that include active drinkers, and maintaining anonymity, especially in smaller towns and other small communities.[24]

Insufficient motivation to change
The motivation to change any health behavior is a balance between the potential benefits and subjective inconveniences/disadvantages. To reach abstinence, patients

must consider ending drinking-related social relationships or abstaining from the various effects (eg, rewarding, euphoric, sedative, anxiolytic, and pain-relieving) of alcohol. This decision-making is influenced by the person's preferences and core values.[20,33] The behavioral change begins with precontemplation, followed by contemplation, and taking action to change.[34] Many patients with ALD are in the pre-contemplation phase, and they have to go through the 3 steps mentioned earlier to become able to change their behavior and cut down alcohol consumption.[20] That shows how difficult it may be to accept the advice of immediate abstinence. Most benefits are long-term, but disadvantages, such as withdrawal symptoms or the disappearance of drinking-related social networks, are instantaneous.

Lack of social and family support

The main driver for maintaining abstinence is support from the family as identified by 66% of LT patients in a survey study.[29] Accordingly, those who relapsed blamed the lack of social and family support, which often drops after a successful LT.[29] If patients with ALD are not ready to reduce drinking or become abstinent, it can destroy family relationships.[20] They may also miss their drinking partners; however, such social networks may place the patient at risk for relapse.[20,29]

Strategies to Surmount Patient-Level Barriers

Appropriate screening is key to timely identify which patient needs AUD treatment and those who are abstinent with a high risk of relapse. The use of the AUD identification test (AUDIT) is highly recommended by the US Preventive Services Task Force to diagnose AUD with a sensitivity of 70% and a specificity of 85% and to assess the severity of AUD.[35] AUDIT is validated widely across different demographic groups. A score of 8 or greater is considered to indicate hazardous or harmful alcohol use. Before and after LT, evaluation of risk factors helps early intervention to prevent or at least mitigate the effects of alcohol relapse. The risk of relapse is higher with younger age, family history of AUD, history of previous treatment of AUD, shorter length of pretransplantation abstinence, poor social support, smoking, comorbid mental health and substance use disorders, and noncompliance with clinic visits.[12] For a proper risk evaluation, clinicians can use the Sustained Alcohol Use Post-Liver Transplant (SALT) score (range 0–11) based on the abovementioned risk factors. The SALT score includes 4 points for greater than 10 drinks per day at initial hospitalization, 4 points for multiple prior rehabilitation attempts, 2 points for prior alcohol-related legal issues, and 1 point for previous substance use. This score has a good sensitivity, but its specificity is low. A SALT score of less than 5 has a 95% negative predictive value, and a score of 5 or greater has only a 25% positive predictive value for sustained alcohol use after LT.[36] However, SALT scoring is a convenient tool to evaluate the chance of a relapse; it also has a disadvantage, namely the portion of false positives is high, thereby potentially stigmatizing numerous patients with ALD.

Underreported alcohol use can be addressed by measuring biomarkers of alcohol consumption. Indirect markers, like serum levels of γ-glutamyltransferase, mean corpuscular volume, aspartate aminotransferase, or carbohydrate-deficient transferrin are widely used by clinicians, but their specificity is low.[12] Direct markers of alcohol metabolism are more specific, and enhancing their availability would alleviate the detection of relapse and getting proper information about actual alcohol consumption. Ethyl glucuronide (EtG) and ethyl sulfate (EtS) are nonvolatile, water-soluble metabolites produced during the elimination of ethanol, and they are detectable in urine up to 90 hours after alcohol consumption.[37] Urinary EtG shows an 89.3% sensitivity and a

98.9% specificity for actual alcohol drinking,[38] and EtG can also be measured in hair and fingernails as markers of long-term alcohol use.[39,40] Phosphatidylethanol can be identified in whole blood samples and is formed only in the presence of alcohol. Therefore, its detection indicates alcohol consumption in the last 28 days, with a sensitivity of 90% to 99% and specificity of 100%.[41] A promising state-of-the-art technology is to use ankle bracelets containing a transdermal electrochemical sensor that detects alcohol vapors closely to the skin.[42,43]

Reducing stigma can also help to overcome many patient-level barriers. Patients with ALD are sensitive to shame, guilt, and judgment about their alcohol use,[24] which leads to underreporting it and rejecting treatment when it is offered. An important step to reduce stigma was the recent name change from "alcoholic" liver disease to ALD, because of the disgrace associated with the word "alcoholic."[44] Clinicians encountering patients with ALD need to behave with a nonthreatening, nonjudgmental approach in order to gain the patient's confidence. Such demeanor facilitates candid conversations with the patient about alcohol use, and psychoeducation about AUD.[45,46] To overcome misconceptions and false beliefs about AUD, education about alcohol-related harms and amounts of alcohol, which can cause liver damage, is essential. Furthermore, providing information about the chronic relapsing-remitting course of AUD and treatment options (both pharmacologic and behavioral) need to be included in the counseling, since many patients are not aware of them.[20] Regarding the gender disparities in misconceptions about AUD, women-targeted motivational interventions need to address stronger reluctance of acknowledging problematic use of alcohol, higher risk for ALD and need for treatment.[28]

Integrated care with a multidisciplinary team of hepatologists and addiction specialists, showed higher efficacy in the treatment of AUD in patients with ALD.[12,16,17] Mental health specialists are able to provide motivational interviewing and recommend the type of AUD treatment. Patients with a tendency for high self-confidence in maintaining abstinence may work collaboratively with addiction specialists without feeling their self-sufficiency threatened.[29] Social workers and case managers can provide help with insurance and transportation issues. Recovery from AUD and ALD includes not just abstinence from alcohol but also aspects of patients' self-image, functional status, social relationships, life goals, and coping skills.[24]

Clinician-Level Barriers

Inadequate identification or quantification of alcohol use

An accurate history of quantity, frequency, and duration of alcohol use is required for the diagnosis of ALD and also to detect the comorbid AUD. A significant barrier is that clinicians who first encounter the patient (eg, primary care providers [PCPs]), may not be trained enough to collect all this detailed information. They may feel uncomfortable asking those questions, be preoccupied and overwhelmed with other medical issues, or simply forget to ask, since many PCPs do not screen routinely for AUD. Even if information is gathered from the patient, the clinician may not contact family members, friends, or significant others asking about alcohol-related patient history.[47,48] Time pressure, and lack of space, clinical knowledge, and training are the most frequent reasons for inadequate screening and identification of AUD. Still, most patients and providers think that PCPs should play a key role in AUD screening and treatment.[48] After the appropriate screening, AUD diagnosis is the next step, which requires a structured clinical assessment of behavioral, physiologic, and social consequences of alcohol consumption, including harm to users and others. Diagnostics and treatment planning takes significant time, because of the comprehensive interview addressing the severity of AUD, prior alcohol use, possible AUD treatment history and social environment of the patient. This needs to be conducted by trained mental health care providers, who are specialized and devote enough time and resources for the examination.[20]

Insufficient knowledge about alcohol use disorder treatment or inadequate therapy for alcohol use disorder

A recent retrospective cohort study found that only 37% of hepatology notes documented discussions about AUD treatment options.[49] In addition, when discussed, treatment recommendations are often not evidence-based and rarely include pharmacotherapy options.[49] In a survey of 408 health care providers (the majority were hepatologists and gastroenterologists, and 80% worked in a tertiary LT center), 60% reported referring the patient to an addiction specialist for behavioral therapy, but 71% never prescribed AUD pharmacotherapy, and 77% complained about the lack of education in addiction medicine.[50] Clinicians often recommend abstaining from alcohol, which is important to reach any improvement in ALD, but they provide no clear directions about how to achieve it. Having a candid conversation about alcohol use and educating the patient about the importance of abstinence is critically important, but it is only the starting point, not the treatment of AUD. Without any behavioral or pharmacologic therapy or help from a mental health care provider, it is entirely up to the patient to comply with the doctor's advice.[20,49] If a patient with ALD has a moderate-to-severe AUD, it requires specific AUD treatment from addiction experts.[20] On one hand, some internists may feel uncomfortable about treating any psychiatric issue and tend to stigmatize patients with AUD for "their responsibility for becoming ill," or feel they morally do not deserve the treatment, which is a waste of time and resources. On the other hand, some mental health care providers may be enormously afraid of admitting patients with any severe somatic illness and tend to prioritize medical stabilization of the patient before providing any AUD treatment, even though they should be simultaneous.[19]

Strategies to Surmount Clinician-Level Barriers

Lack of knowledge among clinicians about how to diagnose and treat AUD properly is one of the main reasons behind clinician-level barriers. Educational symposia and campaigns by addiction experts are required to address this problem. Propagable, concise educational materials containing up-to-date information need to be developed. The distributed documents must include the most important points that a general medical staff should know about harmful alcohol use, ALD, and pharmacologic and behavioral therapy options. Earlier, we discussed the AUDIT questionnaire among patient-level barriers. AUDIT use needs to be used routinely and broadly by clinicians, and it should be included in patient examinations. Knowledge about AUD can be increased by incorporating addiction medicine training in the hepatology fellowship curriculum. That way, hepatologists would also become more comfortable discussing alcohol-related issues with the patient and providing them with adequate help. In addition, they can acquire motivational interviewing and assess how open the patient is to a behavioral change regarding alcohol drinking. However, using all these skills, screening for AUD, and discussing therapy during a medical visit require significant time commitment; therefore, current practices need to be changed to provide additional time for health care providers for an adequate and thorough examination.

The appropriate and meaningful definition of relapse is also required for the adequate treatment of patients with ALD. After a consensus, 3 levels of relapse were defined: mild relapse with occasional "slips" (less than once per month); moderate relapse with continuous drinking within the recommended weekly and daily National Institute on Alcohol Abuse and Alcoholism (NIAAA) standards ($\leq$14 drinks per week for men, and $\leq$7 drinks per week for women); and severe relapse with regular use of alcohol above the NIAAA standards, or appearance of alcohol-related morbidity (eg, pancreatitis, graft loss, and alcohol-associated hepatitis).[12] However, any drinking with liver-related decompensation and/or alcohol-associated hepatitis and even in patients with compensated cirrhosis should be considered harmful[4]; after LT, there is no evidence that mild relapse is associated with patient or graft survival.[12,51] In summary, relapse to drinking is not the same as relapse to AUD, and it is possible that harm reduction (eg, reducing the episodes of heavy drinking) would be a valuable end point, at least in patients with early stages of ALD.

System-Level Barriers

Organizational and logistic barriers

Even if appropriate training is provided, no medical specialty can handle alone comorbid ALD and AUD; therefore, integrated care is required. Nevertheless, a significant barrier for integrated care is the lack of support from health care systems.[20] Separate and isolated care, with no collaboration between different specialists, results in piecemeal care and mixed/conflicting messages to the patient.[19] In a disintegrated system, referrals to other specialists do not happen on a regular basis, and even if they happen, they are not sufficient to create an integrated treatment plan. During these types of referrals, there is always a great risk to miss important information, which again can be overcome by an integrated model.[52] The profit-oriented business health care model pushes to see as many patients as possible per day. This time pressure does not allow to dedicate sufficient time for thorough examination or meaningful consultation with other specialists.[20] Mental health care providers, especially those in addiction units, are often logistically disconnected from the acute medical environments. Hepatology and addiction medicine are often separated in different departments and buildings (eg, Medicaid mental health care and liver specialty care are commonly distant), resulting in difficult collaboration and access to both services.[19,53] The travel distance also negatively affects AUD treatment utilization.[54] A possible reason for this isolation is that addiction services are stigmatized, and other departments want them to be separate and distant. The latter also means that hepatology and addiction medicine services may utilize different electronic system and have different administrative teams.[19,53]

Health insurance barriers

Systems based on private health insurances do not facilitate integrated care. Combined billing is difficult, administrative staff must know a wide range of medical and psychiatric diagnostic codes and encounter types, many of which require separate insurance authorization.[19] A possible strategy to overcome physical distance of hepatology and addiction services would be telehealth, but it is currently underdeveloped.[20] Public health care and socialized health care systems better provide services for socially deprived populations (eg, homeless people), where AUD and ALD may be more frequent.[55] While the first multidisciplinary ALD clinic in the United States was launched in 2018,[19] such approaches have been developed much earlier in European countries with socialized health care systems like Italy[13,16] and France.[56] There are significant racial/ethnic disparities in the effects of structural barriers. African Americans and Latinx are more likely than Whites to underutilize AUD treatment because of structural barriers.[28] That means, Whites are more likely than Latinx or African Americans to receive treatment (37.6%, 22.4%, and 25.0%, respectively).[57]

Strategies to Surmount System-Level Barriers

The development of more integrated care centers is essential to overcome the structural barriers mentioned earlier. National policies are required to increase federal and state-level funding for mental health care and integrated care of AUD and ALD. Funding for attending multidisciplinary conferences and for getting multidisciplinary board certifications (eg, addiction medicine for a hepatologist) would facilitate integrated care and collaboration between medical specialties.[19] Closer collaboration would be important between professional societies and organizations across the hepatology and addiction fields. Research funding needs to target developing new AUD relapse prevention medications and diagnostic practices (eg, biomarkers), relapse risk evaluation, cost-effectiveness of integrated care and implementation of multidisciplinary clinics. Addressing health insurance barriers, coverage should also include specialty AUD and ALD care. Combined billing and integrated administration and electronic systems are also required for an appropriate multidisciplinary care. Health inequities and racial disparities are such system-level barriers that need to be addressed by federal or state social programs and local initiatives.

SUMMARY

AUD is the underlying etiology that leads to the development of ALD; hence, these patients have a dual pathology whose optimal treatment requires both hepatology and addiction specialists involved in their care. However, unfortunately, a synergistic hepatology/addiction integrated management of these patients is more the exception than the rule. Indeed, there are patient-level, clinician-level, and organization-level barriers that prevent the effective development of hepatology/addiction multidisciplinary integrated care approaches to treat these patients. Of note, at least some of the reasons why these barriers exist reflect the strong influence that stigma plays on AUD and addictions in our society. Therefore, it is imperative to develop multidisciplinary integrated care approaches where both hepatology and addiction specialists manage these patients together and synergistically. Investments aimed at developing effective and sustainable multidisciplinary integrated approaches are much needed for patients with this dual AUD/ALD pathology.

CLINICS CARE POINTS

- AUD treatment is often suboptimal or absent in individuals with ALD; however, addressing, managing, and treating AUD is essential to reduce the risk of hepatic decompensation, relapse to drinking after LT, and long-term mortality.
- Integrative care models, like multidisciplinary AUD/ALD integrated clinics, reduce dramatically morbidity and mortality.
- Appropriate screening is crucial to detect which patient needs AUD treatment. AUDIT is useful for diagnosing AUD, and SALT scoring for evaluating the risk of relapse after LT.
- Underreported alcohol use can be addressed by measuring highly specific, direct biomarkers of alcohol consumption, for example, EtG, EtS, or phosphatidylethanol.
- Reducing stigma around AUD is important to facilitate patients' confidence and compliance and the acceptance of AUD treatment.
- Education of the patients about alcohol-related harms and the chronic course of AUD is required to overcome popular misconceptions, which are serious barriers to AUD treatment.
- Education of clinicians can help them properly diagnose and treat AUD.

- National policies are required to increase federal and state-level funding for integrated care of AUD and ALD and for facilitating collaboration between hepatology and addiction medicine.

DISCLOSURE

The authors have nothing to disclose. This study was supported by the National Institutes of Health, United States (NIH) intramural research program funding (ZIA-DA000635) (Section on Clinical Psychoneuroendocrinology and Neuropsychopharmacology, PI: Dr L. Leggio), jointly supported by the National Institute on Drug Abuse, United States (NIDA) Intramural Research Program and the National Institute on Alcohol Abuse and Alcoholism, United States (NIAAA) Division of Intramural Clinical and Biological Research.

REFERENCES

1. Jophlin LL, Singal AK, Bataller R, et al. ACG clinical guideline: alcohol-associated liver disease. Am J Gastroenterol 2024;119:30–54.
2. Penninti P, Adekunle AD, Singal AK. Alcoholic hepatitis: the rising epidemic. Med Clin North Am 2023;107:533–54.
3. Lee MR, Leggio L. Management of alcohol use disorder in patients requiring liver transplant. Am J Psychiatr 2015;172:1182–9.
4. Crabb DW, Im GY, Szabo G, et al. Diagnosis and treatment of alcohol-associated liver diseases: 2019 practice guidance from the American Association for the study of Liver Diseases. Hepatology 2020;71:306–33.
5. Altamirano J, López-Pelayo H, Michelena J, et al. Alcohol abstinence in patients surviving an episode of alcoholic hepatitis: prediction and impact on long-term survival. Hepatology 2017;66:1842–53.
6. Louvet A, Labreuche J, Artru F, et al. Main drivers of outcome differ between short term and long term in severe alcoholic hepatitis: a prospective study. Hepatology 2017;66:1464–73.
7. Peeraphatdit TB, Kamath PS, Karpyak VM, et al. Alcohol rehabilitation within 30 Days of hospital discharge is associated with reduced readmission, relapse, and death in patients with alcoholic hepatitis. Clin Gastroenterol Hepatol 2020; 18:477–85.e475.
8. Pessione F, Ramond MJ, Peters L, et al. Five-year survival predictive factors in patients with excessive alcohol intake and cirrhosis. Effect of alcoholic hepatitis, smoking and abstinence. Liver Int 2003;23:45–53.
9. Chuncharunee L, Yamashiki N, Thakkinstian A, et al. Alcohol relapse and its predictors after liver transplantation for alcoholic liver disease: a systematic review and meta-analysis. BMC Gastroenterol 2019;19:150.
10. Kodali S, Kaif M, Tariq R, et al. Alcohol relapse after liver transplantation for alcoholic cirrhosis-impact on liver graft and patient survival: a meta-analysis. Alcohol Alcohol 2018;53:166–72.
11. Rogal S, Youk A, Zhang H, et al. Impact of alcohol use disorder treatment on clinical outcomes among patients with cirrhosis. Hepatology 2020;71:2080–92.
12. Arab JP, Izzy M, Leggio L, et al. Management of alcohol use disorder in patients with cirrhosis in the setting of liver transplantation. Nat Rev Gastroenterol Hepatol 2022;19:45–59.

13. Attilia ML, Lattanzi B, Ledda R, et al. The multidisciplinary support in preventing alcohol relapse after liver transplantation: a single-center experience. Clin Transplant 2018;32:e13243.
14. Magistri P, Marzi L, Guerzoni S, et al. Impact of a multidisciplinary team on alcohol recidivism and survival after liver transplant for alcoholic disease. Transplant Proc 2019;51:187–9.
15. López-Pelayo H, Miquel L, Altamirano J, et al. Treatment retention in a specialized alcohol programme after an episode of alcoholic hepatitis: impact on alcohol relapse. J Psychosom Res 2019;116:75–82.
16. Addolorato G, Mirijello A, Leggio L, et al. Liver transplantation in alcoholic patients: impact of an alcohol addiction unit within a liver transplant center. Alcohol Clin Exp Res 2013;37:1601–8.
17. Leggio L, Lee MR. Treatment of alcohol use disorder in patients with alcoholic liver disease. Am J Med 2017;130:124–34.
18. Singal AK, Bataller R, Ahn J, et al. ACG clinical guideline: alcoholic liver disease. Am J Gastroenterol 2018;113:175–94.
19. Winder GS, Fernandez AC, Klevering K, et al. Confronting the crisis of comorbid alcohol use disorder and alcohol-related liver disease with a novel multidisciplinary clinic. Psychosomatics 2020;61:238–53.
20. DiMartini AF, Leggio L, Singal AK. Barriers to the management of alcohol use disorder and alcohol-associated liver disease: strategies to implement integrated care models. Lancet Gastroenterol Hepatol 2022;7:186–95.
21. Spector AY, Remien RH, Tross S. PrEP in substance abuse treatment: a qualitative study of treatment provider perspectives. Subst Abuse Treat Prev Pol 2015; 10:1.
22. Chang C, Wang TJ, Chen MJ, et al. Factors influencing readiness to change in patients with alcoholic liver disease: a cross-sectional study. J Psychiatr Ment Health Nurs 2021;28:344–55.
23. Weinrieb RM, Van Horn DH, McLellan AT, et al. Alcoholism treatment after liver transplantation: lessons learned from a clinical trial that failed. Psychosomatics 2001;42:110–6.
24. Mellinger JL, Scott Winder G, DeJonckheere M, et al. Misconceptions, preferences and barriers to alcohol use disorder treatment in alcohol-related cirrhosis. J Subst Abuse Treat 2018;91:20–7.
25. Weinrieb RM, Van Horn DH, Lynch KG, et al. A randomized, controlled study of treatment for alcohol dependence in patients awaiting liver transplantation. Liver Transplant 2011;17:539–47.
26. Saunders SM, Zygowicz KM, D'Angelo BR. Person-related and treatment-related barriers to alcohol treatment. J Subst Abuse Treat 2006;30:261–70.
27. Grüner Nielsen D, Andersen K, Søgaard Nielsen A, et al. Consistency between self-reported alcohol consumption and biological markers among patients with alcohol use disorder - a systematic review. Neurosci Biobehav Rev 2021;124: 370–85.
28. Verissimo AD, Grella CE. Influence of gender and race/ethnicity on perceived barriers to help-seeking for alcohol or drug problems. J Subst Abuse Treat 2017;75:54–61.
29. Heyes CM, Schofield T, Gribble R, et al. Reluctance to accept alcohol treatment by alcoholic liver disease transplant patients: a qualitative study. Transplant Direct 2016;2:e104.
30. Vaughn-Sandler V, Sherman C, Aronsohn A, et al. Consequences of perceived stigma among patients with cirrhosis. Dig Dis Sci 2014;59:681–6.

31. Room R. Stigma, social inequality and alcohol and drug use. Drug Alcohol Rev 2005;24:143–55.
32. Schomerus G, Holzinger A, Matschinger H, et al. [Public attitudes towards alcohol dependence]. Psychiatr Prax 2010;37:111–8.
33. Zuckoff A. "Why won't my patients do what's good for them?" Motivational interviewing and treatment adherence. Surg Obes Relat Dis 2012;8:514–21.
34. Willoughby FW, Edens JF. Construct validity and predictive utility of the stages of change scale for alcoholics. J Subst Abuse 1996;8:275–91.
35. O'Connor EA, Perdue LA, Senger CA, et al. Screening and behavioral counseling interventions to reduce unhealthy alcohol use in adolescents and adults: updated evidence report and systematic review for the US preventive services Task Force. JAMA 2018;320:1910–28.
36. Lee BP, Vittinghoff E, Hsu C, et al. Predicting low risk for sustained alcohol use after early liver transplant for acute alcoholic hepatitis: the sustained alcohol use post-liver transplant score. Hepatology 2019;69:1477–87.
37. Allen JP, Wurst FM, Thon N, et al. Assessing the drinking status of liver transplant patients with alcoholic liver disease. Liver Transplant 2013;19:369–76.
38. Staufer K, Andresen H, Vettorazzi E, et al. Urinary ethyl glucuronide as a novel screening tool in patients pre- and post-liver transplantation improves detection of alcohol consumption. Hepatology 2011;54:1640–9.
39. Iglesias K, Lannoy S, Sporkert F, et al. Performance of self-reported measures of alcohol use and of harmful drinking patterns against ethyl glucuronide hair testing among young Swiss men. PLoS One 2020;15:e0244336.
40. Paul R, Tsanaclis L, Murray C, et al. Ethyl glucuronide as a long-term alcohol biomarker in fingernail and hair. Matrix comparison and evaluation of gender bias. Alcohol Alcohol 2019;54:402–7.
41. Arnts J, Vanlerberghe BTK, Roozen S, et al. Diagnostic accuracy of biomarkers of alcohol use in patients with liver disease: a systematic review. Alcohol Clin Exp Res 2021;45:25–37.
42. Alessi SM, Barnett NP, Petry NM. Experiences with SCRAMx alcohol monitoring technology in 100 alcohol treatment outpatients. Drug Alcohol Depend 2017; 178:417–24.
43. Gurvich EM, Kenna GA, Leggio L. Use of novel technology-based techniques to improve alcohol-related outcomes in clinical trials. Alcohol Alcohol 2013;48: 712–9.
44. Lucey MR, Im GY, Mellinger JL, et al. Introducing the 2019 American association for the study of liver diseases guidance on alcohol-associated liver disease. Liver Transplant 2020;26:14–6.
45. Moriarty KJ. Collaborative liver and psychiatry care in the Royal Bolton Hospital for people with alcohol-related disease. Frontline Gastroenterol 2011;2:77–81.
46. Weinrieb RM, Van Horn DH, McLellan AT, et al. Interpreting the significance of drinking by alcohol-dependent liver transplant patients: fostering candor is the key to recovery. Liver Transplant 2000;6:769–76.
47. McCormick KA, Cochran NE, Back AL, et al. How primary care providers talk to patients about alcohol: a qualitative study. J Gen Intern Med 2006;21:966–72.
48. McNeely J, Kumar PC, Rieckmann T, et al. Barriers and facilitators affecting the implementation of substance use screening in primary care clinics: a qualitative study of patients, providers, and staff. Addict Sci Clin Pract 2018;13:8.
49. Alexandre W, Muhammad H, Agbalajobi O, et al. Alcohol treatment discussions and clinical outcomes among patients with alcohol-related cirrhosis. BMC Gastroenterol 2023;23:29.

50. Im GY, Mellinger JL, Winters A, et al. Provider attitudes and practices for alcohol screening, treatment, and education in patients with liver disease: a survey from the American Association for the Study of Liver Diseases Alcohol-Associated Liver Disease Special Interest Group. Clin Gastroenterol Hepatol 2021;19:2407–16.e2408.
51. Kollmann D, Rasoul-Rockenschaub S, Steiner I, et al. Good outcome after liver transplantation for ALD without a 6 months abstinence rule prior to transplantation including post-transplant CDT monitoring for alcohol relapse assessment - a retrospective study. Transpl Int 2016;29:559–67.
52. Dom G, Peuskens H. Addiction specialist's role in liver transplantation procedures for alcoholic liver disease. World J Hepatol 2015;7:2091–9.
53. Beste LA, Harp BK, Blais RK, et al. Primary care providers report challenges to cirrhosis management and specialty care coordination. Dig Dis Sci 2015;60:2628–35.
54. Fortney JC, Booth BM, Blow FC, et al. The effects of travel barriers and age on the utilization of alcoholism treatment aftercare. Am J Drug Alcohol Abuse 1995;21:391–406.
55. Dionisi T, Mosoni C, Di Sario G, et al. Make mission impossible feasible: the experience of a multidisciplinary team providing treatment for alcohol use disorder to homeless individuals. Alcohol Alcohol 2020;55:547–53.
56. Donnadieu-Rigole H, Jaubert L, Ursic-Bedoya J, et al. Integration of an addiction team in a liver transplantation center. Liver Transplant 2019;25:1611–9.
57. Wells K, Klap R, Koike A, et al. Ethnic disparities in unmet need for alcoholism, drug abuse, and mental health care. Am J Psychiatr 2001;158:2027–32.

Integrated Multidisciplinary Care Model to Manage the Dual Pathology of Alcohol Use Disorder and of Liver Disease

Ashwani K. Singal, MD, MS, AGAF[a],*, Vatsalya Vatsalya, MD[a],
Ruchita Agrawal, MD[b]

KEYWORDS

- Alcohol-associated hepatitis • Alcohol • Alcohol-associated liver disease
- Alcohol use disorder • Cirrhosis • Depression • Liver transplantation

KEY POINTS

- Patients with alcohol-associated liver disease (ALD) receive treatment for alcohol use disorder (AUD) in 10% to 30% patients only, with only 1% to 10% receiving pharmacologic treatment.
- Several patient, clinician, and system level barriers limit treatment of AUD in patients with ALD.
- Observational studies have shown that treating AUDr in patients with aALD improves liver related outcomes and patient survival.
- Well-designed randomized studies are needed to examine the safety and benefit of medications for AUD in patients with ALD.
- Strategies are needed to overcome barriers and promote integrated multidisciplinary treatment of AUD with addiction medicine and hepatology.

INTRODUCTION

Alcohol-associated liver disease (ALD) is the most common cause of advanced liver disease worldwide and in the United States (US). The most important risk factor for ALD is chronic and harmful alcohol use (≥ 2 drinks/d or >7/wk in women and ≥ 3 drinks/d or >14/wk in men), which puts such individuals at risk of liver disease. Alcohol use disorder (AUD) is diagnosed independently using the Diagnostic Statistical Manual-5 (DSM-5) criteria, focusing on the negative effects of alcohol on personal

[a] University of Louisville, 505 South Hancock Street, Louisville, KY 40202, USA; [b] Department of Psychiatry and Behavioral Sciences, Seven Counties Services, Inc, 530 South Jackson Street, Louisville, KY 40202, USA
* Corresponding author.
E-mail address: ashwanisingal.com@gmail.com

Clin Liver Dis 28 (2024) 793–807
https://doi.org/10.1016/j.cld.2024.06.013   **liver.theclinics.com**
1089-3261/24/© 2024 Elsevier Inc. All rights reserved, including those for text and data mining, AI training, and similar technologies.

or social responsibilities and on physical or mental health.[1] Moderate to severe AUD by the DSM-V criteria (≥ 4 of 11 criteria) is frequently observed in 75% to 80% of individuals suspected of ALD.[2,3] Clearly, patients with ALD have 2 concomitant diseases with significant overlapping pathology. Such a landscape of comorbidity for liver disease and for AUD requires concurrent and combined care by hepatology to manage liver disease and addiction team to manage the AUD.

Multidisciplinary collaborative care is a model in which members of different disciplines and expertise contribute to the patient care to achieve a common goal of improving patient outcomes.[4] The concomitant care for AUD and for liver disease can be delivered in their siloed respective practices of mental health providers and hepatologists (*collaborative*) or in a unified single clinic under 1 roof (*integrated*). Collaborative multidisciplinary care is known for other chronic diseases including metabolic dysfunction-associated steatotic liver disease, obesity, and liver transplantation (LT) evaluation process.

In this review article, we will discuss (a) the health care burden of ALD and of AUD highlighting the rationale and need for integrated multidisciplinary care for ALD patients; (b) benefits of AUD therapies (behavioral and pharmacotherapies) and of integrated multidisciplinary care model in both pre- and post-transplant settings; (c) structure and specific roles of team members; and (d) working components of integrated model with long-term goal. Finally, we will conclude and highlight the unmet clinical needs and strategies on promoting implementation of these models in real world clinical practice on the management of patients with ALD.

MAGNITUDE AND HEALTH CARE BURDEN OF ALCOHOL USE DISORDER AND ALCOHOL-ASSOCIATED LIVER DISEASE

AUD is a prevalent disorder in the general population.[5,6] In 2016, 55% of individuals worldwide and 53% in the US have had alcohol at some time point in their lifetime.[7] About 7% to 8% of individuals worldwide report harmful alcohol use; with AUD in 5.1% worldwide and 8.2% in the US.7 Further, alcohol contributes to 6.7% of disability-adjusted life-years (DALY) and 5.5% of deaths in the general population.[7] Alcohol contributed to 3 million deaths in 2016 or 5.3% of all deaths worldwide and 5.5% in the US.

About 35% of at-risk individuals develop various spectra of ALD including cirrhosis or alcohol-associated hepatitis (AH) and associated complications.[5,8,9] Alcohol contributes to over 50% of the attributable fraction of cirrhosis in the US, Europe, and South America.7 In 2017, there were a total of 2.79 million reported cases of cirrhosis worldwide (2.45 million decompensated), with 172116 cases of cirrhosis in the US (153144 decompensated).[10] A total of 67346 individuals died due to cirrhosis in the US, and ALD contributed to 28.2% of these deaths.[10] Over 4000 LTs were performed in 2019 for end-stage liver disease from alcohol.[11,12]

Recent studies have shown an increasing shift in the prevalence of ALD toward younger individuals less than 35 to 40 years and in the female sex.[13–17] ALD contributes to 5.1% of DALY worldwide and 6.7% in the US.[7] The ALD and AUD-related morbidity has further accentuated since the coronavirus disease 2019 (COVID-19) epidemic in March, 2020. This impact has not reached its peak yet, albeit it is highly anticipated that the health care community will continue to encounter the after-effects of COVID-19's impact on the ALD burden.[18]

The AUD-related morbidity and health care burden remains significant in patients who have been hospitalized for advanced ALD. In a more challenging population of severe AH although not in an LT setting, only 45% of patients were abstinent at

3 months and 30% at 1 year after hospital discharge.[19] Limited data on alcohol use recurrence in ALD patients awaiting LT show a prevalence of 11% to 50%.[20–25] The risk of relapse to alcohol use continues even after LT with 8% to 20% recipients at 1 year and up to 50% at 5 years of LT.[26,27] Two meta-analyses on LT recipients for ALD, with pooled data from 7 studies in one,[28] and from 50 studies in another,[29] showed annual alcohol use recurrence rates of 4.7% to 5.6% for any alcohol use and 2.5% to 2.9% for heavy alcohol use. In a retrospective study on 146 recipients of early LT, 70% remained abstinent in the long-term, with 6.2% of recipients reporting late onset alcohol use recurrence.[30] Heavy alcohol use negatively impacts long-term patient survival after 5 to 10 years of LT. In a meta-analysis of 7 studies on LT recipients for ALD, heavy alcohol users versus abstainers had greater than 8- to 9-fold higher risk for AH and advanced fibrosis.[28] Recurrent cirrhosis and malignancy cause mortality in only 2% to 3% of LT recipients for ALD, but this rate could go up to 35% among those who continue with excessive alcohol abuse.[28,31] Malignancy especially upper aero-digestive tract (oral cavity, larynx, esophagus, and lungs) is another common cause of patient mortality among the heavy alcohol users.[28,32]

RATIONALE AND NEED FOR ALCOHOL USE DISORDER TREATMENT IN ALCOHOL-ASSOCIATED LIVER DISEASE PATIENTS

AUD treatment including behavioral or pharmacologic therapies is rarely used in ALD patients including those with cirrhosis.[33–36] For example, in a retrospective cohort of over 35682 veterans with ALD cirrhosis and a diagnosis of AUD, only less than 14% were treated for AUD within 6 months from diagnosis, with only 0.4% receiving some pharmacotherapy.[33] Barriers and gaps at the level of patients, clinicians, and health care ecosystems may be encountered in treating patients with ALD and AUD **(Fig. 1)**.[35,37,38] One of the important barriers at the level of the clinician is lack of adequate time in clinic to address AUD and more importantly the perception of providers that they do not have optimal comfort and training to address AUD in ALD patients.[39,40] For example, in a survey of hepatologists and gastroenterologists, only

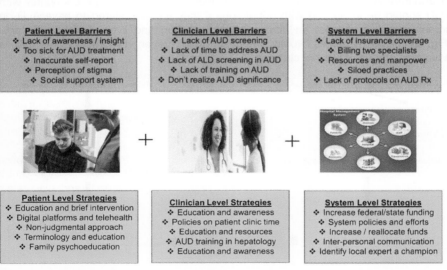

Fig. 1. Strategies to overcome barriers in implementation of model with efforts from hepatology, addiction team, and the organization administration.

60% would refer ALD patients to addiction specialists, 77% reported a lack of training in addiction medicine, and 84% felt uncomfortable in writing prescriptions for AUD medications.[39]

The clinician level barriers also exist among non-hepatology providers on screening for underlying ALD when they see patients for AUD treatment or other alcohol-induced target organ damage like pancreatitis, road traffic accidents, neuropathy, and cardiomyopathy.[6,14,41] Screening for ALD at any health care encounter helps identification at an early stage, identifies patients with asymptomatic advanced fibrosis or cirrhosis, allows referral to hepatology, and improves compliance to AUD treatment after abnormal liver tests are discussed with patients. Incorporating addiction medicine training in residency and fellowship curricula is critical to better prepare future specialists to provide comprehensive care to ALD patients, including treatment of AUD.[35] The National Institute on Alcohol Abuse and Alcoholism has developed "*The Healthcare Professional's Core Resource on Alcohol*" educational resource with 14 articles on alcohol and health, covering principles, clinical impact, and patient-care from screening through recovery. With free continuing medical education credits, the resource aims to fill training gaps and streamline the workflow for providers who are not addiction specialists.[42]

INTEGRATED CARE MODEL FOR OUTSIDE LIVER TRANSPLANT SETTING

Psychoeducation for patients with ALD and AUD comorbidity about the stage of complete abstinence is not enough. Recognizing the clinical presentation of the dual pathology in ALD-AUD patients, effective management of ALD will require management by a hepatologist for liver disease along with an addiction team to manage AUD. Although an intervention for AUD is beneficial in reducing alcohol consumption and outcomes among individuals without liver disease, the data among patients with liver disease are scanty,[43,44] especially at the early stage of ALD.

Ideally the integrated care is not only for established ALD patients including those with cirrhosis and AH but is also relevant for those who have AUD but no diagnosed or apparent liver disease. Identifying individuals at any health care encounter with AUD should be integrated with hepatology if they are discovered to have ALD on screening using at least an ultrasound examination and liver biochemical panel (**Fig. 2**). Such measures would potentially help prevent progression of ALD to advanced stages of alcohol cirrhosis (AC) and of AH.

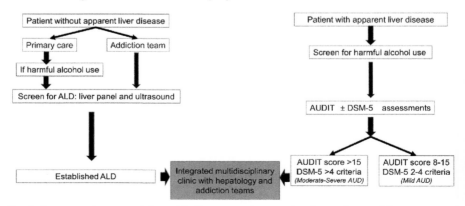

Fig. 2. Integrated care model outside liver transplant setting for patients without apparent liver disease (*left panel*) and those with apparent liver disease (*right panel*).

Benefits of Alcohol Use Disorder Treatment in Non-transplant Settings

Behavioral therapies

Randomized studies. Polyenylphosphatidylcholine in 789 Veterans biopsy characterized ALD patients reduced use of alcohol from 16 to 2.5 drinks per day as compared to patients receiving placebo.[45] All patients in both groups received 12-step-based treatment for AUD. In another randomized study on 60 ALD patients, mobile health application as compared to enhanced usual care increased AUD treatment engagement (27.3 vs 13.3%) and a trend toward greater than or equal to 1 level reduction in WHO drinking risk levels, odds ratio (OR) 2.25 (95% confidence interval [CI]: 0.51–9.97). With recruitment and retention rates of 46% and 65%, respectively, mobile health application was acceptable in over 90% of patients.[46]

Non-randomized studies. Among patients hospitalized for ALD or severe AH, early alcohol rehabilitation within 30 days from discharge or just identification of AUD diagnosis at discharge reduces the readmission rate.[34,47] In a prospective study on 294 hospitalized AH patients, early alcohol rehabilitation in 46 patients was associated with a reduction of 70% to 84% for 30-day readmission, 89% to 91% for 30-day relapse to alcohol, and 80% for patient mortality.[47] Hospitalized patients need to be involved with the addiction team during the hospitalization as soon as they are cognitively ready to engage in a conversation. Studies are needed to examine the benefit of behavioral intervention/s in improving liver-related and patient-reported outcomes.

Pharmacologic therapies

Retrospective cohort studies. Among ALD patients outside of LT setting, several retrospective cohorts using national databases have confirmed low rates of AUD pharmacotherapy (1.0%–9.7%). AUD treatment when used has been shown to be beneficial with improvement of liver disease, reduction in complications, and mortality.[33,48,49] In a cohort of 1135 ALD patients, receiving AUD pharmacotherapy (N = 105) was associated with a 65% reduced incidence of hepatic decompensation.[48] Treatment benefits are seen with pharmacotherapy, as well as behavioral psychotherapy.[48,50] In another retrospective study from a single center, use of naltrexone (Food and Drug Administration [FDA]-approved drug for AUD treatment) in 100 patients with liver disease (47 with cirrhosis, 23 decompensated). Naltrexone use of less than 30 days was associated with a risk of alcohol-related hospitalization over 2 years, with other predictors being liver disease and cirrhosis. The use of naltrexone was observed to be safe including in those with compensated cirrhosis, as assessed by liver enzymes assessment on follow-up.[51]

Randomized studies. Two studies have investigated baclofen (a non-FDA-approved drug for AUD) in ALD patients.[52,53] In one study on 84 patients with ALD cirrhosis, baclofen (N = 42) versus placebo increased the abstinence rate by over 6-fold (71 vs 29%, $P = .001$).[52] Further, cumulative number of abstinence days was over 2-folds higher with baclofen (62.8 vs 30.8 days, $P = .001$).[52] In another study on 104 AUD patients including those with liver disease, the percentage abstinent days were 43%, 69%, and 65% with placebo, baclofen 30 mg per day, and baclofen 75 mg per day, respectively, $P<.05$. Baclofen was found to be safe in both studies.

Gut microbiome and dysbiosis play a critical role in mediating ALD and AH, with modifying gut microbiota being an important therapeutic target in ALD patients.[54] In a study on 46 patients with moderate AH (model of end-stage liver disease [MELD] <20), the use of *Lactobacillus rhamnosus* GG or LGG (N = 24) for 6 months reduced heavy drinking to social or abstinence levels versus those receiving a placebo (N = 22). In a phase-1 pilot randomized clinical trial (RCT) on 20 ALD cirrhosis patients

(MELD score <15), fecal microbiota transplant from healthy donors in 10 patients versus placebo-reduced alcohol craving score, cytokine levels, and urinary ethyl glucuronide (eTG) levels. This was associated with an improved cognitive psychosocial profile and quality of life in patients receiving fecal microbiota transplant.[55]

In a meta-analysis of 8 studies (4 RCT), medications for AUD treatment were beneficial in reducing alcohol use by 32%, P = .03. Although, adverse effects were observed, only 3% could be possibly or probably related to the medications.[56] Clearly, well-designed randomized studies are needed to examine the FDA approved pharmacologic therapies for AUD in ALD patients, and examine their safety and benefit on liver disease and on AUD.

INTEGRATED CARE MODEL WITHIN LIVER TRANSPLANT SETTING

The ideal integrated model in an LT setting is where the addiction team is built into the LT center and follows every patient from the time of consideration for LT, through the evaluation process, on the waitlist, and long-term after LT (**Fig. 3**).

BENEFITS OF ALCOHOL USE DISORDER TREATMENT IN LIVER TRANSPLANT SETTINGS

Data are emerging on behavioral therapies for AUD in ALD patients both before and after LT.

Intervention and Follow-Up in the Pre-liver Transplantation Phase

Randomized studies

Two studies before LT following a collaborative non-integrated approach are described here. In one study on 91 patients with AC and listed for LT, 46 received motivational enhancement treatment. Alcohol relapse occurred in 23 patients, 12 in the intervention arm, P = NS. The intervention of motivational therapy was associated with a reduced number of drinks (3.75 vs 4.3 drinks) and median days (2 vs 7) of drinking.[57] In another study, 8 patients awaiting LT were randomized to receive daily digital text messages on cravings, triggers, and coping strategies as an adjunct to AUD

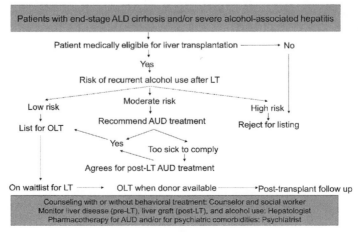

Fig. 3. Integrated care model within liver transplant setting, with the addiction team embedded within the transplant program and following patients through evaluation, waiting period, and after liver transplantation.

treatment compared to 7 receiving AUD treatment alone.[39] At week 8, the text message group had lower alcohol relapse (0 vs 33.3%) based on urinary eTG measurement.[39]

Intervention in Pre- or Post-Liver Transplantation Phase and Follow-up in Post-Liver Transplantation Phase

Studies using a non-integrated model of alcohol use disorder treatment

In a study, 235 LT recipients for ALD (2008–2014) who had met an addiction team before LT were studied. Based on the workup or follow-up, those at risk of relapse were closely followed by the addiction team. Post-LT relapse to alcohol over a mean follow-up period of 3.5 years was observed in 9% of recipients,[40] lower than 11% to 50% in historic controls.[20–25] In another retrospective study on 102 LT at one center in Europe (2000–2017), a multidisciplinary management for AUD including alcohol use assessment by eTG was established in 2014. LT recipients after (n = 28) vs. before (n = 74) 2014 were associated with reduced patient mortality, $P = .02$.[41]

Studies using an integrated model of alcohol use disorder treatment

The best prototype model for an integrated care model in LT settings was reported in 2013 from Italy by *Addolorato and colleagues* In this study, 92 ALD patients undergoing LT (1995–2010), 55 transplanted since 2002 with the implementation of an integrated model versus 37 before 2002 showed lower alcohol use (16.4 vs 35.1%, $P = .038$) and patient mortality (14.5 vs 37.8%, $P = .01$).[58] An integrated model for AUD management has recently also reported benefits among LT recipients for severe AH,[59] a rapidly growing indication for LT in ALD. In this study, of 44 early LT for ALD since the introduction of the integrated AUD treatment model in 2018, only 3 returned to alcohol use within an average follow-up period of 339 days.[59] In another recent retrospective study on 611 LT at one center, those transplanted since the implementation of an integrated model with an addiction team embedded within the LT program showed a lower alcohol relapse rate, $P = .022$.[60]

Albeit limited, data on long-term survival among LT recipients are also favorable for integrated care during the pre-and post-transplant period.[36] In a recent systematic review, the pooled data from 649 LT recipients showed that reduced alcohol relapse and patient mortality by 44% and 71% with a respective OR (95% CI) of 0.56 (0.36–0.87) and 0.29 (0.08–0.99) after AUD treatment using an integrated versus non-integrated model.[36]

Integrated Care Model for Alcohol-Associated Liver Disease Patients in the Real World

Although an integrated multidisciplinary care model is the preferred approach,[35,37] implementation in clinical practice is challenging,[33,35,37] and such a model is more of an exception than the rule in the real world both within and outside LT settings. Despite national and international organizations recommending integrated care models to manage ALD patients,[61,62] widespread adoption of these recommendations is poor.[33] Within the LT setting in most centers, patients are seen by the addiction team during the LT evaluation phase only, and irrespective of the outcome of the patient selection process for LT listing, further follow-up is by the hepatology team during the pre-LT period for listed patients and post-LT for LT recipients.

One of the several barriers to a multidisciplinary integrated approach (**Fig. 1**) is the lack of provider time, especially in a private health insurance-based model. This challenge adds to the other logistical issues like different provider locations and electronic health systems. A system based on private health insurance is an independent predictor of lack of access to LT,[63] and contributes to health disparities in LT access and listing.[63,64] The success of the multidisciplinary model improves the confidence of patients in the providers and the system,[59] and is also more cost-effective saving money to payers and organizations.[65] For example, a recent study showed that implementing pharmacologic treatments (naltrexone and acamprosate) in ALD patients leads to benefits in patient outcomes for liver and non–liver-related comorbidities associated with AUD. Further, it was shown that such an approach is expected to yield cost savings to health care systems.[49] Other studies have also shown the benefits of integrated care in ALD patients to reduce alcohol relapse and improve patient outcomes,[36,44,66,67] due to improved engagement of patients and providers in the health care system. Clearly, studies are urgently needed to validate the benefits of an integrated multidisciplinary model in ALD patients both with and without LT settings, and to address the social determinants of health to overcome administrative and system barriers in the establishment of the multidisciplinary integrated care models.

COMPONENTS AND MODIFICATIONS OF INTEGRATED MULTIDISCIPLINARY MODEL

An ideal integrated multidisciplinary care model for AUD and ALD is where providers depend on individual expertise, yet at the same time have the freedom to provide constructive criticism to each other with the aim being patient-centered care. A healthy discussion and feedback on each patient are critical in developing a formal comprehensive plan for patient management. The final goal of this symbiotic relationship is to maximize the expertise and output of each provider.

Providers should also be flexible to accommodate if the resources and workforce are limited and not ideal. For example, a psychiatrist is an important member of the care plan who may not be available for regularly coming to the clinics due to financial constraints or lack of time because of other clinical or administrative commitments. The providers, especially the leadership of the model, must be flexible and take the collective ownership of the patient-care. The model may be modified with the psychiatrist being consulted on telehealth or phone for a specific issue related to pharmacotherapy for AUD or psychiatric comorbidities like depression, anxiety, or insomnia.

Among patients who are being evaluated for or listed for LT, the multidisciplinary integrated care model should be implemented in the pre-LT phase, for the patients to develop rapport with the addiction team members and have an expectation to be followed closely by the same team members in the post-LT period when they come for their regular follow in the post-transplant clinic (see **Fig. 3**). Following up on these patients in the post-LT without regular pre-LT follow-up is not an effective strategy, as in one such RCT, only 5 patients out of 50 reached out in the post-LT were available for regular follow-up using the integrated approach.[68]

STRUCTURE AND TEAM MEMBERS

An integrated care model overcomes the clinician-level barrier of perceived lack of addiction training and increases the comfort level of hepatologists in addressing AUD and of the addiction team in managing AUD in ALD patients.[35] However, this model may not completely overcome the stigma attached to the diagnosis of ALD.[35] Contact with the addiction team should be sooner than later as patients have maximum motivation for change and reduce alcohol use. For sick patients, this contact should be established during admission, whenever the treatment assesses that the mental and cognitive status is stable enough for a conversation with the counselor or social worker.[34,69]

Hepatologist

It should be recognized that patients with AUD may have liver disease due to causes other than alcohol.[70] A thorough assessment with clinical, biochemical, and radiologic evaluation for (a) liver fibrosis in non-cirrhotic patients; and (b) decompensation (ascites, hepatic encephalopathy, varices, and portal hypertension, and hepatocellular carcinoma), MELD score, nutritional status and need for intervention, and need for LT.[71] Among LT recipients, assessment of graft function and cause for any abnormalities.

Addiction Counselor

Assessment for diagnosis and severity of AUD, alcohol use, barriers are limiting access to treatment and motivation to change. The addiction counselor assists in recovery and relapse prevention strategies or resources,[72] and determination of care level using the American Society of Addiction Medicine's (ASAM) assessment of 6 dimensions: intoxication and risk of withdrawal, medical conditions that can interfere with treatment, coexistent psychiatric or cognitive issues, motivation or readiness to change, relapse risk, social support, and living environment. The counselor then uses this comprehensive evaluation to recommend a level of treatment as (a) outpatient (individual therapy or group therapy), (b) intensive outpatient treatment (administered as the primary treatment with flexible timing, developing recovery skills, and incorporating community support), and (c) inpatient treatment (acute care setting with staff to manage associated medical issues), the best example of integrated multidisciplinary comprehensive care. The comprehensive assessment by the counselor and team on an ongoing basis using the ASAM criteria helps transition and continuity of care.[73,74]

Alcohol use is monitored using the Timeline Follow Back (TLFB) tool (https://www.nova.edu/timeline/index.html), which is self-reported by patients over a given period of up to 12 months. Self and provider feedback on alcohol use patterns from the analysis of the TLFB data increases self-motivation to change.[75] TLFB also allows quantifying alcohol use over time with assessment of the WHO risk level stratification to abstinent (0 gm in both males and females), low risk (1–40 gm in males and 1–20 gm in females), medium risk (41–60 gm in males and 21–40 gm in females), high risk (61–100 gm in males and 41–60 gm in females), and very high risk (>100 gm in males and >60 gm in females). A more than or equal to 2 level reduction of alcohol use is usually considered a successful outcome, but whether this also applies to ALD patients remains a testable hypothesis. Remission is defined as not meeting AUD criteria for more than or equal to 3 months, with sustained remission with no AUD criteria for more than or equal to 12 months. Biomarkers may be used to complement self-reported alcohol use for better accuracy in determining active ongoing alcohol consumption.[76] Biomarkers related to end-organ damage (aspartate aminotransferase, alanine aminotransferase, carbohydrate-deficient transferrin, gamma-glutamyl transpeptidase, and mean corpuscular volume) are limited due to low sensitivity and specificity. Of alcohol metabolites, commercially available phosphatydylethanol levels are most accurate, not confounded by endogenous alcohol exposure, and can pick up alcohol use within the previous up to 3 weeks from the last drink.[76,77]

Social Worker

To assess the biologic, psychologic, and social assessment of the patients to highlight the importance of self-determination and assist them to develop realistic goals that support their health and provide a holistic approach to patient-care.[78] The social

---

Box 1
Areas of clinical unmet need and prospects

1. Randomized double-blind placebo-controlled integrated clinical trials to assess the safety and efficacy of pharmacotherapies for AUD in ALD patients.

2. Derive an objective protocol and criteria of selection for early LT in patients with liver disease and AUD.

3. Examine cost-efficacy of AUD treatment in ALD patients, and integrated versus non-integrated AUD treatment care models.

4. Randomized clinical trials using smart or adaptive design to examine multiple drugs at the same time targeting liver disease or AUD, with an integrated approach to examining benefits on the long-term liver-related mortality and outcomes.

5. Develop uniform definitions of the recurrence of alcohol use among liver transplant recipients.

6. Derive uniform definitions of endpoints on alcohol use, which translate to patient survival and outcomes in patients with ALD.

7. Evaluate biomarkers of alcohol use among patients awaiting liver transplant for the impact of using biomarker monitoring in reducing alcohol use after transplantation.

---

worker also provides resources and guides patients to achieve these goals and coordinates patient's management for patients attending the emergency rooms or admitted to outside hospitals in between the clinic visits.[79]

Psychiatrist

To assess (a) AUD and alcohol use, (b) associated comorbidities like depression (Patient Health Questionnaire-9 or PHQ-9), anxiety (Generalized Anxiety Disorder-7 or GAD-7), (c) provide pharmacotherapy for AUD and for psychiatric comorbidities (later section on pharmacotherapies) and ongoing complications, and (d) manage alcohol withdrawal symptoms and post-withdrawal syndrome, which can last for a long time.[80]

Clinic Nurse

To (a) schedule patient visits and appointments, with time management of providers, (b) establish continuity of care in between follow-up appointments, especially on counseling sessions with an addiction counselor, and (c) coordinate with providers on phone calls from the patients on test results and any questions the patients may have.

SUMMARY

ALD contributes significantly to health care and economic burden. Clearly, the treatment of both liver disease and of AUD is crucial. However, several barriers at the level of patient, clinician, and system limit in receiving treatment for AUD in ALD patients (**Fig. 2**). Evidence-based data demonstrate that models where addiction and hepatology are integrated synergistically may be more effective approach. Hepatologists, psychiatrists, addiction counselors, social workers, and clinic nurses work together under one roof and provide holistic care for the dual pathology of AUD and liver disease in this integrated approach. Furthermore, clinical research and strategies are needed (**Box 1**) to overcome AUD treatment barriers and promotion of an integrated multidisciplinary care model and uniform homogeneous management and follow-up of patients with AUD and ALD.

CLINICS CARE POINTS

- Alcohol use is the most important determinant of long-term outcomes in patients with ALD.
- Several patient, physician, and system barriers limit the use of AUD treatment in real world practice in patients with ALD.
- Self-stigma is the single most important barrier for AUD treatment in ALD patients.
- Integrated multidisciplinary treatment model should be promoted to improve long-term outcomes in ALD patients.

DISCLOSURE

The authors have nothing to disclose.

REFERENCES

1. Hasin DS, O'Brien CP, Auriacombe M, et al. DSM-5 criteria for substance use disorders: recommendations and rationale. Am J Psychiatry 2013;170:834–51.
2. Beresford TP. Predictive factors for alcoholic relapse in the selection of alcohol-dependent persons for hepatic transplant. Liver Transpl Surg 1997;3:280–91.
3. DiMartini A, Weinrieb R, Lane T, et al. Defining the alcoholic liver transplant population: implications for future research. Liver Transplant 2001;7:428–31.
4. Lennon-Dearing R, Florence J, Garrett L, et al. A rural community-based interdisciplinary curriculum: a social work perspective. Soc Work Health Care 2008;47: 93–107.
5. Singal AK, Mathurin P. A review of the diagnosis and treatment of alcohol-associated liver disease reply. JAMA, J Am Med Assoc 2021;326:1976.
6. Devarbhavi H, Asrani SK, Arab JP, et al. Global burden of liver disease: 2023 update. J Hepatol 2023;79:516–37.
7. Global status report on alcohol and health. Switzerland: World Health Organization; 2018.
8. Bataller R, Arab JP, Shah VH. Alcohol-associated hepatitis. N Engl J Med 2022; 387:2436–48.
9. Huang DQ, Mathurin P, Cortez-Pinto H, et al. Global epidemiology of alcohol-associated cirrhosis and HCC: trends, projections and risk factors. Nat Rev Gastroenterol Hepatol 2023;20:37–49.
10. The global, regional, and national burden of cirrhosis by cause in 195 countries and territories, 1990-2017: a systematic analysis for the Global Burden of Disease Study 2017. Lancet Gastroenterol Hepatol 2020;5:245–66.
11. Wong RJ, Singal AK. Trends in liver disease etiology among adults awaiting liver transplantation in the United States, 2014-2019. JAMA Netw Open 2020;3:e1920294.
12. Singal AK, Leggio L, DiMartini A. Alcohol use disorder in alcohol-associated liver disease: two sides of the same coin. Liver Transplant 2023;30(2):200–12.
13. Wong T, Dang K, Ladhani S, et al. Prevalence of alcoholic fatty liver disease among adults in the United States, 2001-2016. JAMA 2019;321:1723–5.
14. Tapper EB, Parikh ND. Mortality due to cirrhosis and liver cancer in the United States, 1999-2016: observational study. BMJ 2018;362:k2817.
15. Singal AK, Arora S, Wong RJ, et al. Increasing burden of acute-on-chronic liver failure among alcohol-associated liver disease in the young population in the United States. Am J Gastroenterol 2020;115:88–95.

16. Singal AK, Arsalan A, Dunn W, et al. Alcohol-associated liver disease in the United States is associated with severe forms of disease among young, females and Hispanics. Aliment Pharmacol Ther 2021;54:451–61.

17. Wong MCS, Huang JLW, George J, et al. The changing epidemiology of liver diseases in the Asia-Pacific region. Nat Rev Gastroenterol Hepatol 2019;16:57–73.

18. Deutsch-Link S, Curtis B, Singal AK. Covid-19 and alcohol associated liver disease. Dig Liver Dis 2022;54:1459–68.

19. Thursz MR, Richardson P, Allison M, et al. Prednisolone or pentoxifylline for alcoholic hepatitis. N Engl J Med 2015;372:1619–28.

20. Erim Y, Böttcher M, Dahmen U, et al. Urinary ethyl glucuronide testing detects alcohol consumption in alcoholic liver disease patients awaiting liver transplantation. Liver Transplant 2007;13:757–61.

21. Vollmar J, Stern F, Lackner K, et al. Urinary ethyl glucuronide (uEtG) as a marker for alcohol consumption in liver transplant candidates: a real-world cohort. Z Gastroenterol 2020;58:30–8.

22. Carbonneau M, Jensen LA, Bain VG, et al. Alcohol use while on the liver transplant waiting list: a single-center experience. Liver Transplant 2010;16:91–7.

23. Berlakovich GA, Soliman T, Freundorfer E, et al. Pretransplant screening of sobriety with carbohydrate-deficient transferrin in patients suffering from alcoholic cirrhosis. Transpl Int 2004;17:617–21.

24. Piano S, Marchioro L, Gola E, et al. Assessment of alcohol consumption in liver transplant candidates and recipients: the best combination of the tools available. Liver Transplant 2014;20:815–22.

25. Faulkner CS, White CM, Manatsathit W, et al. Positive blood phosphatidylethanol concentration is associated with unfavorable waitlist-related outcomes for patients medically appropriate for liver transplantation. Alcohol Clin Exp Res 2022;46:581–8.

26. Arab JP, Izzy M, Leggio L, et al. Management of alcohol use disorder in patients with cirrhosis in the setting of liver transplantation. Nat Rev Gastroenterol Hepatol 2022;19:45–59.

27. DiMartini A, Day N, Dew MA, et al. Alcohol consumption patterns and predictors of use following liver transplantation for alcoholic liver disease. Liver Transplant 2006;12:813–20.

28. Kodali S, Kaif M, Tariq R, et al. Alcohol relapse after liver transplantation for alcoholic cirrhosis-impact on liver graft and patient survival: a meta-analysis. Alcohol Alcohol 2018;53:166–72.

29. Dew MA, DiMartini AF, Steel J, et al. Meta-analysis of risk for relapse to substance use after transplantation of the liver or other solid organs. Liver Transplant 2008;14:159–72.

30. Lee BP, Im GY, Rice JP, et al. Patterns of alcohol use after early liver transplantation for alcoholic hepatitis. Clin Gastroenterol Hepatol 2022;20:409–418 e405.

31. Dumortier J, Dharancy S, Cannesson A, et al. Recurrent alcoholic cirrhosis in severe alcoholic relapse after liver transplantation: a frequent and serious complication. Am J Gastroenterol 2015;110:1160–6, quiz 1167.

32. Watt KD, Pedersen RA, Kremers WK, et al. Evolution of causes and risk factors for mortality post-liver transplant: results of the NIDDK long-term follow-up study. Am J Transplant 2010;10:1420–7.

33. Rogal S, Youk A, Zhang H, et al. Impact of alcohol use disorder treatment on clinical outcomes among patients with cirrhosis. Hepatology 2019;71(6):2080–92.

34. Singal AK, DiMartini A, Leggio L, et al. Identifying alcohol use disorder in patients with cirrhosis reduces 30-days readmission rate. Alcohol Alcohol 2022;57: 576–80.
35. DiMartini AL,L, Singal AK. Barriers to the management of alcohol use disorder and alcohol-associated liver disease: strategies to implement integrated care model. Lancet Gastroenterol Hepatol 2021;7(2):186–95. In Press.
36. Elfeki MA, Abdallah MA, Leggio L, et al. Simultaneous management of alcohol use disorder and of liver disease: a systematic review and meta-analysis. J Addict Med 2022;17(2):e119–28.
37. Mellinger JL, Scott Winder G, DeJonckheere M, et al. Misconceptions, preferences and barriers to alcohol use disorder treatment in alcohol-related cirrhosis. J Subst Abuse Treat 2018;91:20–7.
38. Im GY, Mellinger JL, Winters A, et al. Provider attitudes and practices for alcohol screening, treatment, and education in patients with liver disease: a survey from the American association for the study of liver diseases alcohol-associated liver disease special interest group. Clin Gastroenterol Hepatol 2020;19(11): 2407–16.e8.
39. DeMartini KS, Schilsky ML, Palmer A, et al. Text messaging to reduce alcohol relapse in prelisting liver transplant candidates: a pilot feasibility study. Alcohol Clin Exp Res 2018;42:761–9.
40. Donnadieu-Rigole H, Jaubert L, Ursic-Bedoya J, et al. Integration of an addiction team in a liver transplantation center. Liver Transplant 2019;25:1611–9.
41. Magistri P, Marzi L, Guerzoni S, et al. Impact of a multidisciplinary team on alcohol recidivism and survival after liver transplant for alcoholic disease. Transplant Proc 2019;51:187–9.
42. In.
43. O'Connor EA, Perdue LA, Senger CA, et al. Screening and behavioral counseling interventions to reduce unhealthy alcohol use in adolescents and adults: updated evidence report and systematic review for the US preventive services task force. JAMA 2018;320:1910–28.
44. Leggio L, Lee MR. Treatment of alcohol use disorder in patients with alcoholic liver disease. Am J Med 2017;130:124–34.
45. Lieber CS, Weiss DG, Groszmann R, et al. Veterans Affairs Cooperative Study of polyenylphosphatidylcholine in alcoholic liver disease: effects on drinking behavior by nurse/physician teams. Alcohol Clin Exp Res 2003;27:1757–64.
46. Park LS, Kornfield R, Yezihalem M, et al. Testing a digital health app for patients with alcohol-associated liver disease: mixed methods usability study. JMIR Form Res 2023;7:e47404.
47. Peeraphatdit TB, Kamath PS, Karpyak VM, et al. Alcohol rehabilitation within 30 Days of hospital discharge is associated with reduced readmission, relapse, and death in patients with alcoholic hepatitis. Clin Gastroenterol Hepatol 2020; 18:477–485 e475.
48. Vannier AGL, Shay JES, Fomin V, et al. Incidence and progression of alcohol-associated liver disease after medical therapy for alcohol use disorder. JAMA Netw Open 2022;5:e2213014.
49. Rabiee A, Mahmud N, Falker C, et al. Medications for alcohol use disorder improve survival in patients with hazardous drinking and alcohol-associated cirrhosis. Hepatol Commun 2023;7(4):e0093.
50. Vannier AGL, Przybyszewski EM, Shay J, et al. Psychotherapy for alcohol use disorder is associated with reduced risk of incident alcohol-associated liver disease. Clin Gastroenterol Hepatol 2022;21(6):1571–80.e7.

51. Ayyala D, Bottyan T, Tien C, et al. Naltrexone for alcohol use disorder: hepatic safety in patients with and without liver disease. Hepatol Commun 2022;6: 3433–42.
52. Addolorato G, Leggio L, Ferrulli A, et al. Effectiveness and safety of baclofen for maintenance of alcohol abstinence in alcohol-dependent patients with liver cirrhosis: randomised, double-blind controlled study. Lancet 2007;370:1915–22.
53. Morley KC, Baillie A, Fraser I, et al. Baclofen in the treatment of alcohol dependence with or without liver disease: multisite, randomised, double-blind, placebo-controlled trial. Br J Psychiatry 2018;212:362–9.
54. Singal AK, Shah VH. Therapeutic strategies for the treatment of alcoholic hepatitis. Semin Liver Dis 2016;36:56–68.
55. Bajaj JS, Gavis EA, Fagan A, et al. A randomized clinical trial of fecal microbiota transplant for alcohol use disorder. Hepatology 2021;73:1688–700.
56. Gratacos-Gines J, Bruguera P, Perez-Guasch M, et al. Medications for alcohol use disorder promote abstinence in alcohol-associated cirrhosis: results from a systematic review and meta-analysis. Hepatology 2023;79(2):368–79.
57. Weinrieb RM, Van Horn DH, Lynch KG, et al. A randomized, controlled study of treatment for alcohol dependence in patients awaiting liver transplantation. Liver Transplant 2011;17:539–47.
58. Addolorato G, Mirijello A, Leggio L, et al. Liver transplantation in alcoholic patients: impact of an alcohol addiction unit within a liver transplant center. Alcohol Clin Exp Res 2013;37:1601–8.
59. Carrique L, Quance J, Tan A, et al. Results of early transplantation for alcohol-related cirrhosis: integrated addiction treatment with low rate of relapse. Gastroenterology 2021;161:1896–1906 e1892.
60. Daniel J, Dumortier J, Del Bello A, et al. Integrating an addiction team into the management of patients transplanted for alcohol-associated liver disease reduces the risk of severe relapse. JHEP Rep 2023;5:100832.
61. Lucey MR, Im GY, Mellinger JL, et al. Introducing the 2019 AASLD guidance on Alcohol-related liver disease. Liver Transplant 2019.
62. Singal AK, Bataller R, Ahn J, et al. ACG clinical guideline: alcoholic liver disease. Am J Gastroenterol 2018;113:175–94.
63. Nguyen GC, Segev DL, Thuluvath PJ. Racial disparities in the management of hospitalized patients with cirrhosis and complications of portal hypertension: a national study. Hepatology 2007;45:1282–9.
64. Rivera MN, Jowsey S, Alsina AE, et al. Factors contributing to health disparities in liver transplantation in a Hispanic population. P R Health Sci J 2012;31:199–204.
65. Avancena ALV, Miller N, Uttal SE, et al. Cost-effectiveness of alcohol use treatments in patients with alcohol-related cirrhosis. J Hepatol 2021;74:1286–94.
66. Lucey MR, Singal AK. Integrated treatment of alcohol use disorder in patients with alcohol-associated liver disease: an evolving story. Hepatology 2020;71(6): 1891–3.
67. Caputo F, Domenicali M, Bernardi M. Diagnosis and treatment of alcohol use disorder in patients with end-stage alcoholic liver disease. Hepatology 2019;70: 410–7.
68. Weinrieb RM, Van Horn DH, McLellan AT, et al. Alcoholism treatment after liver transplantation: lessons learned from a clinical trial that failed. Psychosomatics 2001;42:110–6.
69. Kann AE, Jepsen P, Madsen LG, et al. Motivation to reduce drinking and engagement in alcohol misuse treatment in alcohol-related liver disease: a national health survey. Am J Gastroenterol 2022;117:918–22.

70. Russ KB, Chen NW, Kamath PS, et al. Alcohol use after liver transplantation is independent of liver disease etiology. Alcohol Alcohol 2016;51(6):698–701.
71. Moreno C, Mueller S, Szabo G. Non-invasive diagnosis and biomarkers in alcohol-related liver disease. J Hepatol 2019;70:273–83.
72. Ford HB. What is an addiction counselor? In.
73. Morey LC. Patient placement criteria: linking typologies to managed care. Alcohol Health Res World 1996;20:36–44.
74. Chuang E, Wells R, Alexander JA, et al. Factors associated with use of ASAM criteria and service provision in a national sample of outpatient substance abuse treatment units. J Addict Med 2009;3:139–50.
75. Sobell LC, Sobell MB. Timeline follow-back. Totowa, NJ: Humana Press; 1992.
76. Wozniak MK, Wiergowski M, Namiesnik J, et al. Biomarkers of alcohol consumption in body fluids - possibilities and limitations of application in toxicological analysis. Curr Med Chem 2019;26:177–96.
77. Singal AK, Kwo P. Blood phosphatidylethanol testing and liver transplant eligibility selection: a step closer. Alcohol Clin Exp Res 2022;46:702–4.
78. Papadimitriou G. The "biopsychosocial model": 40 years of application in psychiatry. Psychiatriki 2017;28:107–10.
79. Saxe Zerden L Msw P, Lombardi Bm Msw P, Jones A, et al. Social workers in integrated health care: improving care throughout the life course. Soc Work Health Care 2019;58:142–9.
80. Ford HB. Post-acute withdrawal syndrome. In; 2019.

Liver Transplantation in Alcohol-Associated Liver Disease: Current Status and Future Landscape

Alexandre Louvet, MD, PhD

KEYWORDS

- Alcohol • Alcohol-associated liver disease • Alcohol-associated hepatitis
- Liver transplantation • Relapse • Survival

KEY POINTS

- The 6 month rule should no longer be used to select candidates for liver transplantation.
- Significant data are now available to consider early transplantation in patients with a short duration of alcohol abstinence.
- Survival after transplantation is driven by alcohol relapse, cancers, and cardiovascular diseases.

INTRODUCTION

Alcohol-associated liver disease (ALD) has now become the first indication of liver transplantation in Europe over the last years[1] when considering together decompensated alcohol-associated cirrhosis, alcohol-associated hepatocellular carcinoma (HCC), and the attributable fraction of alcohol in patients with mixed etiologies. In the absence of specific pharmacologic treatment, liver transplantation (LT) is the only treatment susceptible to improve the outcome of patients with ALD and liver decompensation who have not shown sufficient improvement after alcohol cessation. Post-LT has improved in recent years and survival at 5 and 10 years is now close to 80% and 60%, respectively.[2–4] Though encouraging, the development of LT for ALD is hampered by organ shortage, but also by the risk of relapse which is a barrier to access to LT in many transplantation centers.

Survival following LT in patients with ALD is now similar to other etiologies,[5] even better at 5 years, while the outcome at longer term (ie, 10 years) is slightly lower. Indeed, the probability of developing extrahepatic malignancies after LT for ALD has been shown to be higher compared to other liver diseases, mostly because of

Service des Maladies de L'appareil Digestif, Hôpital Huriez, Rue Polonowski, Lille Cedex 59037
E-mail address: alexandre.louvet@chru-lille.fr

Clin Liver Dis 28 (2024) 809–817
https://doi.org/10.1016/j.cld.2024.06.015   **liver.theclinics.com**

the direct carcinogenic effect of alcohol and of the strong association with smoking.[6,7] Long-term outcome is also affected by an increase in cardiovascular diseases and several studies have underlined that patients with ALD are prone to develop consequences of the metabolic syndrome and cardiovascular events like patients transplanted for nonalcoholic fatty liver disease.[8,9]

THE COMPLEX INTERPLAY BETWEEN ALCOHOL WITHDRAWAL AND LIVER FUNCTION

Apart from special indications like very severe liver dysfunction threatening life in a very short term (eg, alcohol-associated hepatitis [AH] and sudden liver disease worsening), LT is often considered in patients who have not shown any improvement in liver failure despite alcohol cessation. Indeed, it is expected that patients with ALD and recent use of alcohol will improve once alcohol is stopped.

As an example, a French study has observed that improvement in liver function is mostly seen after 3 months, a plateau being seen after this time point.[10] Thus, patients still having decompensated liver disease after 3 months of alcohol cessation should be referred to a transplantation center. In fact, the relationship between alcohol cessation and liver outcomes varies a lot according to the severity of liver cirrhosis. Patients with moderate liver dysfunction will largely benefit from abstinence: a monocentric cohort has shown that survival at 5 years is much better in patients with Child-Pugh A or B cirrhosis stopping alcohol than patients with persistent drinking.[11] Conversely, in the same study, patients with Child-Pugh C cirrhosis had a similar 5 year survival regardless of alcohol cessation, which demonstrates that an important proportion of patients with significant liver insufficiency will remain at a decompensated stage despite abstinence because the magnitude of improvement will not be sufficient. A large study performed in Spain has confirmed these data by showing that among 420 patients listed for decompensated alcohol-associated cirrhosis, 92 of them (ie, 36.9%) will be delisted before LT because of an improvement in liver function.[12] The model for endstage liver disease (MELD) score was one of the most predictive factors of the probability of being delisted, a higher score being associated with the need for LT. In the same study, the authors found that the duration of abstinence was also correlated with the probability of improvement (P value very close to significance, ie, $P = .053$). These results show that patients with milder liver dysfunction and a longer abstinence are the most likely to improve without needing LT. Similar data have been found by a study performed in the United States on a large sample size of more than 83,000 patients, among which 23% had ALD as an indication for listing.[13] Compared to other etiologies, patients with ALD had a higher probability of being delisted for improvement and a lower probability of being removed from the waitlist for death or being too sick. Interestingly, this was only observed after 12 months on the waitlist. Because patients still on the waitlist after 12 months (ie, those who have not been transplanted early) are those with milder liver dysfunction, this study confirms that a wait-and-watch strategy can be offered to patients with ALD and no severe liver dysfunction but a short period of abstinence because they may improve along with alcohol cessation.

Theoretically, like for other etiologies, LT should be offered to patients with decompensated cirrhosis beyond a sustained MELD score of 15 to 17.[14] Indeed, LT brings a survival benefit to recipients with at least 15 to 17 MELD score compared to patients with milder liver dysfunction (in the absence of HCC). In other words, when the MELD score is lower than 15, LT is associated with an increased mortality compared to a wait-and-watch strategy.[14] Similarly, before the MELD era, a French multicenter randomized controlled trial has shown that patients with Child-Pugh B decompen-sated cirrhosis related to alcohol did not benefit from LT compared to an absence of LT.[15]

SELECTION OF CANDIDATES TO LT AND LENGTH OF SOBRIETY

Because some patients will improve before LT and will not require placement on the waiting list, a minimum length of sobriety has been proposed for decades to select candidates for LT. Historically, 6 months of abstinence were requested with a double aim: not transplant patients who would improve after alcohol cessation and decrease the risk of alcohol relapse after LT (see later discussion). The cut-off of 6 months had been chosen arbitrarily.[16] This "6 month rule" ie, has restricted access to LT to good candidates who were abstinent for less than 6 months.[13,17] It must also be underlined that physicians (namely gastroenterologists) have played an important role in this restricted access: indeed, in a survey published in 1998 and based on fictive vignettes in the United Kingdom has shown that not only the general public but also doctors (including gastroenterologists) considered negatively patients with ALD.[18] This stigma relates to the fact that ALD is considered by some physicians a self-inflicted disease, while a high number of personal, societal, and genetic factors contribute to excessive alcohol consumption.[19] It is surprising that such a stigma is considered less problem-atic in liver recipients with hepatitis C, metabolic dysfunction-associated steatotic liver disease, or acetaminophen overdose. Fortunately, the way people are viewed by the physicians and the general public has markedly changed over the last years.[19] For instance, a minority of the general public now considers that patients with ALD should not be considered for LT: less than 15% of the respondents of an American survey published in 2015 have indeed a negative opinion toward LT for ALD.[20]

The selection of candidates for LT is a complex process that overtakes the simple question of the medical benefit brought by LT and that carries an important degree of subjectivity.[19,21] In 2011, a prospective evaluation of 4 American transplantation se-lection committees found the absence of written program rules regarding addictions, inconsistent judgments within committees, and a lack of consensus among commit-tee members.[22] Not surprisingly, patients with ALD posed the most difficult dilemmas.

The 6 month rule was felt to bring more objectivity in the selection process even if there exists now a consensus to say that the decision should not be based on this cri-terion alone.[1] Indeed, in patients with a low risk of mortality, the longer the abstinence before LT, the lower the probability of alcohol relapse after LT.[23] In the former study, a sobriety period as long as 36 months and beyond was analyzed with a very low risk of problematic drinking after LT. From an ethical point of view, it is, however, illusory to propose such a long period of abstinence before LT because most patients with a sig-nificant liver insufficiency would have died before reaching this timepoint. The ability of the 6 month rule to predict 6 month abstinence has been evaluated in many studies. While relatively specific, its sensibility is very low and the area under the receiver oper-ating characteristic (ROC) curve does not exceed 0.6, and as an example, more than 50% of patients considered "nonabstinent" according to the 6 month rule before LT had stopped their alcohol consumption after LT.[24]

EARLY LT FOR ALCOHOL-ASSOCIATED LIVER DISEASE, INCLUDING ALCOHOL-ASSOCIATED HEPATITIS

Patients with severe liver dysfunction related to ALD have a high risk of mortality at short term and are theoretic candidates to LT despite the lack of prolonged absti-nence. Indeed, patients with ALD and high MELD often have organ dysfunction with criteria of acute on chronic liver failure (ACLF).[25] In patients with severe AH, the presence of ACLF carries a risk of death of more than 50% in the 6 months following the diagnosis, increasing to more than 80% for ACLF 2 and 3.[26] The subgroup of patients with AH not responding to medical treatment, that is, patients with a Lille score 0.45 or greater,[27] have a risk of death evaluated at 70% to 80% at 6 months. In these patients, no strategy has been proven effective in decreasing mortality.[1] Because of an early risk of mortality—most deaths occur within the first 60 days[27]—the jury of the French consensus for LT has stated that the wait-and-watch strategy based on the 6 month was unfair to nonresponders to corticosteroids and recommended a pilot study to evaluate early LT.[28] French and Belgian centers have thus joined their efforts to propose LT to 26 patients with AH not responding to medical therapy after a consensus meeting within the transplantation team.[29] Survival at 24 months was much higher than non-transplanted controls with an acceptable risk of relapse and has thus encouraged other centers to offer early LT to patients with AH. A retrospective American multicenter consensus[30] has confirmed the good outcome with a survival at 3 years of 84%. Any evidence of alcohol use after LT was found to be 28% in this study. More recently, a retrospective Italian study has also shown excellent results at 3 years with a probability of survival of 100%.[31] A modeling approach has also demonstrated that a scenario offering an early LT to patients with AH was associated with the highest survival advantage over other scenarios offering delayed LT.[32]

Because alcohol relapse after LT is an important concern (see the later discussion), a comparison between patients early transplanted for AH and patients transplanted after a significant period of abstinence is mandatory. A prospective non-inferiority trial performed in France and in Belgium[33] has confirmed that the 2 year survival of patients early transplanted for AH was excellent (ie, >85%) and similar to that of patients undergoing "standard" LT for ALD with at least 6 months of abstinence. Based on the prespecified hypothesis, the study did not conclude to non-inferiority in terms of first recurrence to drinking at 2 years (based on the TLFB: alcohol timeline followback calendar) and the subhazard ratio of alcohol relapse was 1.46. The rate of patients with heavy alcohol consumption at 2 years was higher in patients early transplanted for AH and the time spent with any alcohol consumption was not different between the 2 groups. Longer time data are requested. It should be stressed that among the 102 patients with AH selected for early LT (thanks to a dedicated algorithm), only 7 improved on the waitlist, while 21 died before LT, confirming the need for expedited selection process and referral to the transplantation center. More granular data are needed in terms of drivers of alcohol relapse in the setting of early LT even if the SALT score[34] can help identify patients at higher risk of return to drinking. In most studies, good family support, a mild alcohol-use disorder after a careful addiction evaluation, the absence of comorbid psychiatric illness and of legal issues with alcohol, and good compliance and adherence were required to qualify the patient for early LT.[29,33,35] A past medical history of decompensated cirrhosis is also a contraindication for many centers.[27]

Since AH has now become an indication for early LT in selected patients, it is tempting to broaden the disease spectrum of patients who are candidates to LT for ALD. Recent papers[35,36] have analyzed the pilot program of early LT in patients with ALD of 2 centers in North America, in comparison with patients who underwent a standard LT with 6 months of abstinence. The percentage of patients with AH was 65% in one study and not provided in the second. Both studies concluded that early LT did not result in a higher risk of relapse and that survival was similar to standard LT. This suggests thus that patients with a length of sobriety shorter than 6 months without AH can be offered early LT, but longer data are mandatory. In line with previous work,[21,22,29,33] it must be underlined that the decision of early LT should be made in a consensus meeting involving hepatologists, surgeons, nurses, and social workers. It must also be kept in mind that no consensus exists about the addiction evaluation before LT. Clearer protocols are thus needed even if algorithms for selection exist but need validation at a large scale.[33,37] The impact of early LT on the waitlist must also analyzed carefully. From previous studies, it appears that a limited number of patients will eventually be transplanted for AH: for example, AH accounted for 3% of all LT at the time of the pilot study[29]; early LT was offered to 6% of patients referred to the transplantation center in a study by Carrique and colleagues.[35]

ALCOHOL RELAPSE AFTER LT FOR ALCOHOL-ASSOCIATED LIVER DISEASE

As mentioned earlier, some factors are considered predictors of alcohol relapse after LT, even if some of them have not been investigated in the field of LT but of addiction in general.[17,33–35,38,39] Beside length of abstinence, alcohol dependence, psychiatric comorbidities, and lack of compliance/adherence, the presence of good family support is considered by many centers as mandatory before proceeding with LT. In particular, the presence of relatives drinking alcohol excessively is a detrimental factor that underlines the need for a global evaluation by the addiction specialist and the liver team. Consequently, the process may take time, while the risk of mortality can be very high in some patients with severe liver dysfunction.

Trajectories of alcohol relapse after LT for ALD have been extensively studied and the probability of return to drinking is heterogenous across studies. This is related at least in part to a lack of a consensual definition of relapse, but also to methods to diagnose alcohol consumption after LT. Some studies have demonstrated that a careful interview was as effective as "old" standard markers such as blood ethanol or carbohydrate-deficient transferrin to diagnose relapse[40]; the most recent biomarkers such as blood phosphatidylethanol and urine ethylglucuronide now have excellent diagnostic values and should be preferred.[1,41]

Among alcohol consumption pattern after LT,[40] occasional or moderate drinking does not seem to impact graft survival in short term.[42] However, since alcohol relapse is poorly defined and measured in old studies, this must be taken with much caution and should be reanalyzed in specific studies with more accurate biomarkers. While heavy alcohol relapse after LT leads to significant liver damage resulting ultimately in recurrent cirrhosis with a poor outcome.[43,44] As an example, the risk of developing cirrhosis was estimated to be 32% of patients with severe relapse in a multicenter retrospective French study.[43] In most studies having addressed the consequences of return to heavy drinking, the detrimental impact is not seen in the first 5 years following LT and survival within this time frame is similar to that of patients remaining abstinent.[43,45,46] Conversely, beyond 5 years, the risk of graft loss and of mortality in patients returning to alcohol increases and survival at 10 years is constantly lower than 50%.[43,45,46] Not surprisingly, in patients transplanted for ALD, excessive alcohol relapse and extrahepatic cancers are the most important predictors of long-term survival together with age at LT and cardiometabolic risk factors.[45]

The ideal management of addiction after LT for ALD remains still to be defined because the resources vary a lot across centers. Both the European Association for the Study of the Liver and the American Association for the Study of Liver Diseases state clearly in their guidelines that an integrated approach with specialists in addiction and hepatologists is desirable after LT.[1,47] This statement is based on studies showing that an alcohol addiction unit within the LT center helps manage patients and may decrease the probability of return to alcohol drinking based on monocenter studies with a relatively small sample size.[48,49] This remains to be confirmed in larger studies; such a demonstration would be extremely helpful to recruit specialists in addiction in LT centers.

SUMMARY

Results of LT for ALD have improved over the last decades, together with patient selection. While LT is the best treatment of patients with persistent liver insufficiency, some barriers still exist and access to transplantation center is still suboptimal. Early LT for AH has changed markedly the paradigm of the length of abstinence but data in long term are needed. A close partnership between transplantation teams and specialists in addiction will help manage patients with ALD after LT. Updates in alcohol relapse for early LT and long-term survival are mandatory to adapt guidelines and draw country-based and center-based policies.

DISCLOSURE

The author is a consultant for Glaxo-Smith-Kline.

REFERENCES

1. European Association for the Study of the Liver. Electronic address eee, European association for the study of the L. EASL clinical practice guidelines: management of alcohol-related liver disease. J Hepatol 2018;69(1):154–81.
2. Ntandja Wandji LC, Ningarhari M, Lassailly G, et al. Liver transplantation in alcohol-related liver disease and alcohol-related hepatitis. J Clin Exp Hepatol 2023;13(1):127–38.
3. Singal AK, Bataller R, Ahn J, et al. ACG clinical guideline: alcoholic liver disease. Am J Gastroenterol 2018;113(2):175–94.
4. Ursic-Bedoya J, Dumortier J, Altwegg R, et al. Alcohol consumption the day of liver transplantation for alcohol-associated liver disease does not affect long-term survival: a case-control study. Liver Transplant 2021;27(1):34–42.
5. Burra P, Senzolo M, Adam R, et al. Liver transplantation for alcoholic liver disease in Europe: a study from the ELTR (European Liver Transplant Registry). Am J Transplant 2010;10(1):138–48.
6. Dumortier J, Guillaud O, Adham M, et al. Negative impact of de novo malignancies rather than alcohol relapse on survival after liver transplantation for alcoholic cirrhosis: a retrospective analysis of 305 patients in a single center. Am J Gastroenterol 2007;102(5):1032–41.
7. Watt KD, Pedersen RA, Kremers WK, et al. Long-term probability of and mortality from de novo malignancy after liver transplantation. Gastroenterology 2009; 137(6):2010–7.
8. Anastacio LR, Ferreira LG, Ribeiro Hde S, et al. Metabolic syndrome after liver transplantation: prevalence and predictive factors. Nutrition 2011;27(9):931–7.
9. Piazza NA, Singal AK. Frequency of cardiovascular events and effect on survival in liver transplant recipients for cirrhosis due to alcoholic or nonalcoholic steatohepatitis. Exp Clin Transplant 2016;14(1):79–85.
10. Veldt BJ, Laine F, Guillygomarc'h A, et al. Indication of liver transplantation in severe alcoholic liver cirrhosis: quantitative evaluation and optimal timing. J Hepatol 2002;36(1):93–8.

11. Pessione F, Ramond MJ, Peters L, et al. Five-year survival predictive factors in patients with excessive alcohol intake and cirrhosis. Effect of alcoholic hepatitis, smoking and abstinence. Liver Int 2003;23(1):45–53.

12. Pose E, Torrents A, Reverter E, et al. A notable proportion of liver transplant candidates with alcohol-related cirrhosis can be delisted because of clinical improvement. J Hepatol 2021;75(2):275–83.

13. Giard JM, Dodge JL, Terrault NA. Superior wait-list outcomes in patients with alcohol-associated liver disease compared with other indications for liver transplantation. Liver Transplant 2019;25(9):1310–20.

14. Merion RM, Schaubel DE, Dykstra DM, et al. The survival benefit of liver transplantation. Am J Transplant 2005;5(2):307–13.

15. Vanlemmens C, Di Martino V, Milan C, et al. Immediate listing for liver transplantation versus standard care for Child-Pugh stage B alcoholic cirrhosis: a randomized trial. Ann Intern Med 2009;150(3):153–61.

16. European Association for the Study of L. EASL clinical practical guidelines: management of alcoholic liver disease. J Hepatol 2012;57(2):399–420.

17. Kotlyar DS, Burke A, Campbell MS, et al. A critical review of candidacy for orthotopic liver transplantation in alcoholic liver disease. Am J Gastroenterol 2008; 103(3):734–43, quiz 44.

18. Neuberger J, Adams D, MacMaster P, et al. Assessing priorities for allocation of donor liver grafts: survey of public and clinicians. BMJ 1998;317(7152):172–5.

19. Schomerus G, Leonhard A, Manthey J, et al. The stigma of alcohol-related liver disease and its impact on healthcare. J Hepatol 2022;77(2):516–24.

20. Stroh G, Rosell T, Dong F, et al. Early liver transplantation for patients with acute alcoholic hepatitis: public views and the effects on organ donation. Am J Transplant 2015;15(6):1598–604.

21. Donckier V, Lucidi V, Gustot T, et al. Ethical considerations regarding early liver transplantation in patients with severe alcoholic hepatitis not responding to medical therapy. J Hepatol 2014;60(4):866–71.

22. Volk ML, Biggins SW, Huang MA, et al. Decision making in liver transplant selection committees: a multicenter study. Ann Intern Med 2011;155(8):503–8.

23. Tandon P, Goodman KJ, Ma MM, et al. A shorter duration of pre-transplant abstinence predicts problem drinking after liver transplantation. Am J Gastroenterol 2009;104(7):1700–6.

24. DiMartini A, Day N, Dew MA, et al. Alcohol consumption patterns and predictors of use following liver transplantation for alcoholic liver disease. Liver Transplant 2006;12(5):813–20.

25. Gustot T, Jalan R. Acute-on-chronic liver failure in patients with alcohol-related liver disease. J Hepatol 2019;70(2):319–27.

26. Serste T, Cornillie A, Njimi H, et al. The prognostic value of acute-on-chronic liver failure during the course of severe alcoholic hepatitis. J Hepatol 2018;69(2): 318–24.

27. Louvet A, Naveau S, Abdelnour M, et al. The Lille model: a new tool for therapeutic strategy in patients with severe alcoholic hepatitis treated with steroids. Hepatology 2007;45(6):1348–54.

28. Consensus conference. Indications for liver transplantation, january 19 and 20, 2005, Lyon-Palais Des Congres: text of recommendations (long version). Liver Transplant 2006;12(6):998–1011.

29. Mathurin P, Moreno C, Samuel D, et al. Early liver transplantation for severe alcoholic hepatitis. N Engl J Med 2011;365(19):1790–800.

30. Lee BP, Mehta N, Platt L, et al. Outcomes of early liver transplantation for patients with severe alcoholic hepatitis. Gastroenterology 2018;155(2):422–430 e1.
31. Germani G, Angrisani D, Addolorato G, et al. Liver transplantation for severe alcoholic hepatitis: a multicenter Italian study. Am J Transplant 2022;22(4): 1191–200.
32. Lee BP, Samur S, Dalgic OO, et al. Model to calculate harms and benefits of early vs delayed liver transplantation for patients with alcohol-associated hepatitis. Gastroenterology 2019;157(2):472–480 e5.
33. Louvet A, Labreuche J, Moreno C, et al. Early liver transplantation for severe alcohol-related hepatitis not responding to medical treatment: a prospective controlled study. Lancet Gastroenterol Hepatol 2022;7(5):416–25.
34. Lee BP, Vittinghoff E, Hsu C, et al. Predicting low risk for sustained alcohol use after early liver transplant for acute alcoholic hepatitis: the sustained alcohol use post-liver transplant score. Hepatology 2019;69(4):1477–87.
35. Carrique L, Quance J, Tan A, et al. Results of early transplantation for alcohol-related cirrhosis: integrated addiction treatment with low rate of relapse. Gastroenterology 2021;161(6):1896–18906 e2.
36. Herrick-Reynolds KM, Punchhi G, Greenberg RS, et al. Evaluation of early vs standard liver transplant for alcohol-associated liver disease. JAMA Surg 2021; 156(11):1026–34.
37. Artru F, Louvet A, Mathurin P. Liver transplantation for patients with alcoholic hepatitis. Liver Int 2017;37(3):337–9.
38. Mathurin P, Lucey MR. Liver transplantation in patients with alcohol-related liver disease: current status and future directions. Lancet Gastroenterol Hepatol 2020;5(5):507–14.
39. Perney P, Bismuth M, Sigaud H, et al. Are preoperative patterns of alcohol consumption predictive of relapse after liver transplantation for alcoholic liver disease? Transpl Int 2005;18(11):1292–7.
40. DiMartini A, Day N, Dew MA, et al. Alcohol use following liver transplantation: a comparison of follow-up methods. Psychosomatics 2001;42(1):55–62.
41. Mellinger J, Winder GS, Fernandez AC. Measuring the alcohol in alcohol-associated liver disease: choices and challenges for clinical research. Hepatology 2021;73(3):1207–12.
42. Pageaux GP, Bismuth M, Perney P, et al. Alcohol relapse after liver transplantation for alcoholic liver disease: does it matter? J Hepatol 2003;38(5):629–34.
43. Dumortier J, Dharancy S, Cannesson A, et al. Recurrent alcoholic cirrhosis in severe alcoholic relapse after liver transplantation: a frequent and serious complication. Am J Gastroenterol 2015;110(8):1160–6, quiz 7.
44. Erard-Poinsot D, Guillaud O, Hervieu V, et al. Severe alcoholic relapse after liver transplantation: what consequences on the graft? A study based on liver biopsies analysis. Liver Transplant 2016;22(6):773–84.
45. Faure S, Herrero A, Jung B, et al. Excessive alcohol consumption after liver transplantation impacts on long-term survival, whatever the primary indication. J Hepatol 2012;57(2):306–12.
46. Rice JP, Eickhoff J, Agni R, et al. Abusive drinking after liver transplantation is associated with allograft loss and advanced allograft fibrosis. Liver Transplant 2013;19(12):1377–86.
47. Crabb DW, Im GY, Szabo G, et al. Diagnosis and treatment of alcohol-associated liver diseases: 2019 practice guidance from the American association for the study of liver diseases. Hepatology 2020;71(1):306–33.

48. Addolorato G, Mirijello A, Leggio L, et al. Liver transplantation in alcoholic patients: impact of an alcohol addiction unit within a liver transplant center. Alcohol Clin Exp Res 2013;37(9):1601–8.
49. Donnadieu-Rigole H, Olive L, Nalpas B, et al. Follow-Up of alcohol consumption after liver transplantation: interest of an addiction team? Alcohol Clin Exp Res 2017;41(1):165–70.

Artificial Intelligence, Large Language Models, and Digital Health in the Management of Alcohol-Associated Liver Disease

Neeraj Bhala, DPhil, MSc, FRCP, FRCPE[a,b,*], Vijay H. Shah, MD[a,c]

KEYWORDS

- Machine learning • Deep learning • Large language models • Cirrhosis
- Alcohol-associated liver disease

KEY POINTS

- Artificial intelligence (AI) has the potential to aid in the diagnosis and management of alcohol-associated liver disease (ALD).
- Machine learning algorithms can analyze medical data, such as patient records and imaging results, to identify patterns and predict disease progression.
- Newer advances such as large language models (LLMs) can enhance early detection and personalized treatment strategies for individuals with chronic diseases such as ALD.
- However, it is essential to integrate LLMs and other AI tools responsibly, considering ethical concerns in healthcare applications and ensuring an evidence base for real-world applications of the existing knowledge in conditions such as ALD.

BACKGROUND

There is an increasing burden of alcohol-associated liver disease (ALD) globally[1]: in addition, modern medical care produces large volumes of multimodal patient data,

[a] Division of Gastroenterology and Hepatology, Mayo Clinic, Rochester, MN 55904, USA;
[b] Nottingham Digestive Diseases Centre, Translational Medical Sciences, NIHR Nottingham Biomedical Research Centre, Nottingham University Hospitals NHS Trust and the University of Nottingham School of Medicine, Queens Medical Centre, University of Nottingham, Nottingham NG7 2UH, UK; [c] GI Research Unit, Mayo Clinic, 200 First Street, Southwest, Guggenheim 10-21, Rochester, MN 55905, USA
* Corresponding author. Nottingham Digestive Diseases Centre, Translational Medical Sciences, NIHR Nottingham Biomedical Research Centre, Nottingham University Hospitals NHS Trust and the University of Nottingham School of Medicine, Queens Medical Centre, University of Nottingham, Nottingham, Nottingham NG7 2UH, UK
E-mail address: neeraj.bhala@nottingham.ac.uk

Clin Liver Dis 28 (2024) 819–830
https://doi.org/10.1016/j.cld.2024.06.016
liver.theclinics.com
1089-3261/24/© 2024 Elsevier Inc. All rights reserved, including those for text and data mining, AI training, and similar technologies.

which many clinicians struggle to process and synthesize into actionable knowledge. Artificial intelligence (AI) can contribute to the understanding and management of ALD by analyzing large datasets to identify patterns, predict disease progression, and personalize treatment plans based on individual patient data.[2] Machine learning (ML) models may aid in early detection, risk assessment, and optimizing health care interventions for individuals at risk of or affected by ALD. Large language models (LLMs) are an advance in the field that we will assess with a growing number of studies published that apply AI techniques to the diagnosis and treatment of liver diseases. This study will provide a comprehensive overview of hepatology-focused AI research, discuss some of the barriers to clinical implementation and adoption, and suggest future directions for the field.

In health care, various types of AI learning are employed to enhance diagnostics, treatment, and overall patient care.[3] Some key types include (1) Supervised learning used for tasks like medical image analysis and diagnosis, where the algorithm is trained on labeled datasets with known outcomes; (2) Unsupervised learning applied in clustering patient data to discover patterns and relationships, aiding in personalized medicine; and (3) Reinforcement learning utilized for treatment optimization and personalized therapy plans by learning from patient responses and adjusting strategies over time.

Natural language processing (NLP) enables computers to understand and process human language, facilitating tasks like extracting information from medical records or assisting in clinical documentation. Deep learning, particularly in neural networks, is used for complex tasks such as image recognition, pathology detection, and genomics analysis. Predictive analytics combines various AI techniques to forecast patient outcomes, disease progression, or identify high-risk individuals. The integration of these AI learning methods in LLMs in health care aims to enhance diagnostics, treatment planning, and overall health care delivery of conditions like ALD.

ALCOHOL-ASSOCIATED LIVER DISEASE: MULTIFACTORIAL REASONS FOR POOR ALCOHOL RECORDING

Even before considering AI and digital health approaches, poor alcohol recording in electronic health records (EHRs) prior to ALD diagnosis can be attributed to several factors, be it behavioral, systemic, or educational[4]:

Behaviorally, stigma from parents, their support networks, and health care providers means many patients are likely to feel ashamed or reluctant to disclose their actual current alcohol consumption and bingeing patterns due to the social stigma associated with excessive drinking across many cultures globally. Similarly, patients may underestimate or underreport their alcohol consumption due to various reasons, including forgetfulness, denial, or fear of judgment from health care providers.

Systemically, many health care providers may not routinely screen patients for alcohol use or may use ineffective screening tools with inaccurate recording, leading to missed opportunities for documentation prior or when diagnosed with ALD, especially when considering gaps between distinct services not directly overlapping. Health care providers in busy emergency departments and other settings may prioritize other health concerns during appointments, leaving insufficient time to discuss alcohol consumption and document it accurately.

Educationally, health care providers may lack sufficient training or awareness about the importance of documenting alcohol consumption, leading to oversight or neglect in recording this information. Without standardized tools or protocols for assessing alcohol consumption, documentation practices may vary among health care providers, leading to inconsistencies in recording especially in EHRs, although alcohol use disorders identification test (AUDIT) and alcohol use disorders identification test for consumption (AUDIT)-C scores have proved useful in this setting.[4]

Addressing these challenges requires a multifaceted approach, including improved patient–provider communication, standardized screening protocols, provider education, and enhancements to EHR systems to facilitate accurate and comprehensive documentation of alcohol consumption in conjunction with other AI/digital health approaches.

LARGE LANGUAGE MODELS: CHARACTERISTICS AND ALCOHOL-ASSOCIATED LIVER DISEASE IN PARTICULAR

LLMs are sophisticated AI systems designed to understand and generate human-like text based on the input they receive. These models, often built using deep learning techniques, have a vast amount of parameters and are trained on diverse datasets to capture the nuances of language.

Key characteristics of LLMs include generative pre-trained transformer (GPT) architecture—many LLMs, such as ChatGPT, are based on the GPT architecture. They use transformers to process and generate text. Pretraining occurs on existing large datasets: LLMs are pretrained on massive datasets, learning grammar, facts, reasoning abilities, and contextual understanding. Fine-tuning can then be done on specific tasks or domains: LLMs are versatile and used in various diverse applications, such as natural language understanding, text completion, language translation, and generating creative content.

While in theory, LLMs excel at understanding context and generating coherent responses based on the input they receive. The goal is to generate text that is contextually relevant, coherent, and mimics human language patterns, making LLMs suitable for conversation, content generation, and more. The models can adapt to a wide range of user inputs and are designed to handle diverse topics and queries. Despite their capabilities, it is important to note that these models do not have true comprehension or consciousness, generating responses based on patterns learned during training and not always exhibit real-world understanding.

LLMs can be applied to ALD in various ways to improve understanding, diagnosis, and treatment.[5] Some potential applications include

1. Data analysis and literature review: analyzing extensive medical literature, research articles, and clinical notes to extract valuable insights into ALD risk factors, treatment options, and emerging trends.
2. Clinical decision support: assisting health care professionals by providing relevant information and guidelines for diagnosing and managing ALD, based on the latest research and medical knowledge.[6]
3. Patient education: developing informative content to educate patients about ALD, its causes, symptoms, and preventive measures, and promoting health literacy and awareness.
4. Risk prediction and early detection: applying ML models within the context of ALD to predict individual risk factors, facilitating early detection and intervention strategies.[7]
5. NLP for EHRs: enhancing the extraction of critical information from EHR, enabling more efficient monitoring and management of patients with ALD and liver cirrhosis.[8]
6. Telemedicine support: integrating LLMs into telemedicine platforms to assist in virtual consultations, answer patient queries, and provide additional information on ALD management.[9]

7. Behavioral intervention support: developing digital interventions, such as chatbots or mobile apps, to support individuals in managing alcohol consumption and making lifestyle changes to prevent or mitigate ALD.[10,11]
8. Research collaboration: facilitating collaboration among researchers and health care professionals by summarizing and synthesizing information from diverse sources related to ALD.[1,12]

It is important to approach the application of LLMs in health care, including ALD, with consideration for data privacy, ethical concerns, and ongoing validation against medical standards to ensure accuracy and reliability as well as inherent limitations.

LARGE LANGUAGE MODEL LIMITATIONS

While LLMs show promise in health care, they also come with several limitations. First is a lack of specificity and contextual understanding: LLMs might generate responses that fail to fully understand the nuanced context of medical queries, potentially leading to inaccurate information or recommendations.

Inherent biases may exist in the training data: if that used to build LLMs contains marked biases, these biases can be perpetuated further in health care applications, leading to disparities in diagnosis, treatment, or recommendations. Limited validation exists for clinical use: many LLMs lack specific validation for clinical applications in conditions such as ALD, and their outputs may not always align with established medical guidelines, leading to potential misinterpretation or incorrect advice. Ultimately, LLMs have an inability to replace human expertise as they are tools to support health care professionals, but they cannot replace the expertise and clinical judgment of human practitioners.

The dynamic nature of health care requires continual updates and adaptation to new research and guidelines. LLMs may struggle to keep up with the rapidly evolving medical landscape. Health care scenarios also often involve ambiguity, and LLMs might struggle to handle situations where information is incomplete or conflicting. Overreliance on AI models without expert oversight could be problematic.

Ethical challenges arise in areas like patient consent for AI-driven interventions, disclosure of AI involvement, and addressing potential biases that may impact patient outcomes. Data privacy concerns include processing sensitive health care data with LLMs raising concerns about patient privacy, data security, and compliance with regulatory authorities. It is crucial to approach the integration of LLMs in health care with caution, addressing these limitations through rigorous validation, continuous improvement, transparency, and ethical considerations to ensure patient safety and well-being.

DEEP NEURAL NETWORK ARTIFICIAL INTELLIGENCE: CHARACTERISTICS AND ALCOHOL-ASSOCIATED LIVER DISEASE IN PARTICULAR

A deep neural network AI leverages data-driven ML techniques to analyze complex patterns and make predictions or classifications. Clinicians benefit from these models in diagnosis by providing additional insights from large datasets, aiding in early detection, and potentially reducing diagnostic errors. Moreover, ML models can assist in predicting prognosis by analyzing various patient factors and historical data to forecast disease progression or treatment outcomes, enabling personalized treatment plans and improving patient care.

ML models offer several advantages for clinicians in diagnosing and predicting prognosis in ALD.[13]

1. Early detection: ML models can analyze diverse patient data, including biomarkers, imaging results, and clinical history, to identify early signs of ALD in the natural history. This could be done in EHRs without reported alcoholic intake (eg, repeat emergency room [ER] admissions) in theory, but early detection using alcohol intake data would allow clinicians to intervene sooner, improving ALD treatment outcomes and patient prognosis.
2. Improved accuracy: By analyzing large datasets, ML models can identify subtle patterns and correlations that might be overlooked by human clinicians. This can lead to more accurate diagnoses and prognostic assessments, reducing the risk of misdiagnosis or underestimating disease severity. More studies currently focus on differentiating nonalcoholic (metabolic/steatotic) etiology from alcohol,[14] but future studies could be conducting assessing ALD-specific groups.
3. Personalized treatments: ML models can analyze individual patient characteristics and response to treatment to tailor personalized treatment plans. This personalized approach in structured settings, for example, alcohol use disorder (AUD) treatment and acute alcoholic hepatitis, could optimize therapeutic interventions, minimize adverse effects, and improve patient outcomes.
4. Risk stratification: ML algorithms can stratify patients based on their risk of disease progression or complications, such as age, gender, liver cirrhosis, or liver failure. Clinicians can use this risk assessment to prioritize interventions for high-risk patients and allocate resources more effectively (see "A framework for navigating the impact of technology on work in health care" section).

A deep neural network AI ML model can be continuously updated with new data and insights, allowing them to adapt and improve over time. This iterative learning process enables clinicians to stay abreast of the latest developments in ALD diagnosis and prognosis prediction. Overall, ML models offer clinicians powerful tools for enhancing the diagnosis and prognostic assessment of alcoholic liver disease, ultimately leading to better patient outcomes and improved quality of care.

A FRAMEWORK FOR NAVIGATING THE IMPACT OF TECHNOLOGY ON WORK IN HEALTH CARE

In order to explore the potential impact of technology on particular roles in the health care sector, we first need to consider its impact on the component tasks that make up those roles.[4] The Health Foundation provided a framework to support this thinking in **Fig. 1**. Task delivery and task performance can be affected by several different "modes of automation." In the literature, there is often a basic distinction between "automation" (where technology is replacing workers) and "augmentation" (where technology is assisting workers): the left and right side of the grid, respectively. In the real-world work environment, there is a range of contrasting uses of technology to consider as well. A further distinction is, therefore, needed between technology that is "good enough" for use in a real-world work environment— that is, matching or nearly matching human performance (the bottom half of the grid)—and technology that is deployed because it can exceed human performance (shown in the top half).

These distinctions allow us to identify 4 different "modes of automation":

Substituting—when technology is able to perform a task to a similar level to human workers and is used to replace human workers in performing the task, thereby freeing them up to focus on other work.

Superseding—when technology significantly exceeds particular human capabilities and is used to replace human input in performing a task, thereby providing an

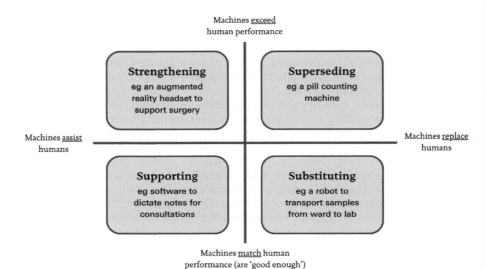

Fig. 1. Different modes of automation. (Hardie T, Horton T, Willis M, Warburton W. Switched on: How do we get the best out of automation and AI in health care? The Health Foundation; 2021 (https://doi.org/10.37829/HF-2021-I03).

opportunity to improve task performance, as well as potentially freeing up staff to focus on other work.

Supporting—when technology is used to provide additional functionality or capacity to assist a worker in performing a task, because the technology effectively increases their capacity or allows them to focus more on other aspects of the task.

Strengthening—when technology designed to assist human task performance extends beyond human capabilities, thereby enabling improved task performance, but is not intended to operate autonomously.

For example, amid all the debate about how LLMs might affect health care work, it should be acknowledged that they could be used in any of these 4 modes, as illustrated in **Fig. 2**.

The impact of a particular technology on work can also shift over time, either as the technology evolves (eg, if it gains greater computing or operational power or combines with other technologies) or as attitudes and norms regarding the use of that technology change (eg, if trust and confidence increase or decrease). **Fig. 3** illustrates how clinical decision support systems with different levels of capability could affect work in different ways. The diagram also highlights the potential for automated systems to shift from decision support to decision-making. Each of these scenarios has its own potential benefits; it is not always the "end goal" for a machine to reach the stage of superseding human labor, and such a situation may not be desirable or feasible.

THE EXAMPLE OF DECENTRALIZED CLINICAL TRIALS, PRESENT ADVANTAGES, DISADVANTAGES, AND ETHICAL CONCERNS

Fueled by adaptations to clinical trial implementation during the coronavirus disease 2019 (COVID-19) pandemic, decentralized clinical trials (DCTs) are burgeoning and highly relevant to liver disease including ALD. DCTs involve many digital tools to

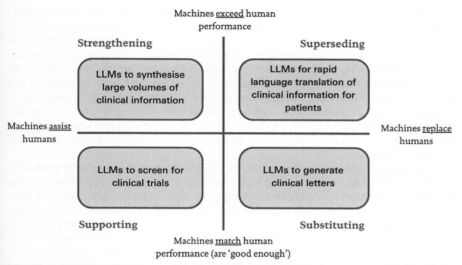

Fig. 2. LLMs could affect work in different ways, depending on their use. (Reproduced with permission by Health Foundation.)

facilitate research without physical contact between research teams and participants at various stages, such as recruitment, enrollment, informed consent, administering study interventions, obtaining patient-reported outcome measures, and safety monitoring.[15] These tools can provide ways of ensuring participants' safety and research integrity, while sometimes reducing participant burden and trial cost.

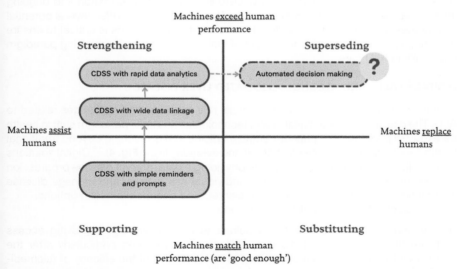

Fig. 3. The impact of technologies on work could evolve as they become more advanced: the example of clinical decision support systems (CDSSs). (Reproduced with permission by Health Foundation.)

Advantages include allowing participation from a broader and more diverse patient population, including those with difficulty accessing traditional clinical trial sites due to geographic or logistical barriers. DCTs have scope for enhanced patient engagement including remote monitoring and digital health technologies enabling real-time data collection and communication between patients and researchers, leading to improved patient engagement and retention. Decentralized approaches offer flexibility in trial design and implementation, allowing researchers to adapt protocols in response to evolving scientific, regulatory, or logistical challenges. Cost and time savings are key pragmatic issues for DCTs, reducing costs associated with site visits, travel expenses, and site infrastructure, leading to more efficient faster trial recruitment and completion timelines.

There are potential disadvantages also as DCTs may exacerbate existing health disparities by excluding individuals who lack access to technology or digital literacy skills required to participate in remote monitoring or telemedicine visits. Remote data collection in DCTs introduces potential risks to patient data security and privacy, particularly with the use of digital health technologies and remote monitoring devices. Ensuring compliance with data protection regulations and safeguarding patient confidentiality is crucial. Remote monitoring may result in decreased oversight of patient safety and data quality compared to traditional clinical trial settings, raising concerns about the reliability and validity of trial results. Challenges in endpoint assessment are also tricky remotely; including virtual assessments may pose challenges in ensuring consistency, accuracy, and reliability, particularly for subjective measures or complex assessments in liver disease.

Ensuring informed consent in DCTs requires careful consideration of how information is presented to participants remotely, as well as mechanisms for verifying comprehension and voluntariness without face-to-face interactions. Ethical considerations arise regarding equitable access to trial opportunities, particularly for vulnerable or underserved populations who may face additional barriers to participation in decentralized trials. DCTs raise questions about patient autonomy and the extent to which participants can make fully informed decisions about trial participation and ongoing involvement in remote monitoring activities. Overall, while DCTs offer several potential advantages, addressing the disadvantages and ethical concerns is critical to ensure the integrity, safety, and ethical conduct of trials conducted in this evolving paradigm especially in ALD care.

DIGITAL HEALTH AND ALCOHOL-ASSOCIATED LIVER DISEASE

Digital health technologies will play a crucial role in addressing challenges related to ALD. The rise in innovative digital health technologies has led a paradigm shift in health care toward personalized, patient-centric medicine that is reaching beyond traditional health care facilities into patients' homes and everyday lives (**Fig. 4**).[16] Digital solutions can monitor and detect early changes in physiologic data, predict disease progression and health-related outcomes based on individual risk factors, and manage disease intervention with a range of accessible telemedicine and mobile health options.

Some applications relevant to ALD include

i. Telemedicine enables remote consultations and monitoring, improving access to health care for individuals with ALD, as we have seen particularly after the COVID-19 pandemic. In a systematic review,[9] studies of the efficacy of telemedicine for remote monitoring interventions to prevent or decrease the risk of decompensation in high-risk patients and those examining improvements in the physical performance and quality of life of patients with cirrhosis through telehealth

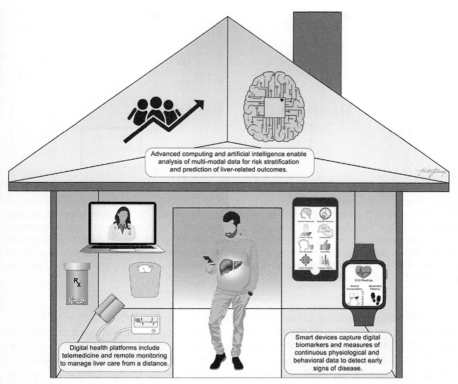

Advanced computing and artificial intelligence enable analysis of multi-modal data for risk stratification and prediction of liver-related outcomes.

R
X

Digital health platforms include telemedicine and remote monitoring to manage liver care from a distance.

Smart devices capture digital biomarkers and measures of continuous physiological and behavioral data to detect early signs of disease.

Fig. 4. The digital transformation of health care defines an innovative model of care delivery for patients with liver disease. (Reproduced with permission from Wu et al. 2022.)

rehabilitation programs have been done, with some expanded during the recent COVID-19 pandemic. Telehealth has the potential to provide and expand treatment access and reduce barriers to care for the most disadvantaged patients[17] and might be able to reduce the need for hospital readmission in ALD, though most practice to test feasibility is still currently in the pilot stage and not scaled up.

ii. Mobile apps can assist in tracking and managing lifestyle factors, such as alcohol consumption/locations for patients with ALD, nutrition, and exercise, helping individuals make informed choices. Smartphone sensors may serve as markers for alcohol craving and mood in patients with ALD and AUD. Findings in smaller proof-of-concept studies suggest that location-based and accelerometer-based features may be associated with alcohol craving.[18] However, data missingness and low participant retention remain challenges, so larger studies are needed for further digital phenotyping of relapse risk and progression of liver disease.

iii. Wearable devices like fitness trackers or smartwatches can monitor vital signs and activity levels, providing valuable data for health care professionals to assess patient health, potentially showing evidence of systemic decompensation. Physical inactivity is a major cause of deterioration in all forms of advanced liver disease.[19] Adoption of wearable activity trackers to measure the moderate-to-vigorous activity, most accurately measured with cardiopulmonary exercise testing is showing promise to identify risk and predict outcomes especially in transplant hepatology with consideration of scale-up into the wider population.

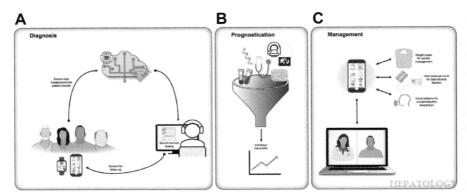

Fig. 5. Examples of applying digital health in the continuum of care for cirrhosis. (*A*) Wearable devices detect biomarkers of compensated cirrhosis and facilitate disease screening and diagnosis in the population. (*B*) AI-based tools predict individual-level disease progression and development of hepatic decompensation or mortality. (*C*) Mobile health applications receive input from digitally connected devices, and longitudinal data on symptoms of decompensated cirrhosis are summarized for clinician review and recommendation. (Reproduced with permission by Wu et al. 2022.)

Thinking ahead beyond observations, digital health also offers scope to actively engage with patients (**Fig. 5**). Behavioral interventions on digital platforms can provide interventions for managing alcohol consumption, particularly offering support and resources to individuals seeking to reduce or quit drinking in those with AUDs, especially relevant to patients with ALD also and demonstrated in text messaging in higher risk groups.[20] Digital biomarkers can use data from these various digital sources (wearables and mobile apps) to create biomarkers for early detection and monitoring of liver disease progression. Remote patient monitoring can continuously check key health metrics allowing for early identification of potential issues and timely intervention, such as if entering licensed premises.

By leveraging digital health tools, there is potential to integrate care, improve patient outcomes, increase engagement, and enhance the overall management of ALD.[21] From a clinician perspective, ML and predictive analytics analyzing larger population health datasets can help predict disease progression, identify risk factors, and personalize treatment plans for individuals with ALD. EHRs and digital health can streamline information sharing among health care providers, including clinical notes, pathology, radiology, and other information to ensure comprehensive and coordinated care for patients, ultimately improving population health of liver disease.

SUMMARY

AI has the potential to aid in the diagnosis and management of ALD even despite some specific challenges such as stigma and reliable recording. Newer AI approaches such as ML algorithms can analyze medical data, such as patient records and imaging results, to identify patterns and predict disease progression. Other AI tools such as LLMs can enhance early detection and personalized treatment strategies for individuals with chronic diseases such as ALD. However, it is essential to integrate AI tools responsibly as part of the wider research agenda,[22] considering ethical concerns in health care applications and ensuring an evidence base for real-world applications.

Digital health solutions also play a crucial role in addressing ALD. Mobile apps and wearable devices can assist individuals in tracking their alcohol consumption, providing real-time data to both patients and health care providers. Additionally, telehealth platforms enable remote monitoring and consultations, enhancing access to health care services for those with ALD. An evidence base for novel AI and digital health tools in hepatology, and ALD in particular, is emerging: however, this needs further augmentation led clinically and applied in real-world practice settings. Integrating digital tools into ALD management with responsible use of LLMs can support prevention, early detection, and ongoing care, ultimately improving patient outcomes at scale.

CLINICS CARE POINTS

Integration of AI in ALD Care
- Predictive Analytics: AI can analyze large datasets to identify patients at risk of developing ALD or progressing to more severe stages, enabling earlier intervention.
- Personalized Treatment Plans: machine learning algorithms can help tailor individualized treatment plans based on patient-specific data, improving efficacy.
- Decision Support Systems: AI-driven clinical decision support systems can provide real-time guidance to clinicians based on the latest evidence.
- Remote Monitoring: AI can facilitate remote monitoring of patients through wearable devices and mobile health applications, ensuring continuous care and early detection of complications.
- Natural Language Processing (NLP): AI can process and analyze large volumes of clinical notes to extract relevant information, enhancing clinical documentation and patient care.
- Large Language Models (LLM): LLMs can be applied to ALD in various ways to improve understanding, diagnosis, and treatment. Incorporating AI into clinical practice requires ensuring data quality, addressing ethical concerns, and validating NLP and LLM tools through rigorous clinical research to ensure safety and effectiveness.

DISCLOSURE

N. Bhala has received the Birmingham Mayo Exchange Collaboration endowed travel fellowship award and receives grant funding from the UK National Institute for Health and Care Research and UK Research and Innovation. V.H. Shah participates on advisory boards for Akaza Bioscience, AgomAb Therapeutics, Generon Shanghai, Intercept Pharmaceuticals, Mallinckrodt, Resolution Therapeutics, and Surrozen and is a consultant for Ambys Medicines, Boehringer Ingelheim, Durect, GlaxoSmithKline, GENFIT, HepaRegeniX, Korro Bio, Novo Nordisk, Novartis, and Seal Rock Therapeutics.

REFERENCES

1. Devarbhavi H, Asrani SK, Arab JP, et al. Global burden of liver disease: 2023 update. J Hepatol 2023;79(2):516–37.
2. Ahn JC, Connell A, Simonetto DA, et al. Application of artificial intelligence for the diagnosis and treatment of liver diseases. Hepatology 2021;73(6):2546–63.
3. Available at: https://www.health.org.uk/publications/long-reads/what-do-technology-and-ai-mean-for-the-future-of-work-in-health-care. [Accessed 1 February 2024].
4. Haroon S, Wooldridge D, Hoogewerf J, et al. Information standards for recording alcohol use in electronic health records: findings from a national consultation. BMC Med Inform Decis Mak 2018;18:36.

5. Zaver HB, Patel T. Opportunities for the use of large language models in hepatology. Clin Liver Dis 2023;22(5):171–6.

6. Ge J, Fontil V, Ackerman S, et al. Clinical decision support and electronic interventions to improve care quality in chronic liver diseases and cirrhosis. Hepatology 2023. https://doi.org/10.1097/HEP.0000000000000583. Online ahead of print.

7. Lee BP, Roth N, Rao P, et al. Artificial intelligence to identify harmful alcohol use after early liver transplant for alcohol-associated hepatitis. Am J Transplant 2022; 22(7):1834–41.

8. Chang EK, Yu CY, Clarke R, et al. Defining a patient population with cirrhosis: an automated algorithm with natural language processing. J Clin Gastroenterol 2016;50(10):889–94.

9. Capuano P, Hileman B, Tigano S, et al. Telemedicine in patients affected by chronic liver disease: a scoping review of clinical outcomes and the devices evaluated. J Clin Med 2023;12(15):5128.

10. Suffoletto B, Scaglione S. Using digital interventions to support individuals with alcohol use disorder and advanced liver disease: a bridge over troubled waters. Alcohol Clin Exp Res 2018;42(7):1160–5.

11. Mellinger JL, Fernandez AC, Winder GS, et al. Management of alcohol use disorder in patients with chronic liver disease. Hepatol Commun 2023;7(7):e00145.

12. Bhala N, Mellinger J, Asrani SK, et al. Tackling the burden of preventable liver disease in the USA -. Lancet Gastroenterol Hepatol 2024;9(1):9–10.

13. Nam D, Chapiro J, Paradis V, et al. Artificial intelligence in liver diseases: improving diagnostics, prognostics and response prediction. JHEP Rep 2022; 4(4):100443.

14. Okanoue T, Shima T, Mitsumoto Y, et al. Artificial intelligence/neural network system for the screening of nonalcoholic fatty liver disease and nonalcoholic steatohepatitis. Hepatol Res 2021;51(5):554–69.

15. Vayena E, Blasimme A, Sugarman J. Decentralised clinical trials: ethical opportunities and challenges. Lancet Digit Health 2023;5(6):e390–4.

16. Wu T, Simonetto DA, Halamka JD, et al. The digital transformation of hepatology: the patient is logged in. Hepatology 2022;75(3):724–39.

17. Sakpal SJ, Holbeck MJ, Wade A, et al. Telemedicine in alcohol liver disease and transplantation care: addiction therapy through video-conferencing-a case report. SAGE Open Med Case Rep 2024;12. 2050313X241235012.

18. Wu T, Sherman G, Giorgi S, et al. Smartphone sensor data estimate alcohol craving in a cohort of patients with alcohol-associated liver disease and alcohol use disorder. Hepatol Commun 2023;7(12):e0329.

19. Dunn MA, Kappus MR, Bloomer PM, et al. Wearables, physical activity, and exercise testing in liver disease. Semin Liver Dis 2021;41(2):128–35.

20. DeMartini KS, Schilsky ML, Palmer A, et al. Text messaging to reduce alcohol relapse in prelisting liver transplant candidates: a pilot feasibility study. Alcohol Clin Exp Res 2018;42(4):761–9.

21. Mellinger JL, Medley S, Kidwell KM, et al. Improving alcohol treatment engagement using integrated behavioral interventions in alcohol-associated liver disease: a randomized pilot trial. Hepatol Commun 2023;7(10):e0181.

22. Singal AK, Kwo P, Kwong A, et al. Research methodologies to address clinical unmet needs and challenges in alcohol-associated liver disease. Hepatology 2022; 75(4):1026–37.

Research Priorities and Future Landscape of Clinical Trials in Alcohol-Associated Liver Disease

Anand V. Kulkarni, MD, DM[a],
Ashwani K. Singal, MD, MS, AGAF[b,c,d,e,f,g,h,i],*,
Patrick S. Kamath, MD[j]

KEYWORDS

- Abstinence • Liver transplantation • MetALD • Noninvasive assessment
- Artificial intelligence

KEY POINTS

- Although there have been advances in research on alcohol-associated liver disease (ALD), several gaps remain in the understanding and management of this disease.
- There are no effective drugs for the management of ALD, and control of alcohol-use disorder (AUD) is the single most important determinant of long-term outcomes.
- Future clinical trials will need to focus on integrated design addressing the dual pathology of ALD and of AUD.
- The primary endpoints of future integrated clinical trials should focus on long-term outcomes and patient survival beyond at least 1 year.

INTRODUCTION

Alcohol use is a leading risk factor for death and disability. The most common organ affected by alcohol-use disorder (AUD) is the liver, with the development of alcohol-associated liver disease (ALD). The morbidity and mortality from ALD are high and

Financial disclosures: None.
[a] Department of Hepatology, AIG Hospitals, Hyderabad, India; [b] Department of Medicine, Division of Gastroenterology Hepatology and Nutrition, University of Louisville, KY, USA; [c] Department of Research, VA Medical Center, Sioux Falls, University of South Dakota, Sioux Falls, SD, USA; [d] American Gastro Association Council (Liver Section); [e] University of Louisville School of Medicine; [f] Clinical Trials in Hepatology, UofL Clinical Trials Unit; [g] University of Louisville Physics Group; [h] University of Louisville Health and Jewish Hospital; [i] Trager Transplant Center; [j] Department of Medicine, Mayo Clinic, Rochester, USA
* Corresponding author. R-505, 505 South Hancock Street, Louisville, KY 40202.
E-mail addresses: ashwani.singal@louisville.edu; ashwanisingal.com@gmail.com

Clin Liver Dis 28 (2024) 831–851
https://doi.org/10.1016/j.cld.2024.06.017
1089-3261/24/© 2024 Elsevier Inc. All rights reserved, including those for text and data mining, AI training, and similar technologies.

increasing in the last few years, with a significant contribution from alcohol-associated hepatitis (AAH), which has a high risk for short-term mortality in its most severe forms. Although several developments in the field of ALD have been made, there remain several knowledge gaps and unmet clinical needs, which the authors discuss in detail here. Over the last decade or so, drug development in the management of ALD has been hampered by an increasing pool of negative clinical trials. Currently, corticosteroids remain the first-line treatment of severe AAH but are a suboptimal treatment option. With the continued emergence of data confirming that alcohol use is the most important determinant of long-term outcomes and patient survival in patients with ALD, there is an increasing need for future clinical trials with a design integrating ALD and AUD treatments, with the primary goal of improving long-term survival of all spectra of ALD. In this review, the authors discuss the research priorities, unmet clinical needs, and future landscape of clinical trials in ALD.

RESEARCH PRIORITIES AND CLINICAL UNMET NEEDS
Alcohol and Metabolic Comorbidities

It is anticipated that 50% of the world's population will be overweight or obese by 2035, and currently approximately 43% of the world's population consumes alcohol (**Table 1**). Therefore, the burden of liver disease secondary to obesity, alcohol use, and the combination will continue to increase. The relationship between alcohol and metabolic comorbidities, especially obesity, is bidirectional. Obesity is a known risk factor for steatosis and cirrhosis, increases the risk of hepatocarcinogenesis, and is a poor predictor of outcomes in patients with AAH.[1] Of all the components of metabolic syndrome, obesity is the strongest predictor of liver-related mortality in patients with ALD.[2],[3] Alcohol is a source of energy (7 kcal/g of alcohol). In addition, there is a positive association between alcohol calories and obesity. Furthermore, alcohol increases subsequent food intake by at least 83 kcal, and daily total energy intake is about 250 kcal higher in drinkers than nondrinkers.[4] A systematic review and meta-analysis of 127 studies reported that drinking is associated with an increased risk of overweight and abdominal adiposity.[1] Therefore, in the new nomenclature of steatotic liver disease, MASLD and ALD (MetALD) has been introduced to characterize patients with dual-risk factors of moderate alcohol use (<2 standard drinks in women; and <3 in men) and one of the metabolic comorbidities.[5] Clinical and translational research is needed to understand the mechanisms of MetALD in regard to the driving force of the disease (alcohol or metabolic issue), safe alcohol limit, if any, in those with metabolic dysfunction associated steatotic liver disease (MASLD), noninvasive tests for disease stratification, and public health strategies to reduce the disease burden like government policy changes such as energy labeling universally of all alcoholic beverages, as suggested by the World Health Organization (WHO).

Spectrum of Alcohol-Associated Liver Disease

The spectrum of ALD varies from simple hepatic steatosis to cirrhosis, with a clinical phenotype unique to ALD of AAH.[6] However, the prevalence and burden of early-stage or non-cirrhotic ALD in the population levels remain unknown. Disease modifiers like female sex, poor nutrition, coexisting viral hepatitis, genetic polymorphisms, epigenetic regulators, and pattern of alcohol consumption (binge drinking outside mealtime) increase the risk and severity of ALD.[7] A large consortium investigated the association of genetic factors with the development of cirrhosis due to alcohol consumption.[8] Three single nucleotide polymorphisms were included in the genetic risk score, which was classified to low (<0), intermediate (0–0.7), and high risk (>0.7). The risk of cirrhosis

Table 1
Research priorities and unmet needs in alcohol-associated liver disease

Research Priorities	What Is Known	What Are Unmet Needs	Strategies to Achieve
Alcohol and Obesity	Alcohol increases risk of obesity and obesity impacts outcomes of ALD	Role of energy labeling of alcohol beverages on obesity. Endpoint in clinical trials for MetALD.	Involvement of government in energy labeling. Trials on MetALD with a composite endpoint of NAS and patient survival
ALD Spectrum	Varying disease severity in individuals with ALD. Role of diabetes as a disease-modifying factor increases the risk of cirrhosis and HCC in ALD	Prevalence of diabetes in ALD and ALD in diabetes Effect of alcohol on non-hepatic malignancies	Awareness in endocrinology and other physicians to identify risky alcohol use in individuals with diabetes. Awareness of using FIB-4 to identify advanced disease. Genetic and epigenetic studies in large diverse cohorts.
Prognostic Scores	MELD, MELD 3.0, mDF, GAHS, ABIC, MIAAH, MAGIC score, and Beclere model can predict short-term survival. Lilles can identify steroid response.	Not all scores can capture extrahepatic organ involvement and performance status	Score inclusive of hepatic and extrahepatic organ indices and performance status. Assess AI and machine learning models in diverse population.
Noninvasive Assessment of AUD and ALD	Blood-based markers can identify AUD and ALD. TAP (trimethylamine and pentane) score, CK 18, M30/M65 ratio, and for diagnosis and prognostication of AAH	Simple noninvasive universally available biomarkers that can identify AUD and ALD simultaneously	Identify pathways of injury and then develop markers Use of smartphone apps for AUD.
ALD and AAH Treatment	Abstinence, nutrition, and steroids are standard of care	Molecules that do not increase the risk of infection/hyperglycemia and target both inflammation and fibrosis are needed	Trials underway and reported in **Table 3**.

(continued on next page)

Table 1
(continued)

Research Priorities	What Is Known	What Are Unmet Needs	Strategies to Achieve
AUD Treatment	Behavioral therapy, naltrexone, and acamprosate are effective	Alcohol-induced polyneuropathy, insomnia, and depression need to be targeted apart from preventing relapse	Need further research in this area regarding prevalence of neuropathy and novel drugs targeting depression, insomnia, neuropathy are needed.
Prevention at Population Level	High prevalence of AUD and ALD is known Misuse of locally brewed alcohol is common in some countries	Prevalence of ALD spectrum at population levels Prevalence of AUD and ALD in populations that consume locally brewed alcohol beverages	Studies like liver screen project to identify the disease prevalence. Involvement of government agencies to curb alcohol use in the population through education and advertisement about harms. Develop public health policies Regulations and labeling of home-made alcohol beverages

Abbreviations: ABIC, age, bilirubin, INR, and creatinine; ALD, alcohol-associated liver disease; AUD, alcohol-use disorder; GAHS, Glasgow alcoholic hepatitis score; HCC, hepatocellular carcinoma; MAGIC, model for alcoholic hepatitis to grade the severity in Asian cohort; mDF, Maddreys discriminant function score; MELD, model for end-stage liver disease; MIAAH, mortality index for alcohol-associated hepatitis.

proportionately increased with the genetic risk score. Although PNPLA3 is known to be associated with the severity of ALD, external validation of such genetic modifiers in other populations is required to identify relevant genetic variants in various populations.[9] The presence of diabetes mellitus increased the risk of cirrhosis in individuals with low-risk and high-risk GRS. Diabetes mellitus is on the rise worldwide and is known to be a significant predictor of the development of cirrhosis and hepatocellular carcinoma (HCC) in patients who consume alcohol, irrespective of their glycemic status.[10] There is a need to assess the population-based prevalence of ALD in diabetes and diabetes in ALD and develop targeted therapy.

AUD and ALD are closely related.[11] The susceptibility to AUD is dependent on several factors, including social, environmental, and psychological factors. Furthermore, early exposure to alcohol, availability of alcohol, and genetic factors also determine the development of AUD.[12] A small study reported that patients with AAH tend to consume large amounts of alcohol due to altered taste and olfactory perception and also carry variants involved in the neutrophil differentiation and DNA damage response, which culminates in AAH.[13] Early identification of at-risk individuals may help prioritize preventive and treatment strategies for such patients.

Like disease modifiers causing ALD in those with harmful alcohol use, it is recognized that alcohol plays a role as a second risk factor in causing cirrhosis and complications in those with other risk factors like MASLD, chronic viral hepatitis, and other liver diseases. Combination of risk factors also increases the risk of HCC, a complication of cirrhosis with an increasing burden globally.[14] Annual incidence of HCC ranges between 1% and 5.6% in patients with cirrhosis due to ALD.[15] Alcohol consumption is underreported among patients with MASLD. Studies are required to assess alcohol's role as a second hit in causing MASLD and HCC.

Prognostication of Patients with Alcohol-Associated Hepatitis

Maddrey's discriminant function (mDF) score, model for end-stage liver disease (MELD), the Glasgow Alcoholic Hepatitis Score, Age, Bilirubin, INR, and Creatinine score, and the Alcoholic Hepatitis Histologic score have been developed to predict 30 day or 90 day mortality in patients with AAH. The Lille score has been used to assess responsiveness to steroids traditionally on day 7, but it is also used to determine response to other medical therapies.[16] A dynamic score combining baseline MELD and Lille score on day 7 is shown to more accurately predict mortality at 2 and 6 months.[17] Another model named Mortality Index for Alcohol-Associated Hepatitis, including age, blood urea nitrogen, albumin, bilirubin, and INR, was reported to be at least as accurate as MELD and mDF in predicting 30 day mortality.[18]

Although there are advantages and disadvantages of these scores, none is an ideal score. Further, presence of organ failures, especially extrahepatic organ failures in most severe forms of AAH, are not captured by these scores. For example, patients with acute-on-chronic liver failure (ACLF) who are on the liver transplant list and have an MELD score less than 25 are disadvantaged in organ allocation based on the MELD score alone which may not capture the true disease severity.[19] Further, frailty, sarcopenia, performance, and functional status of the patient are associated with survival but are not captured by any score. Clearly, there is an unmet need to develop better scores using clinical and/or noninvasive biomarkers for estimating the prognosis of patients with AAH.

Noninvasive Biomarkers

Biomarkers of alcohol use

As self-reported information on alcohol use is not always accurate, there is a need for biomarkers of alcohol use to identify ongoing alcohol consumption in patients with

ALD. More reliable markers of alcohol use include ethyl glucuronide, ethyl sulfate, phosphatidylethanol (PEth), and direct alcohol measurement in urine and blood.[20] Of these, PEth is the most accurate biomarker of alcohol use within a window period of 2 to 4 weeks from last use of alcohol and is commercially available for clinical use in routine practice. However, its use remains heterogeneous across providers and centers with variable cut-off used for a positive test and unclear protocols on persistent discordance between self-report and test results.

Recently, smartphone digital applications have emerged as effective tools to monitor alcohol consumption.[21] These apps help track alcohol consumption anonymously, set goals/limits, assess the number of dry days, assess progress, connect with the sober community, and provide feedback to the patients.[22] The major limitations of these applications are their dependency on self-reporting, lack of availability in developing countries, and risk of data theft. More data are needed on the use, feasibility, and effectiveness of these applications to monitor alcohol use in patients with ALD, especially in monitoring liver transplant candidates on the waitlist.

Biomarkers of alcohol-associated liver disease

Liver biopsy, which helps assess the disease severity, is rarely performed outside clinical trials for AAH. Fibrosis, bilirubinostasis, neutrophil infiltration, and megamitochondria are features of severe AAH and can predict survival at 90 days.[23] National Institute of Alcohol Abuse and Alcoholism (NIAAA) clinical criteria have been developed as consensus criteria for diagnosis of AAH to identify those requiring treatment with corticosteroids or enrollment into clinical trials.[24] In a recently reported meta-analysis, the accuracy of these criteria was good at over 90% in patients with severe AAH but only 65% in those with moderate AAH.[25] Data on noninvasive risk stratification using fibrosis-4 (FIB-4) and transient elastography (TE) for fibrosis in patients with early-stage ALD are evolving.[26] However, the accuracy of these tests, especially of TE, can be confounded with overestimation of fibrosis and liver stiffness in patients who are actively using alcohol due to inflammation, elevated liver enzymes, and hyperbilirubinemia. Extensive work in the area of noninvasive markers has been made in recent years to identify advanced disease.[27] Cytokeratin-18 (CK18) (M65) and cleaved CK18 (M30) correlate with the cell death, and the ratio of M30/M65 has been found to be predictive of severe AAH.[28] Similarly, soluble CD163, interleukin, 1,6, TNF-$\propto$, extracellular vesicles, urinary acrolein metabolite, and blood transcriptome modules have been utilized in diagnosing the severity of alcoholic hepatitis (AH) and response to steroids. These markers have predominantly been assessed from single-center studies with small sample sizes necessitating further validation. Moreover, in the absence of a standardized cut-off for disease identification or prognosis and a lack of universally available facilities, these noninvasive markers are more limited to research laboratories and are far from being integrated into clinical practice.

Alcohol and hepatocellular carcinoma

Alcohol-associated liver cancer estimation score, which consists of age, albumin, and alpha-fetoprotein, may stratify patients with ALD-cirrhosis into the low, intermediate, and high risk of HCC.[29] Another model involving age, gender, body mass index (BMI), diabetes mellitus, platelet count, albumin, aspartate, and alanine transaminase can predict 3 and 5 year HCC risk in ALD-cirrhosis.[30] This model for estimating HCC risk at 3 years is available online (https://www.hccrisk.com/). BMI and diabetes are also strong predictors of HCC in cirrhosis of any etiology, including those with ALD.[30] Studies are needed to validate whether these HCC risk estimating tools apply uniformly across the world given varying causes of HCC, with hepatitis B in the Asian population, hepatitis C in Japan and Egypt, and ALD and MASH in the West.

Alcohol-Associated Liver Disease Treatment

The standard of care for patients with AAH includes alcohol abstinence, adequate nutrition, and corticosteroid therapy in eligible patients to receive these drugs. The treatment of patients with ALD-cirrhosis is like any cirrhosis due to any other etiology. Liver transplant remains the treatment of choice for corticosteroid nonresponders AAH and decompensated cirrhosis patients with MELD score greater than 17.[26]

A daily intake of 30 to 35 kcal/kg and 1.2 to 1.5 g/kg protein is recommended. Screening for mineral and vitamin deficiencies can be performed in those grossly malnourished and appropriate supplementation provided.[6] In a randomized controlled trial, intensive enteral nutrition combined with steroids did not improve overall survival compared to those receiving steroids alone. However, those who received 21.5 kcal/kg/day or more experienced lower mortality versus those receiving less than 21.5 kcal/kg/day, 33% versus 66%.[31] It is unclear from the study whether receiving higher calories resulted in better survival, or whether those patients were more likely to survive consumed more calories. Nonetheless, enteral feeding with at least 21.5 kcal/kg/day must be ensured in patients with AAH. Corticosteroids are recommended for patients with severe AAH (MELD >20), and their use improves short-term survival.[32] About 40% to 50% of patients with severe AAH do not respond to steroids as determined by a Lille score. Liver transplantation remains the only hope for patients not responding to corticosteroids, but this can only be applied to a very small minority of these patients. Clearly, there is a clinical unmet need for effective therapies for ALD and AAH, especially those with moderate AAH who run a risk for up to 10% mortality at 1 year and do not have any pharmacologic therapies. We also urgently need noninvasive biomarkers that can be used in routine clinical practice for personalizing corticosteroid use to those likely to respond to these drugs. Although pentoxifylline is commonly used in clinical practice in those with kidney injury, it has not been reported to provide any survival benefit and can be used for those outside of the therapeutic window of corticosteroids.

Alcohol-Use Disorder Treatment

Control of the risk factor of alcohol use is the most crucial determinant of long-term outcomes in patients with ALD.[33] However, in the real world, several patient clinicians and system-level barriers limit treatment of AUD in patients with ALD.[34,35] There is a need to develop safety and efficacy data on medications for AUD in patients with ALD and determine the safest alcohol use that could be allowed in established ALD, especially those with advanced disease of cirrhosis and AAH. Strategies are also needed to implement and promote integrated multidisciplinary care models with hepatologist, mental health counselor, social worker, and psychiatrist to treat the dual pathology of AUD and of liver disease and provide comprehensive holistic care.[36]

Prevention at Population Level

Alcohol consumption is increasing in the community, especially among younger individuals, female individuals, and minorities.[37] Prevalence of alcohol use in the general population directly correlates with ALD-related morbidity, health care burden, and mortality.[38] Marketing of alcohol use through media has a significant effect on young and adolescent populations who are prone to get influenced.[39] Several federal level policies especially restricting alcohol sales, minimum unit price and increase in taxation, and ban on advertising alcohol at meetings and events have been shown to effectively reduce alcohol use with consequent reduction in ALD morbidity and mortality.[40]

In a recent study, the alcohol preparedness index, which assesses the strength of alcohol-related public health policies, was negatively correlated with outcomes from ALD, cardiovascular disease, and cancer. Clearly, strategies are needed to increase public-level awareness on consequences of harmful alcohol use and promoting implementation of federal-level Public Health Policies (PHP) to reduce alcohol use and improve population health.[40]

FUTURE LANDSCAPE OF CLINICAL TRIALS
Current Landscape of Clinical Trials

Inflammation, fibrosis, and trials in alcohol-associated hepatitis

Over the last decade, several drugs targeting gut–liver axis, inflammation, oxidative stress, and regeneration have been examined (**Table 2**). However, none of these have shown benefit and not progressed beyond phase-2 clinical trials.[41] With the increasing pool of negative trials, there have been several targets that have been shown to be promising.

Drugs with promise and encouraging clinical trials data

Granulocyte colony-stimulating factor (G-CSF) with or without N-acetylcysteine (NAC) in patients with AAH has conflicting reports, with Asian studies reporting improved survival and reduced infection, which could not be replicated in the Western cohort.[42] G-CSF mobilizes CD34+ progenitor cells from the bone marrow, promotes M2 macrophage differentiation in the liver, raises the levels of hepatocyte growth factor, and induces hepatic progenitor cells, which then leads to hepatic regeneration.[43] Conversely, a small study reported granulocyte–monocyte/macrophage apheresis to be effective in reducing MELD scores and improving survival in steroid-ineligible or nonresponsive AAH patients.[44] Another preclinical study reported that a combination of G-CSF and TLR-4 antagonist (TAK-242) ameliorated ACLF induced by lipopolysaccharide that can be extrapolated to AAH.[45] Currently, large clinical trials are underway to investigate the role of G-CSF in the management of AAH (*NCT02442180 and 04066179*).

A recent study on DUR-928, a naturally occurring sulfated oxysterol (larsucosterol) involved in the modulation of gene activities and regulating metabolism, inflammation, and cell survival, was found to be safe in AAH. In a phase-2a clinical trial on 19 patients with AAH (12 severe and 7 moderate AAH), DUR-928 given as intravenous infusion on day 1 led to response as assessed by Lille score in 89% patients with 100% 28 day survival.[46] Following this encouraging data, a larger clinical trial on 300 patients with severe AAH has been just completed; the results seem encouraging based on a press release, with final data awaited. F-652, a recombinant fusion protein of IL-22 and IgG2, was shown to be safe and effective in improving the severity scores in patients with AH in a phase 2 trial.[47] Further randomized controlled trials are needed to assess and confirm its efficacy.

Leaky gut in ALD leads to endotoxemia and hepatic inflammation. Improving gut barrier function, bovine colostrum has shown some efficacy in reducing endotoxemia without affecting survival. Similarly, fecal microbiota transplantation has been shown to be effective in patients with AAH.[48] In fact, a recent small single-center study reported reduction in incidence of infection, encephalopathy, and alcohol relapse.[49] Changing microbiomes through healthy donors seems promising but needs to be validated. Targeting gut microbiome or dual targets of gut and inflammatory pathways may be more beneficial in these patients. In a recently reported clinical trial on 46 patients

Table 2
Current status of clinical trials in alcohol-associated hepatitis with increasing pool of negative trials

Author, Trial Name, Study Type	Sample Size	Interventions	Outcomes	Comments
Inflammation pathway				
Szabo et al,[41] 2022 DASH trial. DB PBO RCT	103	Anakinra 100 mg SC for 14 d + PTX 400 TID for 28 d + zinc 220 mg orally for 6 m	68% survival vs 56% in control arm at 6 m. No difference in other outcomes	Fungal infections higher in prednisolone group
NCT01937130 TB PBO RCT Phase II	10	IDN-6556 5 mg (Emricasan) and 25 mg	Increase in AUC concentration	Terminated
NCT02854631 DB PBO RCT (TLM 2018)	104	Selonsertib 18 mg + Prednisolone for 28 d vs prednisolone	6 month survival: 70.3% vs 81.7% No improvement in liver function	Reduced P38 that contributes to liver injury. No major benefit
Infection pathway				
Nguyen-Khac (AAH-NAC) OL PBO RCT	174	Prednisolone + intravenous NAC for 5 d vs prednisolone	6 month mortality: 27% vs 38% 1 month mortality: 8% vs 24%	NAC provides short-term survival benefit. Cannot be used in outpatients
Stoy et al,[53] Case-control study	31	Vancomycin 500 mg + gentamicin 40 mg + meropenem 500 mg for 7 d	No difference in inflammatory markers or 6 m mortality	Fear of renal injury with nephrotoxic drugs
Kulkarni et al,[54] 2022 DB PBO RCT	33	Prednisolone + norfloxacin for 28 d vs prednisolone	Bacterial infection at day 90: 30% vs 70% No difference at day 30 infection/ survival	Norfloxacin increased the risk of fungal infections.
Jimenez et al,[55] 2022 Case-control study	63	Rifaximin for 90 d vs no rifaximin	Infections: 19% vs 43% in control arm	Small case-control study.
Kimer et al,[57] 2022 OL RCT	31	Rifaximin for 2–4 wk	No reduction in infection, mortality, or inflammatory markers	Only 9 patients in each group received steroids.
Louvet et al,[56] 2023 DB PBO RCT	292	Amoxicillin-clavulanate for 30 d + prednisolone vs prednisolone	Infection at 60 d: 29.7% in drug vs 41.5% in placebo ($P = .02$) No mortality benefit.	Fear of liver injury with amox-clav.

with moderate AAH, use of probiotic LGG (lactobacillus) in 24 patients versus placebo in 22 led to improvement in liver disease at 1 month and reduction in alcohol use at 6 months.[50] Similarly, use of fecal matter transplantation in patients with ALD showed improved liver disease, psychometric profile, and reduced craving for alcohol.[51]

Infection and trials in alcohol-associated hepatitis

Five studies have assessed the efficacy of antibiotics in patients with AAH receiving concomitant corticosteroids.[52–57] All but one reported reduced infection, but none of the studies reported any survival benefit. The antibiotics tested were norfloxacin, rifaximin, and amoxicillin-clavulanate. Of these, the safest appears to be rifaximin, given that rifaximin-α has been reported to reduce the progression of fibrosis.[58] A similar study assessing the efficacy of gut sterilizing antibiotics (vancomycin, gentamicin, and meropenem oral solutions) could not have any major impact on lipopolysaccharide-binding protein, markers of macrophage activation, and systemic inflammation.[53] All these studies employed a dose of 40 mg/day of corticosteroids. It is unknown whether reducing the dose of corticosteroids reduces the risk of infection. Whether a combination of pentoxifylline and low-dose steroids can provide any survival benefit without increasing infection risk needs to be evaluated. Antibiotics are fraught with the risk of the emergence of multidrug-resistant organisms. The infusion of omega-3 fatty acids was shown to be effective in containing the rise in endotoxemia and inflammatory cytokine bursts and preventing infections in patients with alcohol-related ACLF.[59] Such novel nonantibiotic measures are needed to prevent infections in these sick patients.

Extracorporeal liver assist devices and trials in alcohol-associated liver disease

Few studies have reported extracorporeal liver assist devices not to be effective in improving survival in patients with ALD and the studies were prematurely terminated (NCT01471028 and NCT02612428). The use of plasma exchange (PLEX) is quite frequent in Asia, where acceptance of liver transplantation (LT) is poor. Apart from acting as a bridging modality in patients with AH and ACLF, PLEX has been reported to prolong survival in these patients.[60–62] PLEX is most often used for patients who are deemed unfit for corticosteroid therapy, for steroid nonresponders, and for those who are awaiting LT. All these studies are monocentric and have been performed for those who are ineligible for corticosteroid therapy or unfit or awaiting liver transplantation. Further randomized controlled trials are required to assess the efficacy of PLEX in comparison with corticosteroids in patients with AAH.

Liver transplantation and trials in alcohol-associated hepatitis

LT field has moved significantly in the last 10 to 15 years with benefits of early LT (abstinence of <6 months duration) in selected patients with ALD.[63,64] Patient selection for early LT revolves around psychosocial evaluation and excluding those with risk for alcohol relapse after LT. There remains an unmet need for (1) objective criteria and a uniform protocol for patient selection, (2) definition of relapse to alcohol and the amount of use that is associated with harms to the graft and patient survival, and (3) strategies to implement and promote multidisciplinary integrated care models for monitoring alcohol use through the whole process during evaluation, while waiting on the LT list, and during posttransplant follow-up period.[35,36,65]

Trials for alcohol-use disorder

Novel therapies for treating AUD are the need of the hour. Small interfering RNA and gene knockout using clustered regularly interspaced short palindromic reads (CRISPR)/Cas9 have been reported to be useful in preclinical models to reduce alcohol consumption.[66,67] Few studies have reported reduced alcohol intake in pre-clinical models using DNA methylation inhibitors (DNMTi: azacytidine, decitabine), histone deacetylase inhibitors (HDACi: suberoylanilide hydroxamic acid, trichostatin, sodium butyrate, and entinostat), and micro-RNA (miRNA) antagonists (AntagomiR-411, 494).[68]

Targets for treatment of AUD can be informed by studies of Asians who are protected from the harms of alcohol. These individuals who have ALDH do not abuse alcohol and are protected from diseases due to alcohol. This is because deficiency of ALDH leads to the accumulation of acetaldehyde, resulting in flushing syndrome, an uncomfortable situation that prevents individuals from drinking further.[69] A recent study also reported that spironolactone is an effective drug in reducing alcohol intake.[70] Aldosterone levels increase with chronic alcohol consumption due to dehydration, sympathetic nervous stimulation, and hypotension. Aldosterone regulates sodium and water hemostasis by binding it to mineralocorticoid receptors, which are coded by *NR3C2*. These mineralocorticoid receptors are expressed in the central nucleus of the amygdala and prefrontal cortex, which are involved in anxiety and stress-induced alcohol drinking, addiction, and craving.[71] Aldosterone antagonists, which are used for the control of ascites, can also be used for reducing alcohol consumption in patients with ALD. Further studies are needed to assess these drugs in the context of ALD.

Reasons for Failure of Drug Development in Alcohol-Associated Liver Disease

Despite huge efforts and investment into drug development for ALD and AAH, currently effective drugs for improving patient survival and outcomes are not available. One of the main reasons for this is the lack of an animal model that can mimic the human clinical and histologic phenotype of AAH.[72] Second, ALD even in an advanced stage of AAH is a very heterogeneous disease with the clinical picture varying from moderate disease, severe disease, and failure of one of more extrahepatic organs in the most severe form of this disease. Similarly, the pathogenesis is heterogeneous and complex, with simultaneous activation of several pathways in the gastrointestinal tract, hepatic and systemic inflammation, oxidative stress, fibrosis, and hepatic regeneration. There are also challenges that limit recruitment into clinical trials for this disease, including but not limited to (1) unique characteristics of study population like sick patients and focus on liver disease, transportation of patients for research visits, lack of insight, and stigma related to AUD and (2) trial-related issues like complexity of the trial, research coordinators and personnel time, and funding sources.[41,73] This explains discordance on the pace and number of ongoing clinical trials (www.clinicaltrials.gov) for MASLD and ALD, with 1019 and 121 studies for these 2 respective commonest liver diseases (**Table 3**). Another challenge is decreasing mortality due to AAH in more recent clinical trials, which impacts sample calculation for future studies.[74] Finally, clinical trials so far did not examine the control of alcohol use during the study, a factor potentially impacting the study outcomes in both intervention and placebo arms.

Future Landscape of Clinical Trials

Future clinical trials need study designs with strategies to overcome limitations of previous clinical trials. Recognizing the dual pathology of liver disease and of AUD, one of the main strategies for future clinical trials is integrating the liver and alcohol-use components in the clinical trial involving both hepatology and mental health specialists (**Fig. 1**). This integrated study design approach is also promoted by federal organizations like the Food and Drug Administration and the National

Table 3
Ongoing trials on alcohol-associated hepatitis

Serial Number	Trial Number/Phase/Arms/Sample Size	Title	Interventions	Primary Outcome	Status/Tentative Date of Completion
1	NCT01968382 Phase 2a Three arms N = 57 Country—USA	A Multicenter Randomized, Double-Blind, Placebo-controlled, Dosing, Safety and Efficacy Study of IMM 124-E (Hyperimmune Bovine Colostrum) for Patients With Severe Alcoholic Hepatitis	Prednisolone + hyperimmune bovine colostrum (2400 mg/d or 4800 mg/d) vs placebo	Decrease in endotoxin levels	Completed Not published
2	NCT05285592 Phase 4 (?) Two arms N = 84 Country—India	Fecal Microbiota Therapy in Steroid Ineligible Alcoholic Hepatitis: A Randomized Controlled Trial	FMT vs SMT	3 mo mortality	Recruiting Tentative completion March 31, 2024
3	NCT04758806 Phase 3 N = 50 Country—Slovakia	Fecal Microbial Transplantation for Corticosteroids Nonresponders and Non-eligible Patients With Severe Alcoholic Hepatitis	FMT vs SMT	1 y mortality	Recruiting
4	NCT03917407 Phase 2 N = 43 Country—USA	Pilot Trial of DUR-928 in Patients With Moderate and Severe Alcoholic Hepatitis	-	Safety data	Completed
5	NCT05006430 Phase 1 N = 50 Country—USA	Fecal Microbiome Changes Characterization and Safety Evaluation After Oral Administration of Lyophilized Capsules Containing Microbiota Suspension (PRIM-DJ2727) in Severe Alcoholic Hepatitis Patients: Double-blinded, Randomized, Placebo-controlled Study.	Oral lyophilized capsules of healthy microbiota vs placebo for 4 wk	Safety data and survival at 1 y	Recruiting 2025

#	Trial	Title	Intervention	Outcome	Status
6	NCT06159244 N = 200 Country-France	Intestinal Microbiota Profiling in Severe Acute Alcoholic Hepatitis Patients (HepatAlc-IM)	Non-interventional	Bacterial composition of AH on day 0 and day 7	Recruiting May be able to identify bacterial signature suggestive of steroid response/nonresponse.
7	NCT03775109 Phase 2 N = 56 Country—UK	IL-1 Signal Inhibition in Alcoholic Hepatitis (ISAIAH)	Canakinumab 150 mg/mL intravenous vs placebo	Histologic improvement at 28 d	Recruiting May 2024
8	NCT04084522 N = 60 Country—India	Effect of Saturated Fat (Desi Ghee) on Gut-Liver Axis in Alcoholic Hepatitis	Saturate fat vs soyabean oil	Improvement in cirrhosis dysbiosis ratio at 2 mo	Completed
9	NCT02473341 Phase 3 N = 174 Country—India	Comparison of Bovine Colostrum vs Placebo in Treatment of Severe Alcoholic Hepatitis: A Randomized Double-blind Controlled Trial	Bovine colostrum vs Placebo	Survival at 3 mo	Unknown
10	NCT05018481 Phase 1 N = 54 Country—USA	Mechanism of HA35 in Patients with Alcoholic Liver Disease	Hyaluronic acid vs placebo for 3 mo	Percentage change in skeletal muscle mass at 90 d	Recruiting
11	NCT03732586 N = 40 Country—Mexico	Effect of Omega-5 Fatty Acid Supplement on Markers of Inflammation and Oxidative Stress in Patients with Severe Alcoholic Hepatitis Treated With Prednisone	Omega 5 fatty acid with steroids vs placebo with steroids	30 d survival	Completed
12	NCT04066179 N = 126 Country—India	Efficacy of Monotherapy vs Combination Therapy of Corticosteroids with GCSF in Severe Alcoholic Hepatitis Patients—A Randomized Controlled Trial	G-CSF with steroids vs steroids	90 d survival	Unknown status

(continued on next page)

Table 3
(*continued*)

Serial Number	Trial Number/Phase/ Arms/Sample Size	Title	Interventions	Primary Outcome	Status/Tentative Date of Completion
13	NCT02039219 Phase 2 N = 19 Country—USA	A Double-Blind, Placebo-Controlled Trial of Obeticholic Acid in Patients with Moderately Severe Alcoholic Hepatitis (AH)	OCA 10 mg vs placebo for 6 wk	Change in MELD at 6 wk and safety analysis	Terminated No change in MELD score. Serious adverse events 75% in OCA vs 45.5% in placebo
14	NCT05639543 Phase 2 N = 50 Country—USA	FXR Effect on Severe Alcohol-associated Hepatitis (FRESH) Study (FRESH)	INT-787 vs placebo	Lille's score at day 7	Recruiting
15	CTRI/2023/03/050521 N = 250 Country—India	Tapering vs Standard dose of corticosteroids in SAH-A open labeled RCT	Tapering prednisolone (40–30–20–10 mg/d each week) vs prednisolone 40 mg/d for 4 wk	Incidence of infection at day 28 and 90	Recruiting
16	NCT06155760 N = 150 Country—India	Role of Extended Low Dose Prednisolone in Achieving Clinical and Biochemical Remission in Steroid Responsive Severe Alcoholic Hepatitis	Steroid-responsive patients will receive prednisolone 10 mg/day for 90 d	Complete remission of SAH	Not yet recruiting
17	NCT03829683 Phase 2 N = 20 Country—USA	Vitamin C Infusion for TReatment in Sepsis and Alcoholic Hepatitis (CITRIS-AH)	Vitamin C 200 mg/kg/day (in 4 divided doses on day 1) for sepsis in AH	Change in MELD score at day 4	Completed
18	NCT03069300 Phase 3 N = 42 Country—UK	N-Acetylcysteine to Reduce Infection and Mortality for Alcoholic Hepatitis (NACAH)	Prednisolone + 5 d of NAC infusion (as previously described) vs prednisolone alone	Improvement in monocyte oxidative burst at 24 h and 5 d	Recruiting Aimed to understand the mechanism of reduction in infection

19	NCT03845205 N = 200 Country—USA	Alcohol Treatment Outcomes Following Early vs Standard Liver Transplant for SAH	Integrated AUD treatment vs no active intervention	Treatment engagement post-LT and time to alcohol relapse using PEth test and post-LT survival till 1 y	Recruiting
20	NCT05014087 Phase 2 N = 60 Country—USA	Digoxin In Treatment of Alcohol Associated Hepatitis (DIGIT-AlcHep)	Intravenous digoxin for 28 d	Ability to recruit 4 patients/month (feasibility trial)	Recruiting
21	NCT04620148 Phase 2 N = 100	TAK-242 in Patients With Acute Alcoholic Hepatitis	TAK-242 infusion vs placebo	Change in CLIF-C ACLF score at day 8	Unknown status TLR 4 inhibitor may ameliorate inflammation in AAH
22	NCT01922895 N = 45 Triple blind RCT	Novel Therapies in Moderately Severe Acute Alcoholic Hepatitis (NTAH-Mod)	Lactobacillus Rhamnosus GG	Change in MELD score at day 30 Mortality at 6 m	Terminated due to lack of funds

Abbreviations: AH, alcoholic hepatitis; AUD, alcohol-use disorder; FMT, fecal microbiota transplantation; OCA, obeticholic acid; RCT, randomized controlled trial; SMT, standard medical therapy; TLR, toll-like receptor.

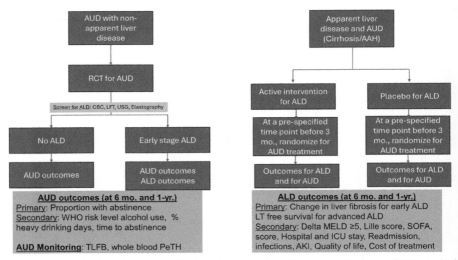

Fig. 1. Proposed integrated clinical trial design to address the dual pathology of AUD and of ALD. AAH, alcohol-associated hepatitis; ACLF, acute on chronic liver failure; AKI, acute kidney injury; CBC, complete blood count; ICU, intensive care unit; LFT, liver function tests; LT, liver transplant; MELD, model for end-stage liver disease; PEth, phosphotidylethanol; SOFA, sequential organ failure assessment; TLFB, time line follow back; USG, ultrasonography; WHO, World Health Organization.

Institute of Health (NIH) in the United States: Clinical Trial Design for Integrated Care for Patients with Alcohol Use Disorder (AUD) and Alcohol-associated Liver Disease (ALD) | National Institute on Alcohol Abuse and Alcoholism (NIAAA; nih.gov). This approach would focus on both liver and alcohol use components with an endpoint of 1 year patient survival as the primary outcome, and several secondary endpoints focusing on alcohol use (AUD endpoints) and on liver disease with accurate surrogate of patient survival (**Table 4**).[75,76] A smart adaptive study design at a certain timepoint during the study period depending on outcomes in one of the arms would be helpful in improving the efficiency of the trial and studying 2 different drugs/targets in the same trial. Apart from the study design, this approach would also have novelty and innovation of examining (1) safety of medications for alcohol-use control in patients with ALD; (2) association of alcohol-use control and WHO risk reduction (see **Table 4**) with liver disease and patient survival; (3) safe alcohol use limit or

Table 4
World Health Organization risk levels for daily alcohol use

Risk Level	Definition in Grams and US Standard Drinks
Low	1–40 g (2.9 drinks) for men and 1–20 g (<1.4 drinks) for women
Moderate	40–60 g (2.9–4.3 drinks) for men and 20–40 g (1.4–2.9 drinks) for women
High	60–100 g (4.3–7.1 drinks) for men and 40–60 g (2.9–4.3 drinks) for women
Very High	>100 g (>7.1 drinks) for men and >60 g (>4.3 drinks) for women

A Reduction in the World Health Organization (WHO) Risk Levels of Alcohol Consumption as an Efficacy Outcome in Alcohol Use Disorder (AUD) Clinical Trials. Compiled By: Alcohol Clinical Trials Infinitive (ACTIVE) & National Institute on Alcohol Abuse and Alcoholism (NIAAA). U.S. Food & Drug Administration,November 09, 2018. Retrieved from: https://www.fda.gov/media/131766/download last accessed on 17.2.2024.

threshold needed for positive outcomes and survival; and (4) noninvasive biomarkers as surrogate for endpoints in the study. In the long term, these studies would help incorporating such an approach in the clinical guidelines as a basis for promoting and implementing integrated care models in routine clinical practice to provide holistic treatment and improve long-term outcomes of patients with ALD.

SUMMARY

AUD and ALD are prevalent conditions globally and, in the United States, with a significant impact on health care burden. Although the field has moved forward in the last 10 to 15 years, there remain several knowledge gaps and unmet research needs. Specifically, drug development for ALD and AAH has recognized several limitations and challenges in patient recruitment and performing clinical trials. One of the major developments in the drug development space is a unified consensus on the role of ongoing alcohol use as a second pathology in patients with ALD. This has accelerated the concept of integrated clinical trial design with a focus on both liver and alcohol use and a goal of improving long-term patient outcomes and survival. The dream and hope of clinicians and researchers in ALD are to have an integrated multidisciplinary approach in the clinic, to provide comprehensive holistic patient care and reduce the health care burden from ALD.

CLINICS CARE POINTS

- Current medical therapies for ALD are limited.
- There is increasing pool of negative clinical trials in ALD.
- Hepatic regeneration based targets are promising.
- Alcohol use disorder treatment is becoming more important in ALD to design integrated clinical trials with assessment of liver and alcohol outcomes.

DISCLOSURE

None.

REFERENCES

1. Golzarand M, Salari-Moghaddam A, Mirmiran P. Association between alcohol intake and overweight and obesity: a systematic review and dose-response meta-analysis of 127 observational studies. Crit Rev Food Sci Nutr 2022;62(29): 8078–98.
2. Chiang DJ, McCullough AJ. The impact of obesity and metabolic syndrome on alcoholic liver disease. Clin Liver Dis 2014;18(1):157–63.
3. McPherson K. Tackling obesities: future choices–modelling future trends in obesity and the impact on health 2nd Edition.
4. Kwok A, Dordevic AL, Paton G, et al. Effect of alcohol consumption on food energy intake: a systematic review and meta-analysis. Br J Nutr 2019;121(5):481–95.
5. Rinella ME, Lazarus JV, Ratziu V, et al. A multisociety Delphi consensus statement on new fatty liver disease nomenclature. J Hepatol 2023;79(6):1542–56.
6. Singal AK, Bataller R, Ahn J, et al. ACG clinical guideline: alcoholic liver disease. Am J Gastroenterol 2018;113(2):175–94.

7. Vishnubhotla R, Kulkarni AV, Sharma M, et al. An update on the genetics of alcoholic liver disease. Frontiers in Gastroenterology 2022;1.

8. Whitfield JB, Schwantes-An TH, Darlay R, et al. A genetic risk score and diabetes predict development of alcohol-related cirrhosis in drinkers. J Hepatol 2022; 76(2):275–82.

9. Salameh H, Raff E, Erwin A, et al. PNPLA3 gene polymorphism is associated with predisposition to and severity of alcoholic liver disease. Am J Gastroenterol 2015; 110(6):846–56.

10. Hsieh PH, Huang JY, Nfor ON, et al. Association of type 2 diabetes with liver cirrhosis: a nationwide cohort study. Oncotarget 2017;8(46):81321–8.

11. Singal AK, Leggio L, DiMartini A. Alcohol use disorder in alcohol-associated liver disease: two sides of the same coin. Liver Transpl 2024;30(2):200–12.

12. Stickel F, Moreno C, Hampe J, et al. The genetics of alcohol dependence and alcohol-related liver disease. J Hepatol 2017;66(1):195–211.

13. Kulkarni AV, et al. Two hit hypotheses of alcohol-associated hepatitis (AAH): the role of genes in AAH. In: Hepatology. Philadelphia: Lippincott Williams & Wilkins Two Commerce SQ; 2023.

14. Xie C, Singal AK. Global burden of cirrhosis and liver cancer due to alcohol: the past, present, and the future. Hepatol Int 2023;17(4):830–2.

15. Huang DQ, Mathurin P, Cortez-Pinto H, et al. Global epidemiology of alcohol-associated cirrhosis and HCC: trends, projections and risk factors. Nat Rev Gastroenterol Hepatol 2023;20(1):37–49.

16. Garcia-Saenz-de-Sicilia M, Duvoor C, Altamirano J, et al. A day-4 Lille model predicts response to corticosteroids and mortality in severe alcoholic hepatitis. Am J Gastroenterol 2017;112(2):306–15.

17. Louvet A, et al. Combining data from liver disease scoring systems better predicts outcomes of patients with alcoholic hepatitis. Gastroenterology 2015; 149(2):398–406, e8; quiz e16-7.

18. Kezer CA, Buryska SM, Ahn JC, et al. The mortality index for alcohol-associated hepatitis: a novel prognostic score. Mayo Clin Proc 2022;97(3):480–90.

19. Abdallah MA, Kuo YF, Asrani S, et al. Validating a novel score based on interaction between ACLF grade and MELD score to predict waitlist mortality. J Hepatol 2021;74(6):1355–61.

20. Kulkarni AV, Singal AK. Screening for alcohol use disorder and monitoring for alcohol use in the liver clinic. Clinical Liver Disease 2023;22(6):219–24.

21. Colbert S, Thornton L, Richmond R. Smartphone apps for managing alcohol consumption: a literature review. Addiction Sci Clin Pract 2020;15(1):17.

22. Singal AK, Kwo P, Kwong A, et al. Research methodologies to address clinical unmet needs and challenges in alcohol-associated liver disease. Hepatology 2022;75(4):1026–37.

23. Altamirano J, Miquel R, Katoonizadeh A, et al. A histologic scoring system for prognosis of patients with alcoholic hepatitis. Gastroenterology 2014;146(5): 1231–9, e1-6.

24. Crabb DW, Bataller R, Chalasani NP, et al. Standard definitions and common data elements for clinical trials in patients with alcoholic hepatitis: recommendation from the NIAAA alcoholic hepatitis consortia. Gastroenterology 2016;150(4): 785–90.

25. Verma NM,R, Haiar JM, Pradhan P, et al. Clinical criteria are accurate for diagnosis of severe but not moderate alcohol-associated hepatitis. Hepatology Communications 2024. In Press.

26. Singal AK, Mathurin P. Diagnosis and treatment of alcohol-associated liver disease: a review. JAMA 2021;326(2):165–76.

27. Im GY. Emerging biomarkers in alcohol-associated hepatitis. J Clin Exp Hepatol 2023;13(1):103–15.

28. Bissonnette J, Altamirano J, Devue C, et al. A prospective study of the utility of plasma biomarkers to diagnose alcoholic hepatitis. Hepatology 2017;66(2):555–63.

29. Lee K, Choi GH, Jang ES, et al. A scoring system for predicting hepatocellular carcinoma risk in alcoholic cirrhosis. Sci Rep 2022;12(1):1717.

30. Ioannou GN, Green P, Kerr KF, et al. Models estimating risk of hepatocellular carcinoma in patients with alcohol or NAFLD-related cirrhosis for risk stratification. J Hepatol 2019;71(3):523–33.

31. Moreno C, et al. Intensive enteral nutrition is ineffective for patients with severe alcoholic hepatitis treated with corticosteroids. Gastroenterology 2016;150(4):903–10.e8.

32. Jophlin LL, Singal AK, Bataller R, et al. ACG clinical guideline: alcohol-associated liver disease. ACG 2024;119(1):30–54.

33. Louvet A, Labreuche J, Artru F, et al. Main drivers of outcome differ between short term and long term in severe alcoholic hepatitis: a prospective study. Hepatology 2017;66(5):1464–73.

34. Lucey MR, Singal AK. Integrated treatment of alcohol use disorder in patients with alcohol-associated liver disease: an evolving story. Hepatology 2020;71(6):1891–3.

35. DiMartini AF, Leggio L, Singal AK. Barriers to the management of alcohol use disorder and alcohol-associated liver disease: strategies to implement integrated care models. Lancet Gastroenterol Hepatol 2022;7(2):186–95.

36. Holbeck M, DeVries HS, Singal AK. Integrated multidisciplinary management of alcohol-associated liver disease. J Clin Transl Hepatol 2023;11(6):1404–12.

37. Singal AK, Arsalan A, Dunn W, et al. Alcohol-associated liver disease in the United States is associated with severe forms of disease among young, females and Hispanics. Aliment Pharmacol Ther 2021;54(4):451–61.

38. Axley PD, Richardson CT, Singal AK. Epidemiology of alcohol consumption and societal burden of alcoholism and alcoholic liver disease. Clin Liver Dis 2019;23(1):39–50.

39. Noel JK, Sammartino CJ, Rosenthal SR. Exposure to digital alcohol marketing and alcohol use: a systematic review. J Stud Alcohol Drugs 2020;19(Suppl 19):57–67.

40. Diaz LA, Idalsoaga F, Fuentes-López E, et al. Impact of public health policies on alcohol-associated liver disease in Latin America: an ecological multinational study. Hepatology 2021;74(5):2478–90.

41. Szabo G, Mitchell M, McClain CJ, et al. IL-1 receptor antagonist plus pentoxifylline and zinc for severe alcohol-associated hepatitis. Hepatology 2022;76(4):1058–68.

42. Marot A, Singal AK, Moreno C, et al. Granulocyte colony-stimulating factor for alcoholic hepatitis: a systematic review and meta-analysis of randomised controlled trials. JHEP Rep 2020;2(5):100139.

43. Spahr L, Lambert JF, Rubbia-Brandt L, et al. Granulocyte-colony stimulating factor induces proliferation of hepatic progenitors in alcoholic steatohepatitis: a randomized trial. Hepatology 2008;48(1):221–9.

44. Kasuga R, Chu PS, Taniki N, et al. Granulocyte-monocyte/macrophage apheresis for steroid-nonresponsive or steroid-intolerant severe alcohol-associated hepatitis: a pilot study. Hepatol Commun 2024;8(2):e0371.

45. Engelmann C, Habtesion A, Hassan M, et al. Combination of G-CSF and a TLR4 inhibitor reduce inflammation and promote regeneration in a mouse model of ACLF. J Hepatol 2022;77(5):1325–38.

46. Hassanein T, McClain CJ, Vatsalya V, et al. Safety, pharmacokinetics, and efficacy signals of larsucosterol (DUR-928) in alcohol-associated hepatitis. Am J Gastroenterol 2024;119(1):107–15.

47. Arab JP, Sehrawat TS, Simonetto DA, et al. An open-label, dose-escalation study to assess the safety and efficacy of IL-22 agonist F-652 in patients with alcohol-associated hepatitis. Hepatology 2020;72(2):441–53.

48. Pande A, Sharma S, Khillan V, et al. Fecal microbiota transplantation compared with prednisolone in severe alcoholic hepatitis patients: a randomized trial. Hepatol Int 2023;17(1):249–61.

49. Philips CA, Ahamed R, Rajesh S, et al. Long-term outcomes of stool transplant in alcohol-associated hepatitis-analysis of clinical outcomes, relapse, gut microbiota and comparisons with standard care. J Clin Exp Hepatol 2022;12(4): 1124–32.

50. Vatsalya V, Feng W, Kong M, et al. The beneficial effects of lactobacillus GG therapy on liver and drinking assessments in patients with moderate alcohol-associated hepatitis. Am J Gastroenterol 2023;118(8):1457–60.

51. Bajaj JS, Gavis EA, Fagan A, et al. A randomized clinical trial of fecal microbiota transplant for alcohol use disorder. Hepatology 2021;73(5):1688–700.

52. Kulkarni AV, Kumar K, Arab JP. Role of prophylactic antibiotics in patients with severe alcohol-related hepatitis. J Clin Exp Hepatol 2023;13(6):1146–8.

53. Støy S, et al. No effect in alcoholic hepatitis of gut-selective, broad-spectrum antibiotics on bacterial translocation or hepatic and systemic inflammation. Clin Transl Gastroenterol 2021;12(2):e00306.

54. Kulkarni AV, Tirumalle S, Premkumar M, et al. Primary norfloxacin prophylaxis for APASL-defined acute-on-chronic liver failure: a placebo-controlled double-blind randomized trial. Am J Gastroenterol 2022;117(4):607–16.

55. Jiménez C, Ventura-Cots M, Sala M, et al. Effect of rifaximin on infections, acute-on-chronic liver failure and mortality in alcoholic hepatitis: a pilot study (RIFA-AH). Liver Int 2022;42(5):1109–20.

56. Louvet A, Labreuche J, Dao T, et al. Effect of prophylactic antibiotics on mortality in severe alcohol-related hepatitis: a randomized clinical trial. JAMA 2023; 329(18):1558–66.

57. Kimer N, Meldgaard M, Hamberg O, et al. The impact of rifaximin on inflammation and metabolism in alcoholic hepatitis: a randomized clinical trial. PLoS One 2022; 17(3):e0264278.

58. Israelsen M, Madsen BS, Torp N, et al. Rifaximin-α for liver fibrosis in patients with alcohol-related liver disease (GALA-RIF): a randomised, double-blind, placebo-controlled, phase 2 trial. Lancet Gastroenterol Hepatol 2023;8(6):523–32.

59. Kulkarni AV, Anand L, Vyas AK, et al. Omega-3 fatty acid lipid emulsions are safe and effective in reducing endotoxemia and sepsis in acute-on-chronic liver failure: an open-label randomized controlled trial. J Gastroenterol Hepatol 2021; 36(7):1953–61.

60. Kumar SE, Goel A, Zachariah U, et al. Low volume plasma exchange and low dose steroid improve survival in patients with alcohol-related acute on chronic

liver failure and severe alcoholic hepatitis - preliminary experience. J Clin Exp Hepatol 2022;12(2):372–8.

61. Kulkarni AV, Reddy R, Sharma M, et al. Healthcare utilization and outcomes of living donor liver transplantation for patients with APASL-defined acute-on-chronic liver failure. Hepatol Int 2023;17(5):1233–40.

62. Vora M, Kulkarni AV, Naik P, et al. Standard volume plasma exchange is safe and effective for patients with severe alcohol-related hepatitis. Journal of Clinical and Experimental Hepatology 2023;13:S14.

63. Lee BP, Im GY, Rice JP, et al. Underestimation of liver transplantation for alcoholic hepatitis in the national transplant database. Liver Transpl 2019;25(5):706–11.

64. Kulkarni AV, Reddy R, Arab JP, et al. Early living donor liver transplantation for alcohol-associated hepatitis. Ann Hepatol 2023;28(4):101098.

65. Elfeki MA, Abdallah MA, Leggio L, et al. Simultaneous management of alcohol use disorder and liver disease: a systematic review and meta-analysis. J Addict Med 2023;17(2):e119–28.

66. Cortínez G, Sapag A, Israel Y. RNA interference against aldehyde dehydrogenase-2: development of tools for alcohol research. Alcohol 2009;43(2):97–104.

67. Wang F, Guo T, Jiang H, et al. A comparison of CRISPR/Cas9 and siRNA-mediated ALDH2 gene silencing in human cell lines. Mol Genet Genomics 2018;293(3):769–83.

68. Rodriguez FD. Targeting epigenetic mechanisms to treat alcohol use disorders (AUD). Curr Pharm Des 2021;27(30):3252–72.

69. Brooks PJ, Enoch MA, Goldman D, et al. The alcohol flushing response: an unrecognized risk factor for esophageal cancer from alcohol consumption. PLoS Med 2009;6(3):e50.

70. Palzes VA, Farokhnia M, Kline-Simon AH, et al. Effectiveness of spironolactone dispensation in reducing weekly alcohol use: a retrospective high-dimensional propensity score-matched cohort study. Neuropsychopharmacology 2021;46(12):2140–7.

71. Aoun EG, Jimenez VA, Vendruscolo LF, et al. A relationship between the aldosterone-mineralocorticoid receptor pathway and alcohol drinking: preliminary translational findings across rats, monkeys and humans. Mol Psychiatry 2018;23(6):1466–73.

72. Mandrekar P, Bataller R, Tsukamoto H, et al. Alcoholic hepatitis: translational approaches to develop targeted therapies. Hepatology 2016;64(4):1343–55.

73. Thursz MR, Richardson P, Allison M, et al. Prednisolone or pentoxifylline for alcoholic hepatitis. N Engl J Med 2015;372(17):1619–28.

74. Gawrieh S, Dasarathy S, Tu W, et al. Randomized-controlled trial of anakinra plus zinc vs. prednisone for severe alcohol-associated hepatitis. J Hepatol 2024.

75. Kamath PS. The need for better clinical trials. Hepatology 2008;48(1):1–3.

76. Sola E, Pose E, Campion D, et al. Endpoints and design of clinical trials in patients with decompensated cirrhosis: position paper of the LiverHope Consortium. J Hepatol 2021;74(1):200–19.

UNITED STATES POSTAL SERVICE ®

Statement of Ownership, Management, and Circulation
(All Periodicals Publications Except Requester Publications)

1. Publication Title	2. Publication Number	3. Filing Date
CLINICS IN LIVER DISEASE	016 – 754	9/18/2024

4. Issue Frequency	5. Number of Issues Published Annually	6. Annual Subscription Price
FEB, MAY, AUG, NOV	4	$339.00

7. Complete Mailing Address of Known Office of Publication *(Not printer)* *(Street, city, county, state, and ZIP+4®)*

ELSEVIER INC.
230 Park Avenue, Suite 800
New York, NY 10169

Contact Person
Malathi Samayan

Telephone *(Include area code)*
91-44-4299-4507

8. Complete Mailing Address of Headquarters or General Business Office of Publisher *(Not printer)*

ELSEVIER INC.
230 Park Avenue, Suite 800
New York, NY 10169

9. Full Names and Complete Mailing Addresses of Publisher, Editor, and Managing Editor *(Do not leave blank)*

Publisher *(Name and complete mailing address)*

Dolores Meloni, ELSEVIER INC.
1600 JOHN F KENNEDY BLVD. SUITE 1600
PHILADELPHIA, PA 19103-2899

Editor *(Name and complete mailing address)*

KERRY HOLLAND, ELSEVIER INC.
1600 JOHN F KENNEDY BLVD. SUITE 1600
PHILADELPHIA, PA 19103-2899

Managing Editor *(Name and complete mailing address)*

PATRICK MANLEY, ELSEVIER INC.
1600 JOHN F KENNEDY BLVD. SUITE 1600
PHILADELPHIA, PA 19103-2899

10. Owner *(Do not leave blank. If the publication is owned by a corporation, give the name and address of the corporation immediately followed by the names and addresses of all stockholders owning or holding 1 percent or more of the total amount of stock. If not owned by a corporation, give the names and addresses of the individual owners. If owned by a partnership or other unincorporated firm, give its name and address as well as those of each individual owner. If the publication is published by a nonprofit organization, give its name and address.)*

Full Name	Complete Mailing Address
WHOLLY OWNED SUBSIDIARY OF REED/ELSEVIER, US HOLDINGS	1600 JOHN F KENNEDY BLVD. SUITE 1600 PHILADELPHIA, PA 19103-2899

11. Known Bondholders, Mortgagees, and Other Security Holders Owning or Holding 1 Percent or More of Total Amount of Bonds, Mortgages, or Other Securities. If none, check box ► ☐ None

Full Name	Complete Mailing Address
N/A	

12. Tax Status *(For completion by nonprofit organizations authorized to mail at nonprofit rates)* *(Check one)*
The purpose, function, and nonprofit status of this organization and the exempt status for federal income tax purposes:
☒ Has Not Changed During Preceding 12 Months
☐ Has Changed During Preceding 12 Months *(Publisher must submit explanation of change with this statement)*

PS Form **3526**, July 2014 [Page 1 of 4 (see instructions page 4)] PSN: 7530-01-000-9931 PRIVACY NOTICE: See our privacy policy on www.usps.com.

---

13. Publication Title	14. Issue Date for Circulation Data Below
CLINICS IN LIVER DISEASE	AUGUST 2024

15. Extent and Nature of Circulation			Average No. Copies Each Issue During Preceding 12 Months	No. Copies of Single Issue Published Nearest to Filing Date
a. Total Number of Copies *(Net press run)*			102	108
b. Paid Circulation *(By Mail and Outside the Mail)*	(1)	Mailed Outside-County Paid Subscriptions Stated on PS Form 3541 (Include paid distribution above nominal rate, advertiser's proof copies, and exchange copies)	54	39
	(2)	Mailed In-County Paid Subscriptions Stated on PS Form 3541 (Include paid distribution above nominal rate, advertiser's proof copies, and exchange copies)	0	0
	(3)	Paid Distribution Outside the Mails Including Sales Through Dealers and Carriers, Street Vendors, Counter Sales, and Other Paid Distribution Outside USPS®	40	61
	(4)	Paid Distribution by Other Classes of Mail Through the USPS (e.g., First-Class Mail®)	7	7
c. Total Paid Distribution *(Sum of 15b (1), (2), (3), and (4))*		►	101	107
d. Free or Nominal Rate Distribution *(By Mail and Outside the Mail)*	(1)	Free or Nominal Rate Outside-County Copies included on PS Form 3541	0	0
	(2)	Free or Nominal Rate In-County Copies Included on PS Form 3541	0	0
	(3)	Free or Nominal Rate Copies Mailed at Other Classes Through the USPS (e.g., First-Class Mail)	0	0
	(4)	Free or Nominal Rate Distribution Outside the Mail (Carriers or other means)	1	1
e. Total Free or Nominal Rate Distribution *(Sum of 15d (1), (2), (3) and (4))*		►	1	1
f. Total Distribution *(Sum of 15c and 15e)*		►	102	108
g. Copies not Distributed *(See Instructions to Publishers #4 (page #3))*		►	0	0
h. Total *(Sum of 15f and g)*		►	102	108
i. Percent Paid *(15c divided by 15f times 100)*		►	99.01%	99.07%

* If you are claiming electronic copies, go to line 16 on page 3. If you are not claiming electronic copies, skip to line 17 on page 3.

PS Form **3526**, July 2014 (Page 2 of 4)

16. Electronic Copy Circulation		Average No. Copies Each Issue During Preceding 12 Months	No. Copies of Single Issue Published Nearest to Filing Date
a. Paid Electronic Copies	►		
b. Total Paid Print Copies (Line 15c) + Paid Electronic Copies (Line 16a)	►		
c. Total Print Distribution (Line 15f) + Paid Electronic Copies (Line 16a)	►		
d. Percent Paid (Both Print & Electronic Copies) (16b divided by 16c × 100)	►		

☒ I certify that 50% of all my distributed copies (electronic and print) are paid above a nominal price.

17. Publication of Statement of Ownership
☒ If the publication is a general publication, publication of this statement is required. Will be printed in the NOVEMBER 2024 issue of this publication. ☐ Publication not required.

18. Signature and Title of Editor, Publisher, Business Manager, or Owner		Date
Malathi Samayan - Distribution Controller	*Malathi Samayan*	9/18/2024

I certify that all information furnished on this form is true and complete. I understand that anyone who furnishes false or misleading information on this form or who omits material or information requested on the form may be subject to criminal sanctions (including fines and imprisonment) and/or civil sanctions (including civil penalties).

PS Form **3526**, July 2014 (Page 3 of 4) PRIVACY NOTICE: See our privacy policy on www.usps.com.

Moving?

Make sure your subscription moves with you!

To notify us of your new address, find your **Clinics Account Number** (located on your mailing label above your name), and contact customer service at:

Email: journalscustomerservice-usa@elsevier.com

800-654-2452 (subscribers in the U.S. & Canada)
314-447-8871 (subscribers outside of the U.S. & Canada)

Fax number: 314-447-8029

Elsevier Health Sciences Division
Subscription Customer Service
3251 Riverport Lane
Maryland Heights, MO 63043

Printed and bound by CPI Group (UK) Ltd, Croydon, CR0 4YY

08/05/2025

01864750-0005